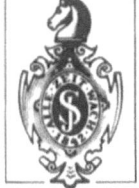

John Martin · Anthony Trowbridge (Eds.)

PLATELET HETEROGENEITY

Biology and Pathology

With 78 Figures

Springer-Verlag
London Berlin Heidelberg New York
Paris Tokyo Hong Kong

John Martin, MBChB, MD
Head, Cardiovascular Research, Wellcome Research Laboratories,
Langley Court, Beckenham, Kent BR3 3BS, UK
and Senior Lecturer and Honorary Consultant Physician,
Department of Medicine, King's College Hospital Medical School,
Denmark Hill, London SE5 9RS, UK

Anthony Trowbridge, MSc, PhD
Senior Lecturer, Department of Medical Physics and Clinical
Engineering, University of Sheffield, Royal Hallamshire Hospital,
Glossop Road, Sheffield S10 2JF, UK

ISBN-13: 978-1-4471-1765-0   e-ISBN-13:978-1-4471-1763-6
DOI:10.1007/978-1-4471-1763-6

British Library Cataloguing in Publication Data
Martin, John
   Platelet heterogeneity.
   1. Man. Blood. Platelets
   I. Title   II. Trowbridge, Anthony
   612.117

Library of Congress Cataloging-in-Publication Data
Platelet heterogeneity: biology and pathology/ John Martin and Anthony
Trowbridge, eds.
   p. cm.
Based on presentation made at the European Society of Clinical Investigation's 23rd
annual scientific meeting in Graz, Austria, in April 1988
   Includes bibliographical references.

   1. Blood platelets – Congresses. I. Martin, John, 1943–   II. Trowbridge,
Anthony, 1942–   . III. European Society of Clinical Investigation. Meeting.
QP97.P535   1990
612.1'17 – dc20   89-26256
                                                                        CIP

Preface

Battle is a practical and sometimes lasting way of solving man's problems. It relies on the strength of the combatants and ignores the truth of the dispute. Discussion face to face can dissolve attitudes which have incorrectly determined judgements. The most striking example of this that I know is a Battle in Ireland in the eleventh century, where the king of Leinster fought a Viking prince. The Icelanders had raided Ireland for several generations in search of women, which they lacked since most of the population of Iceland were men who had arrived there by rowing long-boats from Norway. The prince was leading such a raid for the first time. Standing in the prow of the leading boat he saw Irish cavalry galloping along the beach to meet them. As they approached the shore the Irish king rode out of the band to challenge single combat. The Icelander jumped into the surf to meet him. As they raised their swords each realized that the other's face was like his own. When the Irish king spoke the other recognized the language. It had been spoken in Iceland by his grandmother who had been captured and taken there from Ireland. Swords were dropped and replaced by drinking horns. It was soon established that they were cousins. The battle gave way to a life-time of close co-operation.

However, discussion and co-operation without insight can some-times lead to disaster. Earlier in their history, in 991, the Vikings were raiding the Eastern shore of England. The Anglo-Saxon poem "The Battle of Maldon" tells how they landed hundreds of men from boats onto an island that was linked to the mainland by a narrow causeway. At first the high tide covered the narrow way. For a long time the Vikings and the Saxons faced each other across a short stretch of water. The tide fell, revealing the causeway, and the Vikings ran forward in a thin line. The English killed the Norsemen where the causeway met the mainland. The unnamed Viking leader shouted complaint to the English King Offa that this was not a fair way to fight and Offa agreed (inventing the spirit of cricket), volunteering to withdraw his men so that the Vikings could land and form up on the mainland opposite the English so they could have a fair fight. That was done. Battle recommenced and the English were slaughtered. Offa's discussion was not tempered with a knowledge of the opposition.

Man's investigation of biology is essentially similar to his other enterprises. Dispute from afar can solve problems but is less likely to achieve truth than talking with results in one hand and drinking horn in the other.

The origin of platelet heterogeneity is a unique biological problem. All mammals possess platelets which are peculiarly heterogeneous compared to other cells. They arise from megakaryocytes, not by mitosis but by a unique mechanism not yet understood. The megakaryocyte is the only mature cell in the mammal which is polyploid by its nature. Platelets and megakaryocytes are characteristic features of being a mammal. The control system governing platelet production must also be unique to mammals, since there is no system in lower orders that could give rise to the hormones that must be involved. Such a fundamentally different system in nature when examined by biologists and pathologists is likely to generate dispute, especially in a scientific society where research financing is based upon the successful publication of refereed papers coupled with one's reputation among colleagues. The system of research funding encourages a scientist to be innovative but not audacious. Once a line of study becomes established it is difficult to change direction in the academic world. Although industrial research has many disadvantages in its pragmatic approach to biology, it at least encourages that fruitless research should be stopped.

For twenty years the origin of platelet heterogeneity has been vigorously sought. Sometimes robust debate solves problems. In this case the smoke of battle has occasionally obscured the way forward.

The European Society of Clinical Investigation held its 23rd annual scientific meeting in Graz, Austria, in April 1988. One of the workshops was entitled "Platelet heterogeneity: Biology and pathology". Most of those who had published on the subject were present and took part in debate, which was direct and forceful, yet understanding and constructive. Living, eating and drinking together catalysed the spirit of scientific problem-solving, which was enhanced by the atmosphere of an Austrian–Hungarian provincial capital.

This book contains papers written by the participants after the meeting, but based upon what they said at the meeting. It also contains discussions, slightly edited by Tony Trowbridge, which took place between the papers. Unfortunately it was not possible to include the discussions which took place at the dinner table. Two groups were not able to be present at the meeting: one led by David Penington from Melbourne, the other by Lawrence Harker from La Jolla. However, both groups have contributed chapters. Thus the book stands as a comprehensive definitive statement about a problem whose understanding is essential for anyone working in platelets in particular, and thrombosis and vascular disease in general.

I am grateful to the European Society for Clinical Investigation and its president Alan McGregor for providing the structure within which the meeting was organized and held. Financial help was given by the following companies, for which the participants are grateful: Bayer UK Ltd, Imperial Chemical Industries PLC, Janssen Pharmaceutical Ltd, Sandoz AG, Sanofi UK Ltd and the Wellcome Foundation Ltd. I am most thankful to Annie Higgs whose skilled editorial help has allowed the production of this volume.

The time and money invested in the meeting in Graz was not only humanly and intellectually productive but, I hope, will accelerate an understanding of the meaning of platelet heterogeneity and its involvement in human disease.

Le Soul, Chaudes-Aigues, France, August 1988   John Martin

Contents

8 The Genesis of Platelet Volume and Density Distributions

9 Platelet Heterogeneity in Vascular Disease

Contributors

J. D. Bessman, MD
Associate Professor of Medicine, The University of Texas Medical
Branch at Galveston, Division of Hematology/Oncology, Rm 4.164,
R-E65, Galveston, TX 77550, USA

G. V. R. Born, FRS
Professor William Harvey Research Institute, St Bartholomew's
Hospital Medical College, Charterhouse Square, London EC1M
6BQ, UK

K. G. Chamberlain, BA, BSc
Rm 417, Department of Medicine, Clinical Sciences Building,
University of Melbourne, St Vincent's Hospital, Corner Princes &
Regent St, Fitzroy 3065, Australia

L. Corash, MD
Professor of Laboratory Medicine, Department of Laboratory
Medicine, University of California, San Francisco, CA 94143-0134,
USA

D. Graas, B Pharm
Pharmacist, Laboratory of Hematology, Hôpital du Sart Tilman,
University of Liège, Liège, Belgium

R. Greimers, PhD
Research Associate, Department of Anatomical Pathology, Hôpital
du Sart Tilman, University of Liège, Liège, Belgium

J. C. Grosdent
Assistant, Belgian Fund for Scientific Research, Laboratory of
Hematology, Hôpital du Sart Tilman, University of Liège, Liège,
Belgium

S. R. Hanson, PhD
Hematology-Oncology, Drawer AR, Emory University, Atlanta
GA 30322, USA

L. A. Harker, MD
Hematology-Oncology, Drawer AR, Emory University, Atlanta
GA 30322, USA

C. S. Hunter, MD
US Naval Hospital, San Diego, CA, USA

N. K. Hutson, MS
Research Laboratory Specialist, Department of Hematology/
Oncology, St Jude Children's Research Hospital, 332 N.
Lauderdale, Memphis, TN 38101, USA

C. W. Jackson, PhD
Member, Department of Hematology/Oncology, St Jude Children's
Research Hospital, 332 N. Lauderdale, Memphis, TN 38101, USA

J. A. Jakubowski, PhD
Department of Hemostasis Research, Boston Veteran's
Administration Medical Center, Boston, MA 02130, USA

J. F. Martin, MD, FRCP
Head, Cardiovascular Research, Wellcome Research Laboratories,
Langley Court, Beckenham, Kent BR3 5BS, UK
and Senior Lecturer and Honorary Consultant Physician,
Department of Medicine, King's College Hospital Medical School,
Denmark Hill, London SE5 9RS

R. L. Monroy, PhD
Naval Medical Research Institute, Bethesda, MD 20814, USA

J. F. Mustard, OC, MD, PhD, FRCP(C), FRS(C)
Professor Emeritus, Department of Pathology, McMaster
University, Hamilton, Ontario, Canada L8N 3Z5

M. A. Packham, PhD
University Professor, Department of Biochemistry, University of
Toronto, Toronto, Ontario, Canada M5S 1A8

J. M. Paulus, MD
Director of Research, Belgian Fund for Scientific Research,
Laboratory of Hematology, Hôpital du Sart Tilman, University of
Liège, Liège, Belgium

D. G. Penington, MA, DM (Oxon), FRCP, FRACP, FRCPA
University of Melbourne, Parkville, Victoria 3052, Australia

P. G. Quinn, MD
Department of Medicine, Yale University, New Haven, CT 06510,
USA

M. L. Rand, PhD
Assistant Professor, Department of Biochemistry, University of
Toronto, Toronto, Ontario, Canada M5S 1A8

B. Savage, PhD
Department of Basic and Clinical Research, Scripps Clinic and
Research Foundation, 10666 North Torrey Pines Road, La Jolla,
CA 92037, USA

M. Sequaris, MD
Assistant, Laboratory of Hematology, Hôpital du Sart Tilman,
University of Liège, Liège, Belgium

R. R. Skelly, PhD
Naval Medical Research Institute, Bethesda, MD 20814, USA

S. A. Steward, BS
Research Laboratory Specialist, Department of Hematology/
Oncology, St Jude Children's Research Hospital, 332 N.
Lauderdale, Memphis, TN 38101, USA

C. B. Thompson, MD
Howard Hughes Medical Institute, Departments of Internal
Medicine and Microbiology/Immunology, University of Michigan
Medical Center, Ann Arbor, MI 48109-0650, USA

M. Tong, MD, BS
St Vincent's Hospital, Fitzroy, Victoria, 3065, Australia

E. A. Trowbridge, PhD
Senior Lecturer, Department of Medical Physics and Clinical
Engineering, University of Sheffield, Royal Hallamshire Hospital,
Glossop Road, Sheffield S10 2JF, UK

1 Platelet Density, Heterogeneity and Platelet Ageing

L. Corash

Introduction

The biological significance of platelet heterogeneity has been a controversial topic for two decades (Karpatkin 1969; Penington et al. 1976a; Martin et al. 1982, 1983a; Trowbridge and Martin 1984; Karpatkin and Penington 1984; Martin and Trowbridge 1985; Corash 1985; Mezzano et al. 1987). Two hypotheses have been proposed to explain the origins of platelet heterogeneity: (1) newly produced platelets are released from megakaryocytes with a characteristic set of properties which change with ageing in the circulation; or (2) platelet properties are determined by events during thrombopoiesis and remain unchanged during the platelet life-span. The second hypothesis has been further extended to include the proposition that there is a direct relationship between platelet characteristics and megakaryocyte ploidy, which explicitly implies that megakaryocytes of a specific ploidy class produce platelets with selected properties (Penington et al. 1976a; Martin et al. 1982; Bessman 1982, 1984; Trowbridge and Martin 1984). Among the properties that have been most intensively studied are platelet volume and density. Over the past two decades a vigorous debate has taken place as to whether platelet density decreases (Karpatkin 1969; Amorosi et al. 1971; Corash et al. 1978; Rand et al. 1981, 1983; Corash and Shafer 1982; Mezzano et al. 1984a; Packham et al. 1985), increases (Mezzano et al. 1981; Martin and Penington 1983; Savage et al. 1986) or remains stable (Penington et al. 1976a; Martin and Penington 1983; Martin et al. 1983b), as platelets age. Based on kinetic studies from our laboratory (Corash et al. 1978; Corash and Shafer 1982) and others (Greenberg et al. 1979; Blajchman et al. 1981; Rand et al. 1981, 1983) we have proposed that young platelets are released from megakaryocytes, by an unknown mechanism, with a range of properties which are determined by events during thrombopoiesis. However, as a corollary to this statement, we further propose that the characteristics of newly produced platelets are different from those of average aged platelets, and with time spent in the peripheral circulation these characteristics change further as a reflection of the ageing process. In what direction these properties change, or if they change at all, remains at the centre of the platelet heterogeneity debate.

Based on observations by Aster and Jandl (1964) and Harker and Finch (1976) that platelet removal from the peripheral circulation is approximately linear with minimal random destruction, until the tail-end of the platelet life-span, platelet clearance appears to be a senescent rather than a random process. How removal of aged platelets is effected is unknown but obviously of great interest.

In examining the numerous and diverse studies concerning platelet hetero-geneity it is important to look for common themes and consistency so that a meaningful hypothesis about platelet heterogeneity can be constructed. This is especially difficult since similar experimental models and methods have fre-quently given rise to different results. Some workers have raised the issue of species specificity as an explanation for the divergent results. While possible, this is a very unsatisfying explanation and it would be more satisfying to find that platelet heterogeneity and ageing are similar in all mammals, thus permitting the use of experimental models to ask questions which cannot be asked in human subjects. A great number of studies have been published and it is not possible in this format to review all of them exhaustively. I will focus on those studies which I view as important in helping to elucidate the meaning of platelet heterogeneity, and will provide criticisms where I see problems with the experimental data.

Experimental Models Used to Examine the Significance of Platelet Heterogeneity

One approach used to determine the source of platelet heterogeneity has relied on comparative ultrastructural studies of megakaryocytes and platelets (Pening-ton and Streatfield 1975; Penington et al. 1976b; Martin et al. 1982; Stenberg and Levin 1988). Recently, an analogous design utilizing simultaneous measurement of megakaryocyte and platelet properties, with either flow cytometric or microscopic examination of megakaryocytes and platelets, during normal and perturbed thrombopoiesis has evolved (Bessman 1982, 1984; Martin et al. 1983a; Corash et al. 1987). These studies have largely been restricted to measurement of megakaryocyte ploidy and platelet volume, and have been extensively reviewed elsewhere (Corash 1989).

Ebbe and Jackson have explored the use of animal models in which megakary-ocyte or platelet properties are different from normal, to examine the correlation of abnormalities in either megakaryocytes or platelets with effects on platelet volume, megakaryocyte ploidy, and megakaryocyte and platelet characteristics. This has been informative about the relationships between megakaryocyte properties and platelets, and has yielded some information about subsequent effects during the life-span of these model platelets. This work has been reviewed elsewhere (Jackson 1989).

A number of investigations to determine the source of platelet heterogeneity have utilized physical isolation of platelet cohorts of selected volume or density. Selected cohorts have been isolated, radiolabelled, and re-injected into reci-pients, either animals or humans, and the survival and density distribution have been followed serially (Karpatkin 1969; Ginsburg and Aster 1969; Boneu et al. 1973, 1977, 1982; Corash et al. 1978; Mezzano et al. 1981; Rand et al. 1983; Martin and Penington 1983; Thompson et al. 1983; Savage et al. 1986; Watson and Ludlam 1986). A derivative approach to in vitro physical isolation, radio-labelling, and re-injection of selected platelet cohorts has been the use of in vivo labelling followed by serial isolation of density-dependent platelet cohorts to determine if newly produced platelets change density during circulation (Amor-osi et al. 1971; Charmatz and Karpatkin 1974; Penington et al. 1976a; Rand et al. 1981; Corash and Shafer 1982). Another version of the in vivo labelling model has been the use of aspirin-induced inhibition of circulating platelet prostaglandin production as a means to produce a well-defined cohort of newly released platelets with intact prostaglandin production which can then be serially followed as it enters and exits the peripheral circulation (Leone et al. 1979; Boneu et al. 1980; Mezzano et al. 1981; McDonald and Ali 1983; Packham et al. 1985). Serial measurement of prostaglandin synthesis in density-dependent platelet fractions can then be used to correlate platelet age with density. These studies have produced divergent results depending on the methodologies used and perhaps on the species (Corash 1985; Packham et al. 1985).

Other workers have employed models in which platelet production is either stimulated or inhibited to produce cohorts of young or old platelets whose physical and functional properties can be serially measured (Hirsh et al. 1968; Blajchman et al. 1981). While these models may be useful, the use of non-steady-state thrombopoietic conditions raises questions about the applicability of observations obtained with these models to understanding platelet heterogeneity under normal thrombopoietic conditions.

Potential Problems Associated with Various Experimental Models

Use of the previously discussed experimental models requires that care be taken to ensure that the model is functioning properly without the introduction of artefacts which might influence data generated by these model systems. In our studies of the relationship between platelet heterogeneity and platelet density, we have relied upon the fractionation of complete whole blood platelet populations into density-dependent cohorts (Corash et al. 1977). In order to obtain a total platelet population without selective loss of any subpopulation, we developed a technique using isosmolar arabino-galactan (Stractan®) density gradient centrifugation (Corash et al. 1977) which was based on earlier experience with red cell fractionation studies (Corash et al. 1974). This method provided a technique for high-yield isolation of platelets from whole blood with excellent retention of ultrastructure and function (Corash et al. 1977). It also produced platelets free from erythrocytes and plasma proteins, but not from mononuclear leukocytes. Subsequently, this method was further refined to remove contaminat-ing mononuclear leukocytes so that pure platelet populations could be obtained (Corash and Shafer 1982). This point is particularly important for experiments which are designed to examine the incorporation of radioisotopes, administered in vivo, into newly produced platelets. If the platelet fractions are contaminated with either plasma proteins or leukocytes, then significant amounts of radioactivity incorporated into non-platelet fractions will co-isolate with and contaminate platelet fractions. We have demonstrated that during in vivo labelling experiments, leukocyte contamination will seriously alter data interpretation (Corash and Shafer 1982), and this artefact most likely accounted for the different results obtained by Amorosi et al. (1971) and Penington et al. (1976a). The latter investigators utilized a platelet isolation technique after in vivo isotope administration which produced platelets heavily contaminated with mononuclear leukocytes. A substantial portion of the radioactivity attributed to platelets was probably due to leukocytes which labelled with significantly greater specific activity.

Studies by a number of other investigators, in different laboratories, have confirmed our initial observations concerning the quality and function of platelets isolated by the arabino-galactan density gradient technique (Cieslar et al. 1979; Rand et al. 1981, 1983; Packham et al. 1985; Hill et al. 1988). After isolation of a total platelet population, fractionation into density cohorts was achieved on four-step discontinuous arabino-galactan gradients centrifuged under isopycnic equilibrium conditions (Corash et al. 1977, 1978, 1984; Corash and Shafer 1982). Based on our previous experience with age-dependent red cell density fractionation (Corash et al. 1974), we developed a method for isolation of the density fractions using a tube-slicing technique (Corash et al. 1977). This permitted removal of the respective density fractions without mixing of individual layers which occurs with other types of gradient recovery devices (Corash 1986).

An important aspect of platelet density fractionation is to ensure platelet separation and recovery under conditions which do not produce secretion, since it is well established by a number of laboratories that activated platelets secrete selected subcellular constituents with alteration of platelet density (van Oost et al. 1983, 1984). More importantly, Cieslar and co-workers (1979) have previously demonstrated that degranulated rabbit platelets, with decreased density, circulated normally after re-injection. Thus, studies which rely on density isolation and re-injection of platelet subfractions must ensure that artefactual alteration of platelet density has not occurred, since it would influence interpretation of subsequent in vivo data. To ensure that artefactual platelet density modification has not taken place, it is important to have controls which can verify that platelet density has remained unchanged during fractionation. Two methods can be employed to evaluate the quality of platelet density fractionation. If in vitro radiolabelling of selected density cohorts is performed, after re-injection of the labelled cohort, it is critical to demonstrate that all the label is recovered in the correct density position (Corash et al. 1978). Another approach useful in monitoring the quality of density fractionation is to measure the distribution of a well-established density-dependent platelet property. We have measured the distribution of endogenous serotonin (5-hydroxytryptamine, 5-HT) content in native platelets and fractionated platelet cohorts as an index of density-dependent platelet fractionation (Corash et al. 1984). Endogenous 5-HT is contained in platelet dense bodies which may be secreted during platelet activation. After density fractionation, platelet 5-HT is distributed in a density-dependent fashion, with higher levels in high-density platelets compared to the concentration in low-density platelets (Corash et al. 1984; Mezzano et al. 1984b). Platelet 5-HT concentration can be plotted against position in the gradient (Fig.

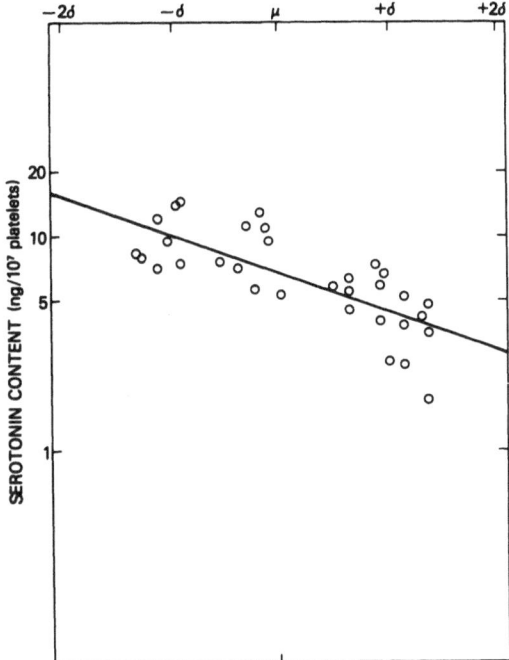

Fig. 1.1. The relationship between platelet position in the gradient and endogenous 5-HT content. Platelets were fractionated into four subpopulations using isopycnic density gradient centrifugation as previously described (Corash et al. 1984). Five separate fractionations of normal human platelets were performed. Endogenous platelet 5-HT content was measured using a sensitive double-isotope dilution assay (Corash et al. 1984). Platelet 5-HT concentration per 10^7 platelets is plotted on a logarithmic scale against position in the gradient where the mid-point (μ) and one and two standard deviations (δ) are indicated on the abscissa. The position of each gradient fraction was based on a cumulative frequency distribution analysis. High-density platelets are located at the left side of the gradient density plot and low-density platelets at the right side.

1.1) and a mid-point value, representative of the average platelet value, can be determined. The mid-point concentration value should match the median 5-HT concentration of native, unfractionated platelets, if no dense body secretion has occurred during the separation process. Subsequently, we have compared mid-point estimates derived from density fractions with the specific organelle activities of native unfractionated platelet populations (Table 1.1). These studies demonstrated that the arabino-galactan density fractionation technique did not produce artefactual platelet density changes due to platelet activation during preparation of density cohorts. Subsequently, we have used these assays, especially for the labile α-granule compartment, to ensure that platelet activation was not induced.

The issue of whether discontinuous gradients do not permit true isopycnic platelet separation has been raised in the literature (Martin et al. 1983b), but evidence obtained from our own studies examining the rebanding of ^{51}Cr-labelled platelets (Corash et al. 1978) and those of others (Cieslar et al. 1979; Rand et al. 1983; van Oost et al. 1984) indicate that valid isopycnic separations are obtained on discontinuous, isosmolar arabino-galactan gradients. This issue has been more fully discussed recently (Corash 1985; Martin and Trowbridge 1985) and I refer the reader to that discussion.

Table 1.1. Comparison of theoretical and observed values for platelet subcellular organelle activities

Compartment/component	N	$II_t{}^a$	Probit estimate[b]
Mitochondria (MAO)	11	9.82±0.44	10.26 (44)
Lysosomes (β-Glu)	14	7.60±0.04	7.10 (56)
Dense Bodies (5-HT)	25	6.48±0.38	6.71 (100)
α-Granules (β-TG)	10	37.42±0.95	37.32 (40)
α-Granules (PF 4)	10	6.47±0.83	6.60 (50)

Platelet constituents were measured in native unfractionated platelets (II_t) and in density-fractionated platelet subpopulations as previously described (Corash et al. 1984).
[a] Indicates a total native platelet population isolated under optimal conditions to prevent activation or secretation.
[b] Indicates the mid-point value of specific subcellular organelle constituents determined using probability plot analysis after density-gradient fractionation into four subfractions (Corash et al. 1984). This value was obtained from probability plot analysis derived from the pooled values of all subfraction measurements. The number of data sets for each probability analysis is indicated in parentheses.
N indicates the number of normal subjects used to measure native platelet properties and to perform density-dependent platelet fractionation. The mean and standard error of the mean are indicated for native platelet measurements. MAO (monoamine oxidase), mmol/10^8 platelets/hour; β-Glu (beta glucuronidase), nmol/10^8 platelets/hour; 5-HT (endogenous serotonin), ng/10^7 platelets; β-TG (β-thromboglobulin), μg/10^9 platelets; PF 4 (platelet factor 4), ng/10^6 platelets.

Ultrastructural Studies and Platelet Heterogeneity

The relationship between platelet density and organelle content is intriguing, particularly in view of the report of van Oost and co-workers (1984) that platelet α-granule content is the major determinant of platelet density. In our initial examination of the ultrastructure of density-dependent platelet cohorts (Corash et al. 1977), we found no difference in the numbers of mitochondria in different platelet density cohorts, but substantial differences in the total granule content of high- and low-density platelets were observed (Table 1.2). In a later study (Corash et al. 1984), we demonstrated that there was a significant difference in both dense body and α-granule content with respect to density, but no difference in lysosomal content. We also measured the frequency of dense bodies in platelet fractions of different densities (Corash et al. 1984). This was done using whole mounts of platelets which were examined under the electron microscope and electron-dense bodies were enumerated (Fig. 1.2). Since platelet dense bodies are not normally distributed, but instead demonstrate a marked positive skew, we measured the cumulative frequency distribution of dense bodies in each density fraction and determined the median dense-body frequency for each density fraction. Unfractionated platelets exhibited an average median dense-body frequency of 5.4 per platelet compared to 3.5 of least dense platelets and 6.8 of most dense platelets. Thus, platelets of various densities exhibited a differential distribution of selected subcellular organelles rather than a uniform distribution of all organelles within a density cohort.

A recent study by Duyvené de Wit et al. (1987) confirmed our previous observations that granules were distributed in a density-dependent fashion

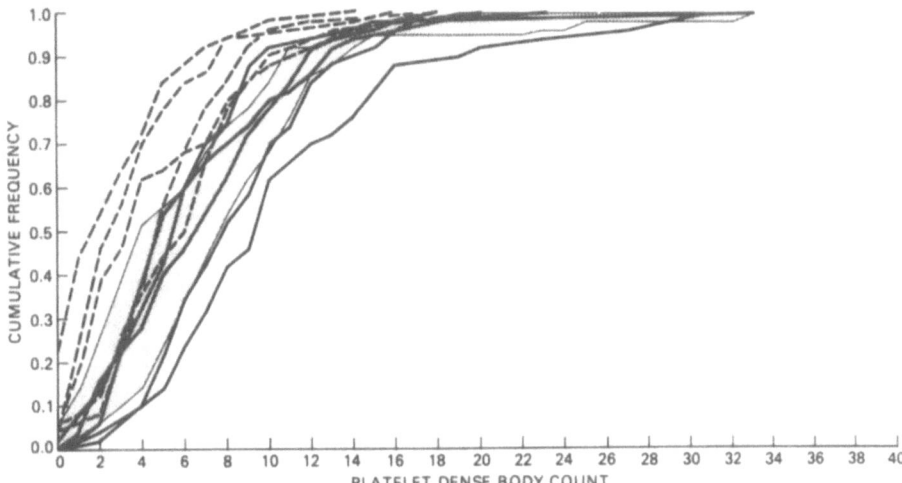

Fig. 1.2. The cumulative frequency distribution of dense bodies in unfractionated, low-density and high-density human platelets. Platelets from five normal subjects were fractionated into density-dependent cohorts on arabino-galactan gradients (Corash et al. 1984). Unfractionated platelets, obtained from whole blood, and platelets from the two density cohorts were prepared as whole-mount electron micrographs and the numbers of dense bodies per platelet were determined. Five hundred platelets were examined in each platelet population. The cumulative frequency distributions of platelet dense body content of unfractionated platelets (*shaded area*), least dense platelets (*broken lines*), and most dense platelets (*solid lines*) are indicated on the ordinate. The numbers of dense bodies per platelet (platelet dense body count) is indicated on the abscissa.

Table 1.2. Ultrastructural analysis of platelet density subpopulations

Subpopulation	n^a	Granules[b]	Mitochondria[c]
I-s	1140	2.03±0.54	0.76±0.45
II-s	1724	3.27±0.82	0.57±0.28
II-s	1604	4.82±1.11	0.57±0.16
IV-s	1669	6.48±1.36	0.66±0.21

Total platelet populations from nine normal subjects were separated into four subfractions (I-s, II-s, III-s and IV-s) using isosmolar discontinuous arabino-galactan gradients centrifuged under isopycnic equilibrium conditions. I-s indicates least dense platelets, II-s and III-s indicate platelets of intermediate density, and IV-s indicates most dense platelets. Platelet subfractions were prepared for thin-section electron microscopy and random sections were obtained for morphological analysis. A large number of sections were examined to minimize the effect of variation in section levels of individual platelets. These studies have been previously reported in detail (Corash et al. 1977).
[a] n indicates the number of platelet sections examined for each density fraction.
[b] Dense bodies, lysosomes and α-granules were counted together to obtain a total granule count for each platelet section. The mean number of granules per platelet section and standard deviation for each density fraction platelet section are indicated.
[c] The mean number of mitochondria per platelet section and the standard deviation were determined for each density fraction.

(Table 1.3). These authors also reported a density-dependent distribution of mitochondria, but the difference among the density fractions was less than that for granules. It is important to note that these authors did not sub-classify different granule types which have been shown to be differentially distributed with respect to density (Corash et al. 1984).

Table 1.3. Number of granules and mitochondria in density-dependent platelet subpopulations

Subpopulations	No. of granules	No. of mitochondria
I	111.7±72.2	23.3±14.28
II	101.1±57.1	16.9± 4.9
III	42.5±27.8	6.5± 2.8
IV	28.8±27.0	9.6± 6.4

These data were obtained from the report of Duyvené de Wit and co-workers (1987). Platelets were separated into four density fractions using arabino-galactan gradients as described by Duyvené de Wit et al. (1987). The most dense platelet fraction is labelled I and the least dense platelet fraction is labelled IV. Each platelet was sectioned serially, and the total number of granules and mitochondria in each platelet examined were tabulated. α-Granules and dense bodies were counted together as a single granule population.

Penington and co-workers (1976a, b) have examined the relationship between the heterogeneity of platelet characteristics and megakaryocyte properties. This approach was based on separating platelets according to density, measuring platelet volume, and examining the ultrastructural subcellular organelle content of different platelet density cohorts. These determinations were correlated with simultaneous ultrastructural analyses of megakaryocytes of different ploidy classes. With this technique, they reported that low-density platelets exhibited a smaller mean platelet volume than high-density platelets. This relationship had previously been established by Karpatkin (1969). A similar correlation between platelet buoyant density and volume was subsequently confirmed in our laboratory with both human and rabbit platelets (Corash and Shafer 1982; Corash et al. 1977). Penington et al. (1976b) also noted that platelet organelle content varied with platelet density and that megakaryocyte organelle content varied with megakaryocyte ploidy class. They did not discriminate among the different types of subcellular granules (α-granules, dense bodies or lysosomes). Based on these findings, Penington and co-workers postulated that low-ploidy (8N) megakaryocytes give rise to high-density, organelle-rich platelets, and high-ploidy megakaryocytes (32N) produce low-density, organelle-poor platelets. Combining their observations of density-dependent platelet organelle content, megakaryocyte ploidy and megakaryocyte ultrastructure, Penington et al. proposed that megakaryocyte ploidy was a major determinant of platelet characteristics, including cell volume. In an earlier study, Penington and Streatfield (1975) had concluded that 32N megakaryocytes produce "large sponge-like" platelets while 8N megakaryocytes produce "compact platelets of relatively constant size with numerous granules". These differing conclusions concerning a differential effect on platelet volume and organelle content with respect to buoyant density were not discussed in their later report (Penington et al. 1976b). Our observations (Corash et al. 1977) and those of Duyvené de Wit and colleagues (1987) are inconsistent with the observations of Penington and colleagues (1976b) that there is uniform variation of all subcellular organelles with respect to platelet density and megakaryocyte ploidy.

Density-Dependent Platelet Properties and Platelet Heterogeneity

Platelet volume, usually measured as mean platelet volume (MPV), has been the most frequently measured density-dependent characteristic. Some workers have fractionated platelets into density-dependent cohorts and used MPV as a means to test density separation validity. Studies from our laboratory have shown that while the mean or median platelet volumes of low-density and high-density platelets are significantly different (Corash et al. 1977) there is substantial overlap in the volume distribution of these two populations (Fig. 1.3). The observation indicates that platelet volume does not correlate specifically with density. Karpatkin and Penington (1984) have also emphasized this point. Thompson et al. (1982) demonstrated that size-dependent platelet cohorts prepared by elutriation exhibited a small but significant ($p<0.01$) difference in mean platelet density. In a later study, Thompson and colleagues (1983) reported that in baboons large platelets have a longer life-span than small platelets and they concluded that platelet size heterogeneity was due to differences in production factors in the bone marrow rather than in the circulation. These studies do not conclusively prove that platelet volume does not change during the cell's life-span. Data from other studies indicate that platelet density, rather than platelet volume, is a more specific age-related characteristic (Corash et al. 1978; Rand et

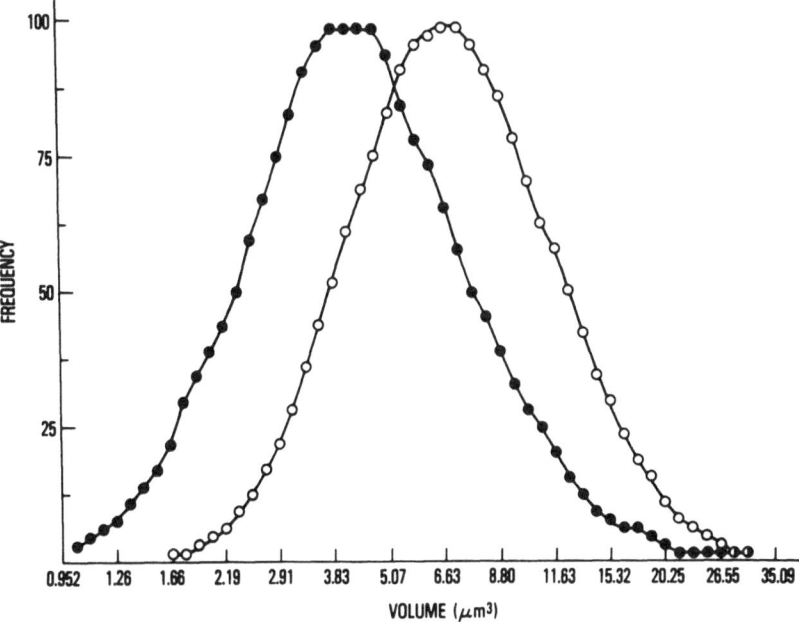

Fig. 1.3. Volume distribution of most dense and least dense platelets. Human platelets were separated into the least dense (*solid circles*) and the most dense (*open circles*) platelet fractions on discontinuous arabino-galactan density gradients (Corash et al. 1977). Relative frequency in per cent is indicated on the ordinate and volume in cubic micrometres is indicated on the abscissa.

al. 1981, 1983; Corash and Shafer 1982; Watson and Ludlam 1986). The substantial overlap in volume distribution of least-dense and most-dense platelets strongly suggests that, even if there is an age difference between these two fractions, events during platelet production must be important determinants of the platelet volume distribution.

In another series of experiments, human platelets were separated into four density-dependent fractions and the specific activities of subcellular organelle associated properties measured (Table 1.4) (Corash et al. 1984). 5-HT measured by a sensitive double isotopic dilution assay, was used as an indicator of dense body content. Monoamine oxidase activity was measured as an index of mitochondrial content and β-glucuronidase was measured as an index of lysosomal activity. Platelet factor 4 and β-thromboglobulin were both measured as indicators of α-granule content. These activities were expressed per milligram of platelet protein to normalize for differences in platelet size between the density fractions (Corash et al. 1984). It is important to note that other investigators have not expressed the concentration of platelet subcellular constituent activities on the basis of protein content (Thompson, 1982, 1983; Martin et al. 1983b), although Thompson has used platelet volume as an indirect means to normalize his measurements of platelet constituents (Thompson et al. 1982). α-Granule activities exhibited the greatest variation among different platelet density cohorts, in agreement with observations by van Oost et al. (1984). A small difference between mitochondrial enzyme activity of high-density and low-density platelets also was observed. This finding was attributed to in vivo decay of a non-renewable protein (Corash et al. 1984), since there is no evidence that mitochondria are secreted during the ageing process.

Table 1.4. Density-dependent platelet subpopulation specific activities

Component	N^a	I-s	II-s	III-s	IV-s	P^b
5-HT[c]	9	0.216	0.299	0.421	0.455	<0.001
Monoamine oxidase[d]	9	0.048	0.053	0.060	0.064	<0.025
β-Glucuronidase[e]	7	41.6	37.4	35.9	38.2	NS[f]
β-Thromboglobulin[g]	6	13.5	11.5	18.3	19.6	<0.001
Platelet factor 4[g]	6	13.3	23.4	32.1	41.0	<0.001

Total human platelet populations were separated into four density-dependent subpopulations using discontinuous arabino-galactan gradients (Corash et al. 1984). I-s indicates the least dense platelets, II-s and III-s indicate intermediate-density platelets and IV-s indicates the most dense platelets.
[a] N indicates the number of individual experiments.
[b] P indicates the p value of one-tailed paired t tests comparing the specific activities of least dense (I-s) with most dense (IV-s) platelets.
[c] ng/μg of platelet protein.
[d] nmol/μg platelet protein/hour.
[e] nmol/mg platelet protein/hour.
[f] NS, not significant.
[g] μg/mg platelet protein.

As discussed earlier, another important aspect of these studies was to establish that there was close agreement between the median biochemical constituent activities of the platelet density gradient subpopulations, determined from the mid-point gradient probit plot analysis, and the independently measured activities of native, unfractionated total platelet populations (Table 1) (Corash 1985;

Corash et al. 1984). A high level of agreement indicates that platelet activation and secretion did not occur during density centrifugation. Poor agreement between these two measurements would indicate that secretion and density modification had taken place during the fractionation procedure. As evidenced from our data (Table 1.1), there is close agreement between these two measurements, indicative of a valid density separation without secretion.

Kinetic Models to Examine the Relationship Between Platelet Density and Age

We have utilized two animal models to examine the relationship between platelet density and age. In the first study we evaluated two hypotheses: (1) high-density platelets have a longer life-span than low-density platelets; and (2) with time spent in the circulation (ageing), high-density platelets become less dense. In order to test these hypotheses, we developed a *Macaca mulatta* monkey model in which selected high-density and low-density platelet cohorts were isolated, labelled with radiochromium (^{51}Cr), re-injected into donor animals, and the survival and density distribution of the labelled cohorts followed with serial density gradient analyses (Corash et al. 1978). These studies demonstrated that the mean life-span of high-density platelets was 313.6 hours ±45.3 (standard error of the mean, SEM) compared to 74.6 hours ±15.3 (SEM) for low-density platelets. When radiolabelled high-density cohorts were re-injected into donor animals, virtually all of the radioactivity was located in the high-density fraction 1 hour after injection. Similarly, when low-density radiolabelled platelets were re-injected into donor animals, they were localized to the low-density gradient fraction.

Serial density gradient analyses following injection of low-density platelets demonstrated that low-density labelled platelets were rapidly cleared from the circulation, and during the entire platelet life-span high-density platelet fractions never became radioactive (Fig. 1.4). This experiment provided strong evidence that low-density platelets did not become more dense with ageing in the circulation, and also that there was not transfer of label in vivo from low-density to high-density platelets. Conversely, when high-density platelets were radio-labelled and re-injected into donor animals (Fig. 1.5), initially, labelled platelets were restricted to the high-density gradient fractions and low-density fractions were non-radioactive. Subsequently, with ageing, the high-density-gradient fractions became less radioactive while the low-density-gradient fractions became progressively more radioactive. In combination with the preceding observation that high-density platelets had a longer survival than low-density platelets, we concluded that the serial density gradient studies supported the hypothesis that high-density platelets have a longer in vivo survival and become less dense during ageing in the peripheral circulation (Corash et al. 1978).

We have also utilized another experimental model to examine the density distribution of newly produced platelets (Corash and Shafer 1982). This model used injection of radiolabelled amino acids into rabbits followed by serial fractionation of platelets into density-dependent platelet cohorts in order to

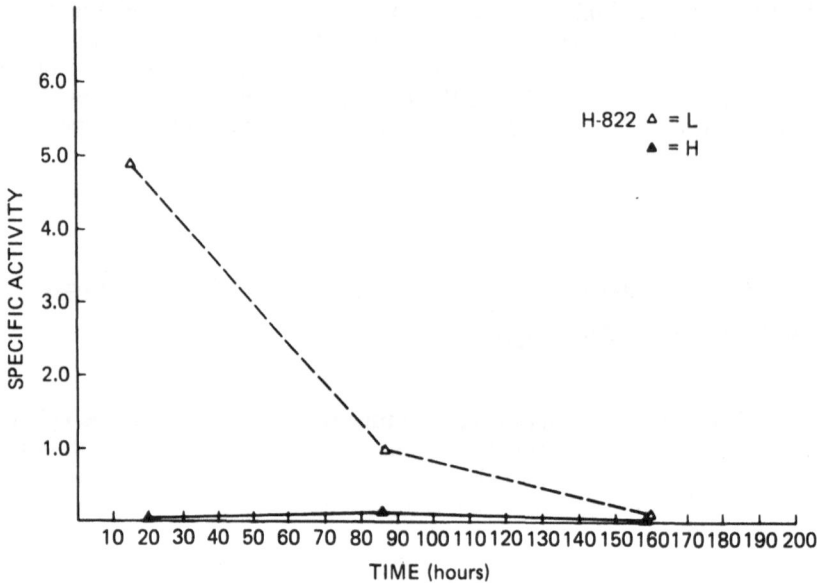

Fig. 1.4. Serial density-dependent distribution of radiolabelled low-density platelets after re-injection into a donor monkey (H-822). A narrow cohort of low-density platelets was isolated using an arabino-galactan gradient, labelled with ^{51}Cr, and infused into the donor animal (Corash et al. 1978). Serial blood samples were obtained following infusion of the labelled platelet cohort and density-gradient analysis was performed. The ordinate indicates platelet specific activity and the abscissa indicates time (hours) after injection.

ascertain the density distribution of newly produced platelets. Evatt and Levin (1969) have shown that parenterally administered radiolabelled amino acids are incorporated into newly produced platelets without uptake by mature platelets and with minimal re-utilization of label after clearance of the labelled cells. Similar models have been described by Karpatkin and his colleagues (Amorosi et al. 1971; Charmatz and Karpatkin 1974), Penington and co-workers (1976a), and Rand et al. (1981). We used splenectomized rabbits for our studies to avoid splenic retention of newly released platelets (Freedman and Karpatkin 1975). In addition, after pulse labelling, platelets for density gradient analyses were prepared free of plasma proteins and mononuclear leukocytes to ensure that radioactive amino acid incorporation into non-platelet fractions did not con-taminate the platelet fractions (Corash and Shafer 1982). Using this experimental model, we observed that radiolabelled, newly produced platelets preferentially appeared in the dense gradient fractions and that peak radioactivity of the most dense and least dense gradient fractions were temporally separated (Fig. 1.6). Examination of the ratios between most dense and least dense platelet specific activities (dpm/µg platelet protein) demonstrated that initially high-density platelets were two to four times as radioactive as low-density platelets, and 4 days later the ratio had declined to less than 0.5 (Fig. 1.7). Comparison of the post-labelling specific activities (dpm/µg cellular protein) of leukocytes and platelets confirmed that leukocytes were 20 times as radioactive as platelets 4 days after injection of labelled amino acids (Corash and Shafer 1982). Thus, if contami-nation of platelet fractions with leukocytes occurred, it would significantly affect

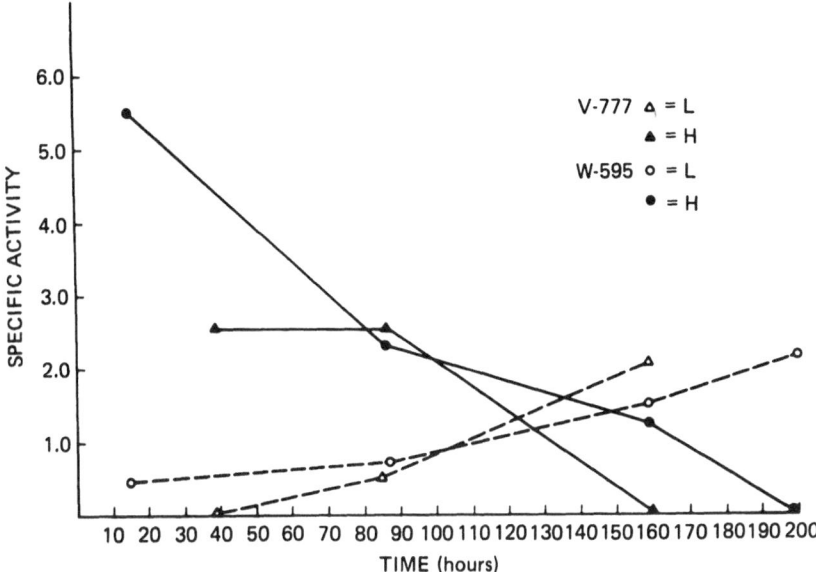

Fig. 1.5. Serial density-dependent distribution of radiolabelled high-density platelets after reinjection into two donor monkeys (V–777 and W-595). A narrow cohort of high-density platelets was isolated using an arabino-galactan gradient, labelled with ^{51}Cr, and infused into the donor animal (Corash et al. 1978). Serial blood samples were obtained following infusion of the labelled platelet cohort and density-gradient analysis was performed. The ordinate indicates platelet specific activity and the abscissa indicates time (hours) after injection.

the radioactivity attributable to the platelet fraction. We concluded from the preceding studies that in asplenic rabbits newly released platelets are more dense than average platelets and that peak radioactivity of low-density platelets occurs 2–3 days after peak activity of dense platelets. The latter observation, in the light of a 4–5-day rabbit platelet life-span, suggests that platelet density declines with platelet ageing.

Not all workers have observed the same results with either in vitro or in vivo cohort labelling studies. Mezzano et al. (1981) measured the survival of ^{51}Cr-labelled unfractionated human platelets and radiolabelled density cohorts. They concluded that newly formed platelets are less dense and become more dense with ageing. Mezzano et al. found the platelet survival of fractions enriched with low-density platelets was significantly longer than that of fractions enriched with high-density platelets. However, in their studies, density cohorts were not produced under isopycnic conditions; and no controls were used to ensure that platelet secretion with density modification during the initial preparation of density cohorts nor during subsequent analytic fractionation studies had been avoided.

In a second study Mezzano et al. (1984a) measured the relative radioactivity of low-density and high-density platelet fractions isolated after injection of autologous unfractionated ^{51}Cr-labelled platelets. These experiments were performed in human volunteers who had recovered from autoimmune thrombocytopenia (ITP) or Hodgkin's disease. The density-dependent fractionation was validated by measurement of endogenous 5-HT content in low-density and high-density

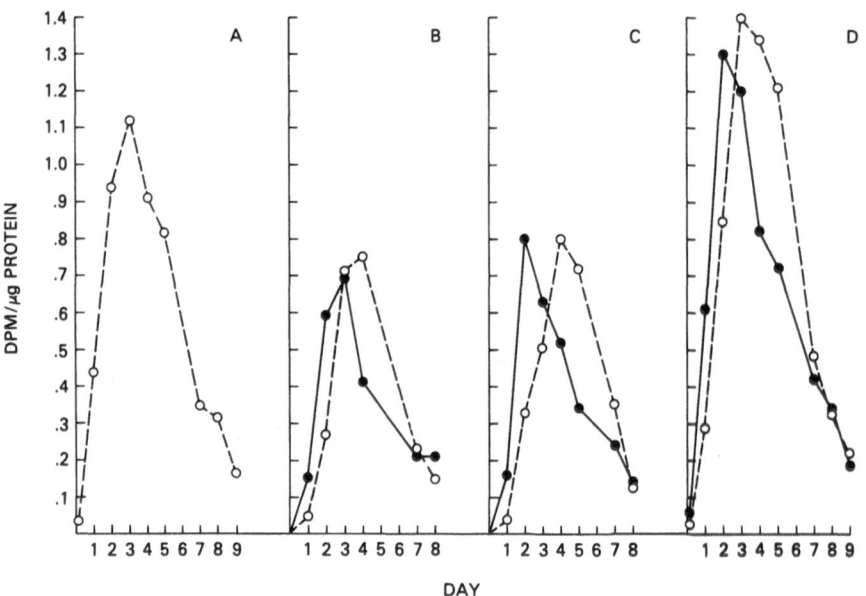

Fig. 1.6. Sequential appearance of newly produced radioactive platelets in a total unfractionated platelet population (**a**), and into the most dense (*solid line*) and least dense (*broken line*) platelet fractions obtained from three asplenic rabbits (**b**, **c** and **d**). Splenectomized rabbits were injected with a pool of ^{3}H amino acids. Following injection, platelets were isolated daily and the specific activities of total platelet population (**a**) and the most dense and least dense platelets were determined (Corash and Shafer 1982).

platelet fractions. Mezzano et al. observed a higher average endogenous 5-HT content in the most dense platelets compared to the least dense platelets, similar to the observations reported by our laboratory (Corash et al. 1984). Platelet density fractions were prepared using one-step discontinuous arabino-galactan gradients, but precise methodological details about preparation of the narrow density cohorts were not described. Moreover, it is not clear from this report why there were differences in the recoveries of radioactivity in the different density fractions, and why there were marked differences between the three experimental subjects.

After injection of a labelled total platelet population, they observed a more rapid decline in the relative specific activity of low-density as compared to high-density platelets. When they examined the 5-HT levels of patients recovering from ITP, they found that endogenous platelet 5-HT increased with recovery of the platelet count (Mezzano et al. 1984b). They have interpreted these findings, in combination with their previous studies (Mezzano et al. 1981), to indicate that platelet density increases with ageing and that accumulation of 5-HT in platelet dense bodies may be the mechanism for platelet density modification. It is of interest that Mishory and Danon (1978) found that rabbit platelet dense body number increased during recovery from experimental thrombocytopenia induced by platelet antiserum. Whether recovery from either ITP in humans or immune-induced thrombocytopenia in rabbits is analogous to events during normal thrombopoiesis remains unclear. Importantly, Illes et al. (1987) found that

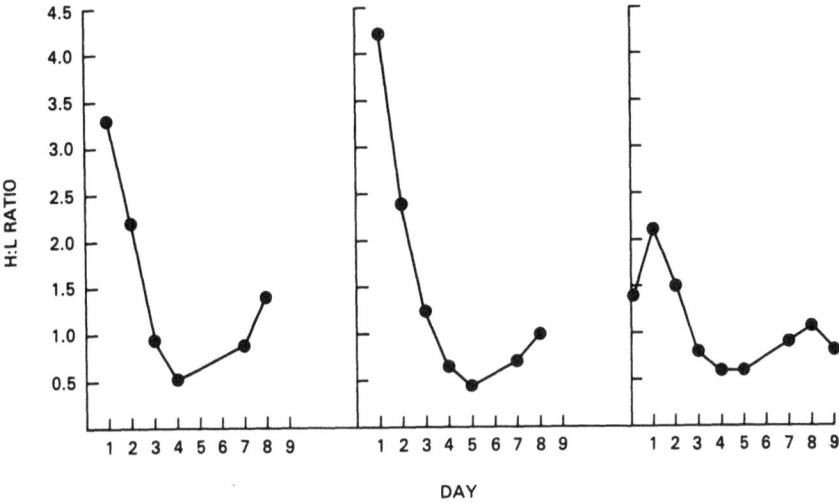

Fig. 1.7.   Ratio of high-density (H) and low-density (L) platelet specific radioactivity after injection of labelled amino acids into three splenectomized rabbits. Platelets were serially fractionated into a high-density and low-density fraction daily after injection of the label. Platelet subfractions were isolated as previously described and the H:L specific activity ratios were determined (Corash and Shafer 1982).

platelet density in ITP patients was similar to that of normal subjects. Thus, the observations of Mezzano et al. and Illes et al. regarding the density and 5-HT content of platelets in ITP and as a platelet ageing model appear discrepant. If newly released, young platelets acquire 5-HT and increase in density as a result of this process, then the density of normal and ITP platelets should be different, rather than similar as reported by Illes et al. (1987).

In a third study, Mezzano and co-workers (1984a) examined the serial density distribution of radiolabelled density-dependent platelet cohorts in splenectomized dogs. In contrast to their earlier studies in humans (Mezzano et al. 1981, 1984b), with this experimental model they reported that high-density platelet cohorts had a significantly longer life-span than low-density cohorts. More importantly, they observed that after injection of labelled high-density cohorts low-density platelet fractions became progressively more radioactive. After injection of labelled low-density platelet cohorts, high-density platelet fractions remained non-radioactive. These observations are similar to our earlier studies with the same model in *Macaca mulatta* monkeys (Corash et al. 1978). Mezzano concluded these findings indicated that in dogs platelet density decreases with ageing in the peripheral circulation, and he speculated that the significant contrast with his earlier studies and those of others (Martin and Penington 1983) was due to species differences.

Martin and Penington (1983) measured the density distribution of ^{51}Cr-labelled total platelet populations after injection into *Macaca fascicularis* monkeys, a close relative to *M. mulatta* used by Corash et al. (1978). They concluded that "lighter platelets" have a slightly shorter life-span than dense platelets, and observed a small but significant ($p<0.001$) increase in density of the labelled platelet population. These studies were not performed with true isopycnic density gradient centrifugation conditions and there were no controls to ensure that valid density separations without secretion were achieved.

More recently, Savage et al. (1986) have reported studies using baboons and autologous ^{111}In-labelled platelets to measure the density distribution following infusion of unfractionated and fractionated density cohorts. They reported that platelet density increased with ageing, but the survival of low-density and high-density cohorts were equal. These studies also were performed with Percoll gradients which may not have achieved isopycnic equilibrium, and there were no measurements of density-dependent properties to validate that true density separation had been effected nor that activation had not occurred. The authors did measure plasma levels of α-granule constituents and observed a slight increase ($p=0.05$) in levels of plasma platelet factor 4 after chronic arteriovenous cannulation used to perform the studies. It is also important to note that Savage et al. (1986) did not observe significant differences between mean platelet volume of the mid-point fractions and the most dense fractions (Fig. 1). This suggests the possibility that complete isopycnic separation was not effected since it has been universally noted that high-density platelets exhibit greater mean platelet volumes compared to average-density platelets.

In a recent study, Watson and Ludlam (1986) measured the in vivo survival of ^{111}In-labelled autologous platelets in normal and splenectomized humans. After injection, samples were divided into density-dependent subfractions on Percoll gradients which were centrifuged at high forces, but most likely not true isopycnic conditions. No measurements of density-dependent properties were reported in order to verify that adequate separation had occurred without secretion. In contrast to the Mezzano studies, Watson and Ludlam concluded that high-density platelets were preferentially retained in the spleen and had longer survivals than low-density platelets, in both normal and splenectomized subjects. Unfortunately these studies did not specifically examine the survival of in vitro labelled density cohorts which were then re-injected to measure survival.

Packham and Mustard have published an extensive series of papers using rabbit platelets and isopycnic arabino-galactan density gradient fractionation techniques, similar to our methods, in which they have consistently observed a relationship between platelet density and platelet ageing (Rand et al. 1981, 1983; Packham et al. 1985). Collectively, their studies and those from our laboratory support the hypothesis that platelet density decreases with ageing in the peripheral circulation. A corollary of these observations is that high-density platelets have a longer survival than low-density platelets. In combination with our observations that α-granule and dense body content varies inversely with platelet density, these studies suggest that selected platelet properties may be modified during ageing.

Is Heterogeneity of Density-Dependent Platelet Properties Significant?

The distribution of platelet density-dependent properties has been determined by events during thrombopoiesis; however, the processes by which these differences in platelet composition arise remain unknown. It has always been intriguing that there is a substantial density-dependent difference in platelet content of α-granule and dense body constituents and little or no difference in mitochondrial or lysosomal constituents (Mezzano et al. 1984b; Corash et al. 1984). The earlier observations by Kaplan et al. (1979) that α-granules are more easily secreted than lysosomes suggests that this difference may be related to platelet density modification in vivo through a process of continuous platelet secretion during ageing. This is consistent with the observations by Sixma and his group that platelet α-granule content is a major determinant of platelet density (van Oost et al. 1983, 1984). Both the Mustard group and the Sixma group have shown that platelet activation leads to a decrease of platelet density, but not necessarily of platelet survival (Cieslar et al. 1979; van Oost et al. 1983). Thus, with ageing in the peripheral circulation and participation in haemostatic events in which platelets are activated, but not removed, platelet density may decrease due to α-granule loss until a limiting point is reached when low-density platelets are cleared.

The signal which initiates clearance of senescent platelets is unknown, although Khansari and Fudenberg (1983) have suggested that accumulation of immunoglobulin on platelets may serve as a clearance signal to monocytes. Lalezari and Driscoll (1982) have noted that haematopoietic cells lose HLA antigens with maturation, and have demonstrated that platelets can absorb HLA antigens from plasma. Pereira et al. (1988) have observed that low-density platelets express 42% more HLA-A2 and 55% more class I HLA antigens than high-density cells. This finding taken with those of Lalezari suggests that low-density platelets may accumulate surface HLA antigens as they age in the circulation, and perhaps this may play a role in signalling platelet senescence.

Contributions of Events During Thrombopoiesis to Platelet Heterogeneity

More recently, we have developed another model with which to determine the contributions of events during thrombopoiesis to platelet heterogeneity. The availability of two-colour fluorescence-activated flow cytometry for analysis of megakaryocyte ploidy makes feasible serial observations during induction and recovery from thrombocytopenia. Using a murine model, our laboratory has serially examined the relationship between bone marrow megakaryocyte ploidy and platelet volume (Corash et al. 1987). In response to acute, severe thrombocytopenia (reduction of the platelet level of $<0.05 \times 10^6/\mu l$) we observed that platelet volume increased 40 hours before a detectable shift in bone marrow megakaryocyte ploidy (Corash et al. 1987). Less severe thrombocytopenia (reduction of the platelet level to $0.150–0.250 \times 10^6/\mu l$) resulted in a delay of the shift in the ploidy distribution from 48 hours to 72 hours after the onset of thrombocytopenia. Moderate thrombocytopenia ($0.300–0.400 \times 10^6/\mu l$) did not result in a ploidy shift, but did produce a significant and prolonged increment in mean platelet volume. In response to moderate thrombocytopenia, mean platelet volume was significantly increased as early as 12 hours after the administration of platelet antiserum and remained increased during the period of thrombocytosis after recovery (Corash et al. 1987).

In contrast to the observations of Martin et al. (1983a) after the induction of acute severe thrombocytopenia, we observed that the peak change in platelet volume occurred at 24 hours, although there was a significant change in platelet volume as early as 8 hours after the onset of thrombocytopenia (Corash et al. 1987). Our studies, compatible with the observations by Ebbe et al. (1988) and Odell et al. (1976), suggest that the early increase (8–36 hours) in platelet volume after either severe or moderate thrombocytopenia occurs prior to an increase in megakaryocyte ploidy, and perhaps in the absence of a sustained increase in megakaryocyte plasma volume. This early increment in platelet volume may arise secondary to a change in the process of platelet release from mature megakaryocytes, perhaps due to increased production of "pro-platelets", which could account for the early increment of platelet volume as described by Tong et al. (1987).

Conclusions

Two decades after the seminal paper by Karpatkin (1969) on platelet heterogeneity, we are still embroiled in an active controversy about the significance of platelet heterogeneity. Despite this controversy, there is agreement on several points:

1. Platelets are heterogeneous with respect to volume, density, functional properties and biochemical composition. A large number of studies have contributed information which establish this conclusion.

2. Under normal conditions, platelet survival appears to be approximately linear in most mammals, consistent with the concept that some form of senescent process rather than random destruction limits platelet life-span.

3. Platelet activation results in secretion of selected subcellular organelles while other organelles, mitochondria for example, are not secreted.

4. Platelets can be separated by density-dependent fractionation and high-density platelets have a greater mean volume than low-density platelets.

5. High-density platelets also exhibit greater protein content and greater amounts of selected subcellular constituents, although there is not universal agreement on the density dependency of all constituents.

6. Events during thrombopoiesis contribute significantly to platelet heterogeneity, but megakaryocyte ploidy does not necessarily affect platelet properties (Corash 1989). This latter point may not be universally accepted at present, but data from several laboratories suggest that this will prove to be the case.

At present we do not have a definitive answer whether platelet heterogeneity is related to in vivo ageing. We are left with three choices since it is highly likely that platelets undergo some "ageing" process in the peripheral circulation. Platelet properties, most notably density, may remain unchanged, increase or decrease during this hypothesized ageing process. One issue which continues to intrigue me, and which I raise in conclusion for those in the field to ponder, revolves around the question of how each of these events may arise. If platelets remain unchanged, then we have no need to postulate an ageing mechanism except to conclude that they are removed by some mysterious process. This is disquieting, since we suspect that some age-related changes must occur with time spent in the circulation, and there is some evidence that during disease platelets may be activated with attendant changes in density. If platelet density increases during ageing, how does this process arise? It is well known that platelets have limited capacity for de novo protein synthesis, thus it seems unlikely that continuing protein synthesis can account for an increase in density. If high-density platelets are old platelets how do we explain the presence of glycogen and ribosomes in them, but not in the postulated low-density young platelets? Recently, Handagama and colleagues (1987) have shown that circulating protein may be incorporated into megakaryocytes and platelet α-granules. However, it was not possible to determine whether platelets could endocytose proteins. They also reported preliminary studies demonstrating that in vivo defibrination of rats resulted in decreased amounts of platelet and megakaryocyte fibrinogen, but platelet α-granule content of platelet factor 4 was normal (Handagama et al. 1988). Thus, it is possible that megakaryocytes may acquire proteins from the plasma. It is unknown whether platelets can endocytose circulating proteins, but if possible then this would be a mechanism to increase platelet protein content and density without protein synthesis.

It is reasonably well established that platelets can secrete α-granules and continue to circulate (Cieslar et al. 1979; van Oost et al. 1983). In addition, there is evidence that in pathological conditions platelet survival may be correlated with the plasma concentration of α-granule proteins (Doyle et al. 1980). In normal subects, the plasma levels of α-granule secretory products have been reported to decline when platelet function is inhibited by aspirin (Kaplan et al. 1979). Thus, it is feasible to entertain the idea that α-granule secretion may occur continuously at a low level as part of the platelet ageing process. This may contribute to a progressive reduction of platelet density with time spent in the circulation. Under pathological conditions, the secretion of α-granules may increase, accelerating the density decline and giving rise to "prematurely aged" platelets. Currently, I find better evidence to support an ageing mechanism by which platelet density decreases with ageing. However, we have yet to design an experiment which provides clear proof of this hypothesis. That will be the challenge for all of us working in this field since we have not yet solved the mystery of platelet heterogeneity.

Supported in part by Research Grant HL 33340 from the National Heart, Lung, and Blood Institute, National Institutes of Health, Bethesda, MD.

References

Amorosi E, Garg SK, Karpatkin S (1971) Heterogeneity of human platelets. IV. Identification of a young platelet population with Se^{75}-selenomethionine. Br J Haematol 21:227–232
Aster RH, Jandl JH (1964) Platelet sequestration in man. I. Methods. J Clin Invest 43:843
Bessman D (1982) Prediction of platelet production during chemotherapy of acute leukemia. Am J Hematol 13:219–227

Bessman JD (1984) The relation of megakaryocyte ploidy to platelet volume. Am J Hematol 16:161–170

Blajchman MA, Senyi AF, Hirsh J, Genton E, George JN (1981) Hemostatic function, survival, and membrane glycoprotein changes in young versus old rabbit platelets. J Clin Invest 68:1289–1294

Boneu B, Boneu A, Raisson CI, Guiraud R, Bierme R (1973) Kinetics of platelet "populations" in the stationary state. Thromb Res 3:605–611

Boneu B, Corberand J, Plante J, Bierme R (1977) Evidence that platelet density and volume are not related to ageing. Thromb Res 10:475

Boneu B, Sie P, Caranobe C, Nouvel C, Bierme R (1980) Malondialdehyde (MDA) re-appearance in human platelet density subpopulations after a single intake of aspirin. Thromb Res 19:609

Boneu B, Vigoni F, Boneu C, Caranobe C, Sie P (1982) Further studies on the relationship between platelet buoyant density and platelet age. Am J Hematol 13:239

Charmatz A, Karpatkin S (1974) Heterogeneity of rabbit platelets. I. Employment of an albumin density gradient for separation of a young platelet population identified with [75]selenomethionine. Thromb Diath Haemorrh 31:485

Cieslar P, Greenberg JP, Rand ML, Packham MA, Kinlough-Rathbone RL, Mustard JF (1979) Separation of thrombin treated platelets by density gradient centrifugation. Blood 53:867

Corash L (1985) Platelet density heterogeneity. Blood 65:779–780

Corash L (1986) Density dependent red cell separation. In: Beutler E (ed) Red cell metabolism. Churchill Livingstone, New York, pp 90–108

Corash L (1989) The relationship between megakaryocyte ploidy and platelet volume. Blood Cells 15:81–107

Corash L, Shafer B (1982) Use of asplenic rabbits to demonstrate that platelet age and density are related. Blood 60:166–171

Corash L, Piomelli S, Chen H, Seaman C, Gross E (1974) Separation of erythrocytes according to age on a simplified density gradient. J Lab Clin Med 84:147–151

Corash L, Tan H, Gralnick HR (1977) Heterogeneity of human whole blood platelet subpopulations. I. Relationship between buoyant density, cell volume, and ultrastructure. Blood 49:71–87

Corash L, Shafer B, Perlow M (1978) Heterogeneity of human whole blood platelet subpopulations. II. Use of a subhuman primate model to analyze the relationship between density and platelet age. Blood 52:726–734

Corash L, Costa JL, Shafer B, Donlon JA, Murphy D (1984) Heterogeneity of human whole blood platelet subpopulations. III. Density-dependent differences in subcellular constituents. Blood 64:185–193

Corash L, Chen HY, Levin J, Baker G, Lu H, Mok Y (1987) Regulation of thrombopoiesis: effects of the degree of thrombocytopenia on megakaryocyte ploidy and platelet volume. Blood 70:177–185

Doyle DJ, Chesterman CN, Cade JF, McCready JR, Rennie GC, Morgan JF (1980) Plasma concentrations of platelet specific proteins correlated with platelet survival. Blood 55:82–87

Duyvené de Wit LJ, Badenhorst PN, du P. Heyns A (1987) Ultrastructural morphometric observations on serial sectioned human blood platelets. Eur J Cell Biol 43:408–411

Ebbe S, Yee T, Carpenter D, Phalen E (1988) Megakaryocytes increase in size within ploidy groups in response to the stimulus of thrombocytopenia. Exp Hematol 16:55–61

Evatt BL, Levin J (1969) Measurement of thrombopoiesis in rabbits using [75]selenomethionine. J Clin Invest 48:1615–1626

Freedman ML, Karpatkin S (1975) Heterogeneity of rabbit platelets. V. Preferential splenic sequestration of megathrombocytes. Br J Haematol 31:255

Ginsburg AD, Aster RH (1969) Kinetic studies with 51-chromium-labeled platelet cohorts in rats. J Lab Clin Med 74:138

Greenberg JP, Packham MA, Guccione MA, Rand ML, Reimers HJ, Mustard JF (1979) Survival of rabbit platelets treated in vitro with chymotrypsin, plasmin, trypsin, or neuraminidase. Blood 53:916

Handagama PJ, George JN, Shuman MA, McEver RP, Bainton DF (1987) Incorporation of a circulating protein into megakaryocyte and platelet granules. Proc Natl Acad Sci USA 84:861–865

Handagama P, Shuman R, Shuman MA, Bainton DF (1988) In vivo defibrination results in markedly decreased levels of fibrinogen in megakaryocytes and platelets in rats. Blood (Suppl 1) 72:323a

Harker LA, Finch CA (1976) Thrombokinetics in man. J Clin Invest 48:963

Hill RJ, Stenberg P, Sullam P, Levin J. Use of arabino-galactan to obtain washed mouse platelets appropriate for functional and morphological studies and free of contaminating plasma proteins. J Lab Clin Med 111:73–83

Hirsh J, Glynn MF, Mustard JF (1968) The effect of platelet age on platelet adherence to collagen. J Clin Invest 47:466

Illes I, Pfueller SL, Hussein S, Chesterman CN, Martin JF (1987) Platelets in idiopathic thrombocytopenic purpura are increased in size but are of normal density. Br J Haematol 67:173–176

Jackson CW (1989) Animal models with inherited hematopoietic abnormalities as tools to study thrombopoiesis. Blood Cells 15:237–253

Kaplan KL, Broekman MJ, Chernoff A, Lesznik GR, Drillings M (1979) Platelet alpha-granule proteins: studies on release and subcellular localization. Blood 53:604–611

Karpatkin S (1969) Heterogeneity of human platelets I. Metabolic and kinetic evidence suggestive of young and old platelets. J Clin Invest 48:1073–1082

Karpatkin S, Penington D (1984) Heterogeneity of platelets. Br J Haematol 56:351–354

Khansari N, Fudenberg HH (1983) Immune elimination of aging platelets by autologous monocytes: role of membrane-specific autoantibody. Eur J Immunol 13:990–994

Lalezari P, Driscoll AM (1982) Ability of thrombocytes to acquire HLA specificity from plasma. Blood 59:167

Leone G, Agostini A, Decrescenzo A, Bizzi B (1979) Platelet heterogeneity: relationship between buoyant density, size, lipid peroxidation and platelet age. Scand J Haematol 23:204

Martin JF, Penington DG (1983) The relationship between the age and density of circulating ^{51}Cr-labelled platelets in the sub-human primate. Thromb Res 30:157

Martin JF, Trowbridge EA (1985) Platelet density heterogeneity. Blood 65:779

Martin JF, Trowbridge EA, Salmon GL, Slater DN (1982) The relationship between platelet and megakaryocyte volumes. Thromb Res 28:447–459

Martin JF, Trowbridge EA, Salmon G, Plumb J (1983a) The biological significance of platelet volume: its relationship to bleeding time, platelet thromboxane B_2 production and megakaryocyte nuclear DNA concentration. Thromb Res 32:443–460

Martin JF, Shaw T, Heggie J, Penington DG (1983b) Measurement of the density of human platelets and its relationship to volume. Br J Haematol 54:337–352

McDonald JWD, Ali M (1983) Recovery of cyclooxygenase activity after aspirin in populations of platelets separated on stractan density gradients. Prostaglandins Leukotrienes Med 12:245–252

Mezzano D, Hwang K, Catalano P, Aster RH (1981) Evidence that platelet buoyant density, but not size, correlates with platelet age in man. Am J Hematol 11:61

Mezzano D, Aranda E, Foradori A, Rodriguez S, Lira P (1984a) Kinetics of platelet density subpopulations in splenectomized mongrel dogs. Am J Hematol 17:373–382

Mezzano D, Aranda E, Rodriguez S, Foradori A, Lira P (1984b) Increase in density and accumulation of serotonin by human aging platelets. Am J Hematol 17:11–21

Mezzano D, Aster RH, Peters AM, Watson HHK, Ludlam CA (1987) Survival of platelet density subpopulations. Br J Haematol 65:505–507

Mishory B, Danon D (1978) Structural aspects of in vivo aging rabbit blood platelets. Thromb Res 12:893–906

Odell TT, Murphy JR, Jackson CW (1976) Stimulation of megakaryocytopoiesis by acute thrombocytopenia in rats. Blood 48:765–775

Packham MA, Guccione MA, O'Brien KM (1985) Duration of the effect of aspirin on the synthesis of thromboxane by density subpopulations of rabbit platelets stimulated with thrombin. Blood 66:287–290

Penington DG, Streatfield K (1975) Heterogeneity of megakaryocytes and platelets. Ser Haematol 8:22–48

Penington DG, Lee NLY, Roxburgh AE, McGready JR (1976a) Platelet density and size: the interpretation of heterogeneity. Br J Haematol 34:365–376

Penington DG, Streatfield K, Roxburgh AE (1976b) Megakaryocytes and the heterogeneity of circulating platelets. Br J Haematol 34:639–653

Pereira J, Cretney C, Aster RH (1988) Variation of class I HLA antigen expression among platelet density cohorts: a possible index of platelet age? Blood 71:516–519

Rand ML, Greenberg JP, Packham MA, Mustard JF (1981) Density subpopulations of rabbit platelets: size, protein, sialic acid content, and specific radioactivity changes following labeling with ^{35}S-sulfate in vivo. Blood 57:741–746

Rand ML, Packham MA, Mustard JF (1983) Survival of density subpopulations of rabbit platelets: use of ^{51}Cr–^{111}In labeled platelets to measure survival of least dense and most dense platelets concurrently. Blood 61:362–367

Savage B, McFadden PR, Hanson SR, Harker LA (1986) The relation of platelet density to platelet age: survival of low- and high-density ^{111}Indium-labeled platelets in baboons. Blood 68:386–393

Stenberg PE, Levin J (1988) Ultrastructural analysis of experimental immune thrombocytopenia in mice: dissociation between alterations in megakaryoctes and platelets. Blood 72 (Suppl 1):340a

Thompson CB, Eaton KA, Princiotta SM. Size dependent platelet subpopulations: relationship of platelet volume to ultrastructure, enzymatic activity, and function. Br J Haematol 50:509–519

Thompson CB, Love DG, Quinn PG, Valeri CR (1983) Platelet size does not correlate with platelet age. Blood 62:487–494

Tong M, Seth P, Penington DG (1987) Proplatelets and stress platelets. Blood 69:522–528

Trowbridge EA, Martin JF (1984) An analysis of the platelet and polyploid megakaryocyte response to acute thrombocytopenia and its biological implications. Clin Phys Physiol Meas 5:263–277

van Oost B, Hien-Hagg IHV, Ans PM, Timmermans PM, Sixma JJ (1983) The effect of thrombin on the density distribution of blood platelet: detection of activated platelets in the circulation. Blood 62:433–440

van Oost BA, Timmermans APM, Sixma JJ (1984) Evidence that platelet density depends on the α-granule content in platelets. Blood 63:482–485

Watson HHK, Ludlam CA (1986) Survival of 111-indium platelet subpopulations of varying density in normal and post splenectomized subjects. Br J Haematol 62:117–124

Technical Questions

Trowbridge: Could you tell me the way that you measured the number of dense granules in the platelets? Did you use electron micrographs through sectioned platelets? What technique did you use to make sure that the size of the platelet was taken into account?

Corash: This technique is called whole mount technique and it was developed by Jonathon Costa at the National Institutes of Health when we were collaborating together. One does not section the platelets. The platelets are suspended in arabino-galactan and are allowed to settle onto a grid. Because the dense bodies are electron-opaque one counts everything in the cell under the transmission-scope, so planar section has really nothing to do with it. In the absence of overlapping cells, when they have settled on the grids, you get a beautifully precise count of dense body content. It is tedious but if you have a dedicated person doing it, it works quite nicely.

Trowbridge: Did you take the size of the platelet into account? Is it dense body per unit volume of platelet, or is it actually dense bodies per platelet, irrespective of size?

Corash: It is dense bodies per platelet, not corrected for unit volume. In our system the difference in volume between the low-density cells and high-density cells, at least in humans, is about 23 or 24%. That correlates very well with the difference in protein content that we find as well. The dense body content, first of all, is not normally distributed. It is very much positively skewed, so that is why we used the cumulative frequency distribution and looked at the median of those distributions. If you compare medians and correct those for unit volume you are still left with very significant differences, if you do a non-parametric test, between the high-density and low-density cells.

Rendu*: I was a bit worried about the α-granule content you described in the four different populations. I think you said 30; I am not sure of the units, was it nanograms or micrograms per 10^8 platelets?

Corash: Actually those values were not adjusted for platelet protein. We would have to go back and look at the appropriate figure. I would refer you instead to

*Dr Francine Rendu, INSERM, U–150, Hôpital Lariboisière, 6 rue Guy Patin, 75010, Paris, France.

my 1984 paper published in *Blood*, where it is expressed both per number of cells and per microgram of protein.

Rendu: If it is expressed per number of cells, I am worried because in high-density platelets with the highest level of β-thromboglobulin, 30 seems to be very low. As you mentioned, α-granules liberate their contents very easily and you may have differences in that release between the different populations. That would interfere with your results.

Corash: We thought a lot about that. At the time we thought the numbers that we had obtained were in good agreement with other values published in the literature. We have studied whether there has been secretion with an extremely sensitive assay, by using the expression of GMP140 on the platelet surface. Work by Paula Stenberg, as well as our own flow cytometric assay, has shown there to be no secretion. GMP140 is a granule membrane protein of 140 kD described by Rod McKiver in some work starting in 1984. There is a monoclonal antibody called S12 which has been raised against this protein. If you get platelet activation, at extremely low levels, then you get expression of GMP140 on the cell surface. We have not seen any expression of GMP140 on the surface of these cells.

Rendu: Even in the light platelets?

Corash: Yes, even in the light platelets, separated in this system. As a matter of fact, we thought that would be a wonderful marker for previous events having taken place. We hoped to isolate platelets from patients and find expression of GMP140 as an index of some sort of ageing process, but that has not been the case.

If you isolate platelets carefully from normal individuals, you find about 1% or so expression of GMP140. Clearly this would be too little to say that these are some sort of old platelets.

2 The Biology of Platelet Volume Heterogeneity

C. B. Thompson, R. L. Monroy, R. R. Skelly,
P. G. Quinn and J. A. Jakubowski

Introduction

Platelet volume heterogeneity has been recognized by haematologists for over 100 years (Bizzozero 1882; Olef 1936). Despite this, the aetiology and the significance of platelet volume heterogeneity continues to be a controversial subject. Several years ago our laboratory developed a technique for the separation of platelets into size-dependent subpopulations using counterflow centrifugation (Thompson et al. 1982). Using this newly devised cell separation technique, we have been able to address a number of questions concerning the aetiology and significance of platelet volume heterogeneity. Platelets separated into size-dependent subpopulations contain platelet granular contents in direct proportion to their volume (Thompson et al. 1982, 1983a). The intrinsic function of size-dependent platelet subpopulations is similar when function is measured as a percentage of granular contents that are released following activation by any of a variety of platelet agonists (Thompson et al. 1983a). However, because of the volume-dependent differences in the absolute amounts of intrinsic granular and membrane components, the ability of platelets to affect each other and their environment as measured by aggregation and total amounts of granular contents released is proportional to their size. These results confirmed that platelet volume correlates with absolute platelet function (Mannucci and Sharp 1967; Karpatkin 1978). In contrast, despite the previously held belief that platelet volume heterogeneity is created by decreases in platelet volume as platelets age in the circulation, our studies reveal that platelet heterogeneity is created primarily during platelet production (Thompson et al. 1983b). During steady-state thrombopoiesis the platelet count and mean platelet volume (MPV) of circulating platelets are inversely correlated, suggesting that platelet production is regulated to maintain a constant circulating functional platelet mass (Thompson and Jakubowski 1988). We have been able to test this hypothesis by observing the platelet count and mean platelet volumes in rhesus monkeys during continuous infusion of granulocyte–macrophage colony-stimulating factor (GM–CSF). The infusion of GM–CSF results in a significant increase in the circulating platelet count and a concomitant decline in the mean platelet volume (Monroy et al. 1989). Other studies (Evatt and Levin 1969; Martin et al. 1982; Bessman 1984; Corash et al. 1987; Tong et al. 1987) have shown that stimulated thrombopoiesis, which occurs under periods of increased haemostatic demand, can induce simultaneous increases in both the number and MPV of the platelets produced. Together these results suggest that the mean platelet volume and number of platelets produced in the bone marrow during a given period of time are under at least partly independent regulatory control during platelet production.

Characteristics of Size-Dependent Platelet Subpopulations

During steady-state haematopoiesis the platelet volume distribution approaches log normality with platelets ranging in size from $<2\ \mu m^3$ to $>15\ \mu m^3$ in volume. This variation in size is considerably greater than that observed for other circulating blood elements and the physiological relevance of this heterogeneity has long been controversial (Paulus 1975). To test directly the characteristics of platelets of different sizes, we have developed a technique for the separation of platelets into size-dependent subpopulations using a counterflow centrifuge (Thompson et al. 1982; Fig. 2.1).

Counterflow centrifugation utilizes a centrifugal force opposed by a flow force to separate particles (Fig. 2.2). The velocity of flow necessary to remove a particle from the centrifugation chamber is proportional to the size of the particle as predicted by Stokes' law. Counterflow centrifugation has proved to be a highly reproducible method to separate platelets into size-dependent subpopulations and the volume distributions of platelets before and after separation into

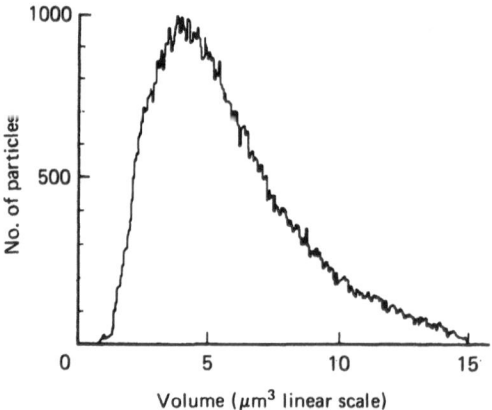

Fig. 2.1. Volume distribution of platelets isolated from the peripheral blood of a normal volunteer. The platelet volume distribution is approximately log-normal and platelets ranging in size from $<2\ \mu m^3$ up to $15\ \mu m^3$ are evident.

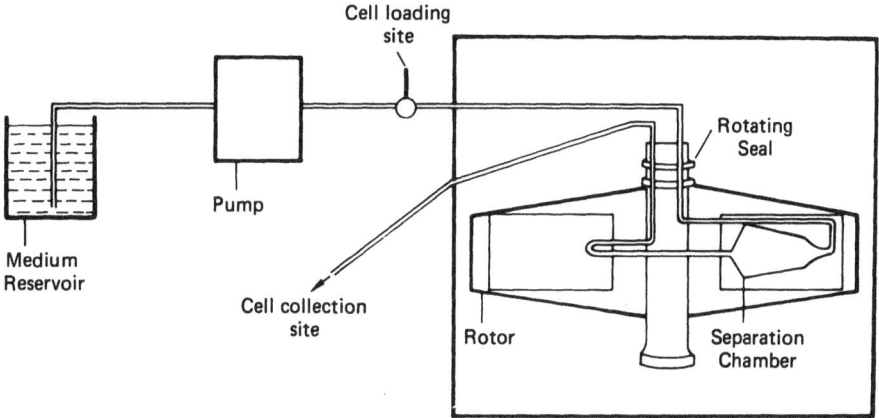

Fig. 2.2. Separation system for the generation of size-dependent subpopulations. The set-up of a basic counterflow centrifugation system is schematically depicted. Cells were loaded at the cell loading site and enter a rotating centrifuge separation chamber by means of a rotating seal. Fluid is pumped through the separation chamber by means of an external pump. The flow of fluid is in opposition to the centrifugal force created by centrifugation of the rotor. Cells are collected distally at the cell collection site following elution from the separation chamber. The velocity at which a particle is removed from the separation chamber is determined by Stokes' law, $V \propto (w^2 r D^2 \rho_{rel})/(kn)$, where V is the velocity, $w^2 r$ is the centrifugal force created by the centrifuge, D is the particle diameter, ρ_{rel} is the density of the particle minus the density of the supporting media, k is a particle shape factor, and n is the viscosity of the supporting media.

subpopulations appear to be unaffected by this separation technique. When size-dependent platelet subpopulations were examined for their content of a variety of platelet-specific and non-specific contents, it was found that the amounts of β-thromboglobulin as an index of α-granule content, adenosine triphosphate (ATP) as an index of dense granule contents, and lactate dehydrogenase (LDH) as a measure of cytoplastic volume were roughly proportional to the platelet volume (Table 2.1). Consistent with this, only slight differences in the mean diversity of small and large platelets were observed (Thompson et al. 1982). When an equivalent number of platelets were resuspended in either citrated

Table 2.1. Characteristics of human size-dependent platelet subpopulations $(n \geqslant 5)$[a]

Fraction no.	MPV (μm^3)	Recovered platelets (%)	Mean platelet density (g/cm³)	LDH (IU/10^{10} plt)	β-TG ($\mu g/10^8$ plt)	ATP (nmol/10^8 plt)
1/2	4.15±0.64	12.9±3.3	1.069±0.002	5.80±0.96	3.05±0.91	1.54±0.50
3	5.08±0.74	16.0±3.8	1.071±0.002	6.94±0.91	4.58±0.77	1.89±0.61
4	5.93±0.75	20.8±2.3	1.071±0.002	8.33±0.82	5.90±1.14	2.41±0.70
5	6.93±0.75	22.6±3.5	1.071±0.002	10.11±0.56	7.99±1.73	3.11±1.09
6/7	7.92±0.68	23.8±4.2	1.072±0.001	12.90±0.83	10.99±2.07	3.79±1.05
[b]U	6.57±0.61	—	1.070±0.001	9.47±1.45	6.43±1.59	2.74±0.87

[a] Data compiled from results previously published in Thompson et al. 1982, 1983a.
[b] U, unfractionated platelet population.

platelet-poor plasma or buffer, and platelet aggregation measured following
addition of either collagen, thrombin, ATP or arachidonic acid (Fig. 2.3), it was
found that the larger platelets aggregated more rapidly and more completely
when submaximal doses of the agonists were used. An explanation for this
observation could not be found in differences in the collision frequencies of the
individual platelets of the subpopulations, because it was found that when
platelet agglutination was induced by ristocetin the rate and extent of aggregation
was equivalent in all subpopulations at all doses tested. In addition, all
subpopulations aggregated to a similar extent when maximal doses of direct
aggregating agents were used. These results suggested that the differences in the
extent of platelet aggregation observed within the size-dependent subpopulations
at submaximal concentrations of aggregating agents was the result of the intrinsic
contents of platelets of different sizes (Thompson et al. 1983a). This hypothesis
was confirmed by the observation that the absolute amount of β-thromboglobu-
lin, ATP or thromboxane A_2 produced by the size-dependent platelet subpopulations was proportional to their mean platelet volume (Fig. 2.4). However, when
the identical data were expressed as a percentage of the initial granular or
membrane contents, it was found that the intrinsic function of size-dependent
platelet subpopulations was similar. These results suggest that the ability of
platelets to affect each other and their environment, as measured by aggregation
and total release, is proportional to their size (Thompson et al. 1983a).
Additional studies have also shown that the ability of platelets to incorporate
serotonin (5-hydroxytryptamine, 5-HT) both in vivo and in vitro also correlates
directly with the platelet volume (Thompson et al. 1982, 1983b). To date, none of
our studies have demonstrated any qualitative differences in platelet activities
between size-dependent platelet subpopulations. All of the observed differences
in platelet physiology of size-dependent platelet subpopulations can be accounted
for by quantitative differences based on size.

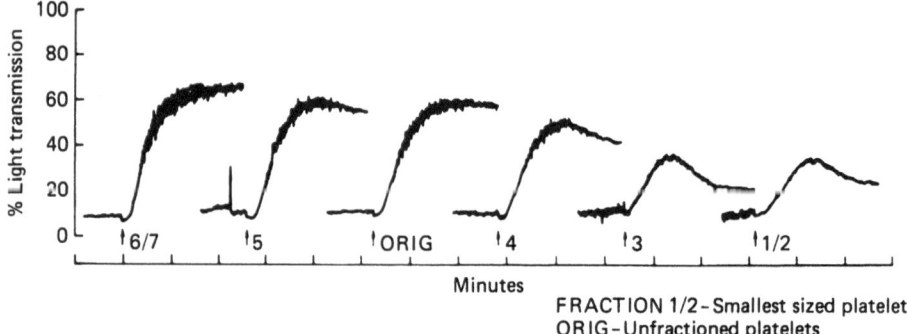

FRACTION 1/2 – Smallest sized platelets
ORIG – Unfractioned platelets
FRACTION 6/7 – Largest sized platelet

Fig. 2.3. Arachidonic acid-induced aggregation of size-dependent platelet subpopulations and
original unfractionated platelets. The platelet count in each fraction was 2×10^8/ml. The stimulating
dose of arachidonic acid was 1 mM. The figure is a representative of three consecutive experiments.
At this submaximal dose of arachidonic acid, a marked discrepancy in the extent of aggregation
induced in each of the size-dependent platelet subpopulations is observed. In the smallest platelets,
represented by fraction 1/2, the rate of aggregation is slower, less extensive, and partially reversible.
In the largest platelets, as represented by fraction 6/7, the aggregation response is more rapid, occurs
to a greater extent, and does not appear to be reversible.

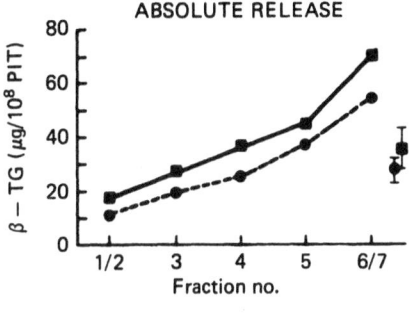

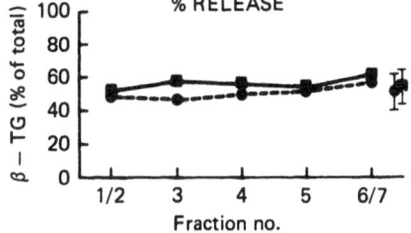

● 10 μg/ml Collagen (mean of 4 Expts., ● Unfractionated Platelets — Mean ± SD)

■ 1 μg/ml Thrombin (mean of 5 Expts., ■ Unfractionated Platelets — Mean ± SD)

Fig. 2.4. Collagen- and thrombin-induced β-thromboglobulin release from size-dependent platelet subpopulations. ●, 10 μg/ml of collagen, ■, 1 unit/ml of thrombin; data from unfractionated platelets (mean ± 1 SD) are presented on the right-hand side of the figure. In the upper panel the absolute release of β-thromboglobulin from platelets resuspended at 2×10^8/ml is plotted. In the lower panel, these data are re-expressed as a percentage of the total β-thromboglobulin present in 2×10^8/ml of platelets of the given fraction. As can be seen from the data, while larger subpopulations release higher absolute quantities of β-thromboglobulin, the percentage release is similar in each fraction. These data were originally presented by Thompson et al. (1983a).

Relationship of Platelet Size to Platelet Age

Previous studies have suggested that the platelet size distribution is determined primarily by ageing of platelets in the circulation (Karpatkin 1969; Ginsburg and Aster 1972; Corash et al. 1978). To test this hypothesis directly in a primate model, we adapted our counterflow centrifugation technique to produce size-dependent platelet subpopulations in the baboon (Thompson et al. 1983b). Platelets were then collected from a baboon and, following ^{51}Cr-labelling, were re-infused to determine autologous survival. In baseline studies it was shown that the extent of chromium labelling of individual platelets was proportional to their volume. At several intervals following reinfusion platelets were re-isolated from the baboons and subjected to counterflow centrifugation to determine the distribution of radioactivity. When the decay of radioactivity in each of the size-dependent platelet subpopulations was observed over time, it was found that the

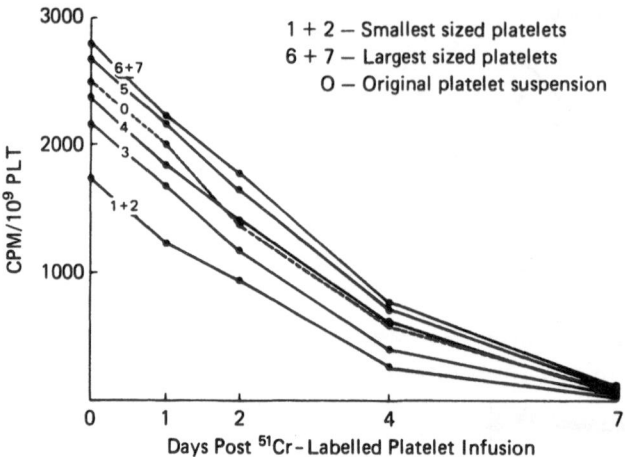

Fig. 2.5. Survival of ^{51}Cr-labelled platelets in an unseparated platelet suspension and in the five size-dependent platelet subpopulations over time following autologous re-infusion. The rate of loss of ^{51}Cr is nearly identical in all size-dependent subpopulations and the unfractionated platelet suspension. These data were originally presented by Thompson et al. (1983b).

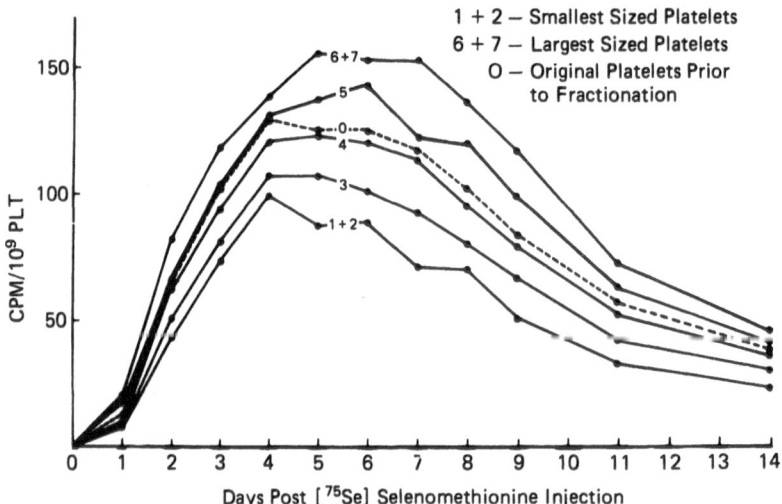

Fig. 2.6. [^{75}Se]Selenomethionine incorporation in unfractionated platelets and in five platelet size-dependent subpopulations following a single intravenous infusion of [^{75}Se]selenomethionine (5.5 μCi/kg) injected on day 0. Blood samples are taken daily from the 1st to 9th day and also on the 11th and 14th day post-injection. Platelets were isolated, size fractionated and the radioactivity per platelet in each fraction determined using a gamma counter. The rate of incorporation of the label in each of the size-dependent subpopulations was identical and the [^{75}Se]selenomethionine label was lost from each subpopulation at an equivalent rate. These data were originally presented by Thompson et al. (1983b).

radioactivity was lost from each subpopulation at an equivalent rate during normal steady-state haematopoiesis (Thompson et al. 1983b; Fig. 2.5). These data suggested that there was no significant shift in the platelet volume distribution during ageing in the circulation, as measured by in vivo chromium survival. These data were confirmed using individually labelled subpopulations (data not shown).

To confirm these results, an independent platelet-labelling technique using [^{75}Se]selenomethionine was utilized. [^{75}Se]Selenomethionine acts as a cohort label for platelets since it is incorporated into platelets only during their production in the bone marrow by megakaryocytes. Following in vivo injection of [^{75}Se]selenomethionine, radioactivity begins to appear in the circulating platelet population within 1–2 days (Thompson et al. 1983b; Fig. 2.6). By separating platelets into size-dependent subpopulations, it was determined that the initial rate of incorporation of [^{75}Se]selenomethionine into each of the size-dependent platelet subpopulations was identical when these data were corrected for known differences in platelet volume. Again, the rate of loss of [^{75}Se]selenomethionine from each of the size-dependent subpopulations suggested that no major differences in platelet size distribution occurred during in vivo ageing. Together these data demonstrate that during normal steady-state haematopoiesis platelet volume distribution is created during platelet production and not during ageing in the circulation (Thompson et al. 1983b). Based on these data, it is probable that the log-normal distribution of platelet volumes during normal steady-state haematopoiesis is merely a normal physiological by-product of the mechanism by which platelets are produced from megakaryocytes.

The Relationship of the Mean Platelet Volume to the Platelet Count

As described above, for a given individual during steady-state haematopoiesis, the platelet volume distribution may be entirely accounted for by factors that determine platelet production. It is possible that platelet volume heterogeneity in a given individual is thus merely the consequence of either megakaryocyte demarcation or fragmentation during platelet production. Interestingly, however, significant differences in MPV also exist between individuals. When the MPV is plotted against the platelet count using data from normal volunteers, one finds a striking inverse correlation between these two parameters of platelet physiology (Thompson et al. 1983c; Fig. 2.7). This inverse correlation has led us and others to hypothesize that during steady-state haematopoiesis the MPV and platelet count within a given individual is maintained in such a way as to maintain a constant functional platelet mass (Frijmovic and Milton 1982; Jakubowski et al. 1983; Thompson 1986; Thompson and Jakubowski 1988). The relationship of the MPV and platelet count in a given individual appears to be stable over long periods of time. Two of the individuals depicted in Fig. 2.7 have been followed for a period of more than 3 years without any significant deviation in their position on this graph. Similar observations have been noted by others (Levin and Bessman 1983; Martin et al. 1983). Von Behrens has suggested that the relationship

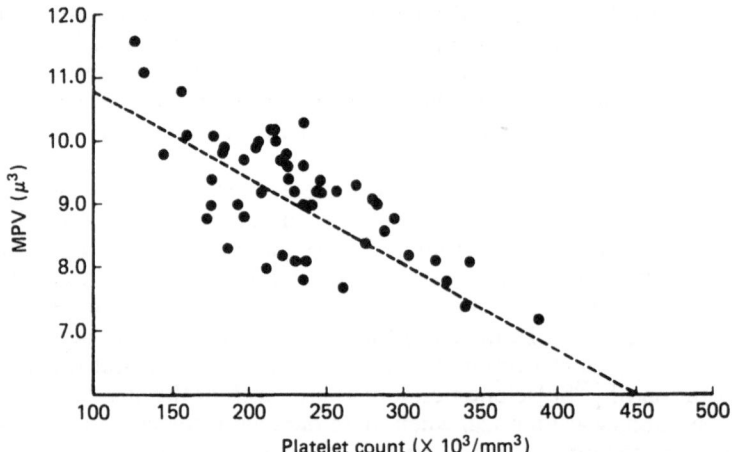

Fig. 2.7. The relationship between the mean platelet volume (MPV) and platelet count in 52 normal volunteers. The relationship between the mean platelet count and MPV displays a significant negative correlation ($r = -0.72$, $p < 0.001$). Similar data have been obtained by a number of investigators. These data were originally presented by Thompson et al. (1983c).

between the MPV and platelet count may be partly inherited (von Behrens 1975). The platelet count and MPV of an individual appears to be either directly or indirectly the result of haemopoietic growth factors, since we have been able to show that continuous infusion of the haemopoietic factor, GM–CSF, can induce an increase in the platelet count and a concomitant decrease in the MPV during the period of GM–CSF infusion in normal rhesus monkeys (Monroy et al. 1989; Fig. 2.8). Despite this inverse correlation between the platelet count and MPV volume during steady-state haematopiesis, others have demonstrated that during stimulated thrombopoiesis there are simultaneous increases both in the number of platelets produced and the MPV of those platelets (Evatt and Levin 1969; Martin et al. 1982; Bessman 1984, Corash et al. 1987; Tong et al. 1987). Together these data suggest that the platelet number and MPV are under at least partly independent control during platelet production.

A number of potentially important regulatory events have been identified in platelet production, as demonstrated schematically in Fig. 2.9 (Thompson 1986). Regulation of platelet production can occur at the level of stem cell commitment and proliferation, the extent of nuclear proliferation within a given megakaryocyte, the rate and extent of cytoplasmic maturation, and the physiological conditions under which platelet release occurs. To gain further understanding of the regulation of both the platelet count and the MPV, we will need a greater understanding of how each of these important events is regulated.

Summary

Our data demonstrate that, in conjunction with the platelet count, the MPV is an important determinant of platelet physiology. During normal steady-state hae-

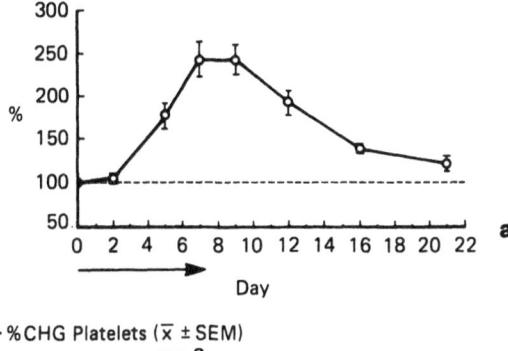

%CHG Platelets ($\bar{x}$ ± SEM)
n = 8

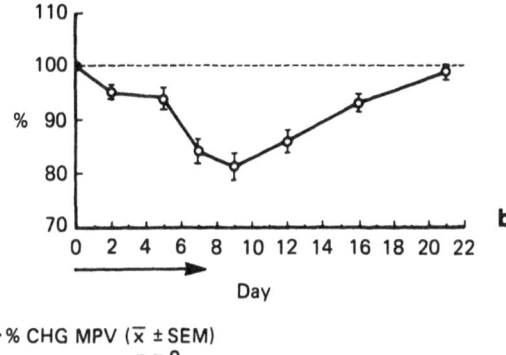

% CHG MPV ($\bar{x}$ ± SEM)
n = 8

Fig. 2.8. Changes in the platelet count and mean platelet volume (**a**) during and (**b**) following a continuous infusion of GM–CSF. Rhesus monkeys were given a continuous infusion of recombinant GM–CSF at a dose of 5.04×10^4 U/kg per day by a continuous infusion pump between days 0 and 7 of study. A platelet count and MPV were determined on days 2, 5, 7, 9, 12, 16 and 21. Changes in the platelet count and MPV are expressed as a percentage. Within 2 days following the initiation of GM–CSF infusion, a gradual increase in the platelet count with a concomitant decrease in MPV is observed. This inverse relationship in the effects on the platelet count and MPV is observed throughout the period of the continuous infusion. Both values return to baseline during the 2 weeks subsequent to GM–CSF infusion.

matopoiesis, platelet production is regulated to maintain a constant functional platelet mass. Both the MPV and the platelet count in a given individual are stable over time, may be partly determined by heredity, and result from events that occur during platelet production. Clinical determinations of platelet function should take into account both the platelet count and MPV of the individual being tested. Failure to account for individual differences in platelet heterogeneity may introduce significant errors in the interpretation of data from both laboratory and clinical investigations.

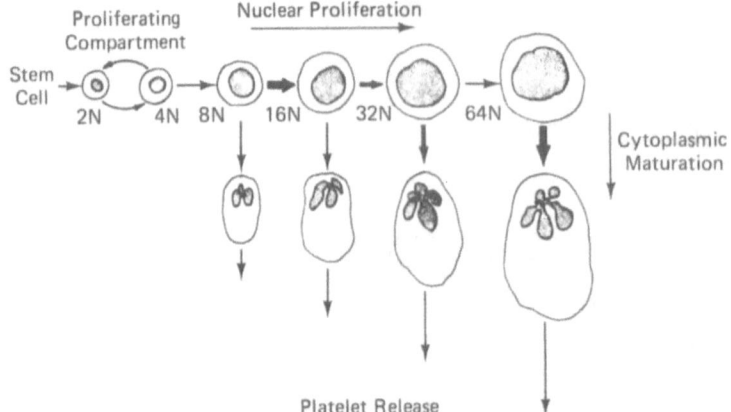

Fig. 2.9. A basic schematic model of platelet production. A number of possible control points are depicted which may regulate the number and/or MPV of platelets produced during thrombopoiesis and platelet release. A similar model has previously been presented by Thompson (1986).

References

Bessman JD (1984) The relation of megakaryocyte ploidy to platelet volume. Am J Hematol 16:161–170

Bizzozero G (1882) Ueber einen neuen Formbestrandtheil des Blutes und dessen Rolle bei Thrombose und der Blutgerinnung. Virch Arch 90:261–332

Corash L, Shafer B, Perlow M (1978) Heterogeneity of human whole blood platelet subpopulations. II. Use of a subhuman primate model to analyze the relationship between density and platelet age. Blood 52:726–734

Corash L, Chen HY, Levin J, Baker G, Lu H, Mok Y (1987) Regulation of thrombopoiesis: effects of the degree of thrombocytopenia on megakaryocyte ploidy and platelet volume. Blood 70:177–185

Evatt BL, Levin J (1969) Measurement of thrombopoiesis in rabbits using ^{75}selenomethionine. J Clin Invest 48:1615–1626

Frojmovic MM, Milton JG (1982) Human platelets size, shape, and related functions in health and disease. Physiol Rev 62:185–261

Ginsburg AD, Aster RH (1972) Changes associated with platelet aging. Thromb Diath Haemorrh 27:407–415

Jakubowski JA, Thompson CB, Vaillancourt R, Valeri CR, Deykin D (1983) Arachidonic acid metabolism by platelets of differing size. Br J Haematol 53:503–511

Karpatkin S (1969) Heterogeneity of human platelets. I. Metabolic and kinetic evidence suggestive of young and old platelets. J Clin Invest 48:1073–1082

Karpatkin S (1978) Heterogeneity of human platelets. VI. Correlation of platelet function with platelet volume. Blood 51:307–316

Levin J, Bessman JB (1983) The inverse relation between platelet volume and platelet number: abnormalities in hematologic disease and evidence that platelet size does not correlate with platelet age. J Lab Clin Med 101:295–307

Mannucci PM, Sharp AA (1967) Platelet volume and shape in relation to aggregation and adhesion. Br J Haematol 13:604–617

Martin JF, Trowbridge EA, Salmon GL, Slater DN (1982) The relationship between platelet and megakaryocyte volumes. Thrombosis Res 28:447–459

Martin JF, Plumb J, Kilbey RS, Kishk YT (1983) Changes in volume and density of platelets in myocardial infarction. Br Med J 287:456–459

Monroy RL, Skelly RR, Thompson CB, Donahue RE, MacVittie TJ (1989) Modulation of platelet production by in vivo infusion of GM–CSF into primates. Manuscript in preparation

Olef I (1936) The differential platelet count: its clinical significance. Arch Int Med 57:1163–1185

Paulus JM (1975) Platelet size in man. Blood 46:321–336
Thompson CB (1986) From precursor to product: how do megakaryocytes produce platelets? In:
   Levine RF, Williams N, Levin J, Evatt BL (eds) Megakaryocyte development and function:
   progress in clinical and biological research, vol 215. Liss, New York, pp 361–371
Thompson CB, Jakubowski JA (1988) The pathophysiology and clinical relevance of platelet
   heterogeneity. Blood 72:1–8
Thompson CB, Eaton KA, Princiotta SM, Rushin CA, Valeri CR (1982) Size dependent platelet
   subpopulations: relationship of platelet volume to ultrastructure, enzymatic activity, and function.
   Br J Haematol 50:509–520
Thompson CB, Jakubowski JA, Quinn PG, Deykin D, Valeri R (1983a) Platelet size as a determinant
   of platelet function. J Lab Clin Med 101:205–213
Thompson CB, Love DG, Quinn PG, Valeri CR (1983b) Platelet size does not correlate with platelet
   age. Blood 62:487–494
Thompson CB, Diaz DD, Quinn PG, Lapins M, Kurtz SR, Valeri CR (1983c) The role of
   anticoagulation in the measurement of platelet volumes. Am J Clin Pathol 80:327–332
Tong M, Seth P, Penington DG (1987) Proplatelets and stress platelets. Blood 69:522–528
von Behrens WE (1975) Mediterranean macrothrombocytopenia. Blood 46:199–208

Technical Questions

Bessman: When you looked at the functional differences between different sized platelets, out of the same population from stratified subpopulations, could you mimic the same results by using whole platelets from a person who had, or an animal that had, the same mean platelet volume to begin with? That is for a given platelet size, if the platelet size is produced as a nominally old, let us say, or a nominally smallest of the group populations, is that going to have the same physiological characteristics as the average of another platelet population or the top of a third population?

Thompson: The best study that has been published that addresses that problem is one by Simon Karpatkin in 1978, where he showed that with a large number of individuals there was a positive correlation between an individual's mean platelet volume and their functional assay. By using a similar kind of assay technique, resuspending them to a set number and then evaluating their aggregation properties he showed that they correlate. We have not studied that extensively, but we did have the good fortune to have two of the physicians in the Naval Blood Research Laboratory, where most of this work was done, who were at the opposite ends of the spectrum. One had a platelet count of 300 000 and the other, who is of Mediterranean descent, had a platelet count of 125 000. Both individuals fit on the normogram. These two basically substantiate just what you have asked. They function as if they were a subpopulation of that size, but that is a population of only two people.

Born: Although I am not working directly in this field, as you may know I have been worried about the Coulter counter idea of volume measurement. The thing is, after this injury, you measure, as you do all the time, basically by the Coulter method for volume distribution. Might it be that the platelets are different, I mean that you have got more activated platelets or that they are different in shape by a certain proportion after this person's injury and then could there be a non-volume explanation for the difference in the curves?

Thompson: The data associated with the rhesus monkey model were collected by Lt.-Commander Rod Monroy. All the volume distributions were obtained in EDTA. This anticoagulant, as everyone knows, causes platelet swelling. Hence measurements were all obtained with a minimal delay of 2 hours. This is an adequate time, I think, for the full shape change to occur. This was for logistical reasons, not because it was planned. The samples were obtained from the primate colony and then had to be analysed on the clinical machine. We wondered whether the only difference was a shape change. In the anticoagulant ACD the platelets are biconcave discs and they do have the normal ACD/EDTA ratio. We have done nothing further. We have not used anything like monoclonal antibodies to investigate for activation. I think that would be a good idea for the future in this model.

Jackson: Would you clarify your remarks on the relationship between platelet volume and shape?

Thompson: Scott Murphy has published the best data on this concept. Platelets circulate essentially as disc-shaped cells. When one stimulates them with EDTA or binds out extracellular calcium one gets a spherical shape change. We have found that in the larger platelets in a population shape change is less important, because they seem to start out as plumper, fatter discs than do the smaller ones. I think Dr Paulus has similar data to support that idea. Hence, there is an artefact, in the sense that we do all of our measurements in ACD and so the shape factor in measuring the absolute volume is different in small platelets from that associated with large platelets. That effect does go away when one treats the platelets with EDTA and allows them to come to a swelling equilibrium, which is probably iso-osmotic.

Corash: In your size-dependent separations, if I recall your papers, there is a difference in the density distributions of your different size populations. Your large cells are slightly denser than your small cells. Is that correct?

Thompson: That is 100% correct. Our measurements in both baboons and humans show that there is a small but measurable difference in the density which is linear through the fractions. The range in humans is 1.067–1.072 g/ml. You can tell me whether that is physiologically significant or not. I think this means that if you have a certain small particle and a certain amount of it has to be occupied by membrane infrastructure to maintain integrity, then the remaining volume is a determinant of density. The difference is not perfectly correlated with the total volume that you measure, but with the cytoplasmic distribution volume. If you take it on that basis, I think the density differences would disappear. However, you are correct. Based on our data, there is a positive correlation between density and volume.

Corash: A brief comment on your observations concerning the old data of Ginsburg and Aster. We have to be very careful to distinguish between normal thrombopoiesis and these stressed states. In the past, we have all been trapped into observations about young platelets after some perturbing event and then we have tried to extrapolate to normal thrombopoiesis. I think we should be cautious about those models and what they really represent.

Thompson: I could not agree more.

Mustard: When you tested the platelet function to arachidonic acid what medium were the platelets suspended in?

Thompson: I cannot remember.

Mustard: Citrated plasma?

Thompson: They have been measured in both citrated plasma and a physiological buffer based on PBS (phosphate-buffered saline) I think, but I would have to check. Those studies were done over 4 years ago.

Mustard: Did you test thrombin?

Thompson: Yes.

Mustard: What medium did you test the thrombin in?

Thompson: We would both have to go back and look at our earlier papers. I understand why you are asking these questions and I agree they are important and that is why we used both citrated plasma and a physiological medium.

Mustard: I will come back to this point in the general discussion. Were all your baboon experiments and volume studies with baboon platelets done after the platelets were taken into EDTA?

Thompson: No, the baboon work was performed in media that were anticoagulated with citrate.

Mustard: But, you said the platelets were taken into EDTA.

Thompson: I am sorry, the baboon studies were only the homeostasis ones. In those we measured platelet survival. The last studies were rhesus monkeys, if I did not make that clear. They were all performed using EDTA.

Mustard: So the selenomethionine experiments were performed with which anticoagulant?

Thompson: Citrate.

Packham: In your aggregation curves, did you normalize those baselines? In our experience the smaller platelets give a different baseline of light transmission.

Thompson: They are all normalized with 10% as the starting point and the maximal response as 90%.

Packham: So those curves are adjusted for the difference in volume, essentially?

Thompson: Yes, there is a slight difference in light scatter properties at baseline.

Packham: When you get the large aggregates, starting with small platelets, they will be smaller also?

Thompson: But they still go on their own individual scale to 90%. In every one of those studies we obtained a maximal stimulation curve.

Packham: In your release data using thrombin and collagen, the concentration of thrombin was given in micrograms per millilitre. I do not translate that readily into units, but if it is a very strong stimulus you may be stimulating all of the platelets maximally. You might not see a difference unless you went down to threshold stimulation. Then you might see a difference in the extent to which the different populations respond.

Thompson: These data were taken from a paper published in the *Journal of Clinical and Laboratory Medicine* in 1983. I agree that that is a strong dose of thrombin, but we have done it with a lower dose and got similar results.

3 Is Platelet Heterogeneity Due to Ageing or Thrombopoiesis?

M. A. Packham and M. L. Rand

Introduction

The question is not just "Is platelet heterogeneity due to ageing or thrombopoiesis?" The question also implies an attempt to understand what happens to platelets as they circulate under normal and abnormal conditions, and why and how they are eventually removed from the circulation. What changes occur in platelets when they interact with an injury site on a vessel wall, or encounter an aggregating agent in the circulation? The petechial haemorrhages that are characteristic of thrombocytopenia indicate that platelets are necessary to maintain the integrity of the endothelium. How do they support the endothelium and are they altered in doing so? No attempt will be made in this review to answer all these questions, but they are posed to illustrate that it is not unreasonable to suggest that platelets may be changed because of their encounters in the circulation.

We began our studies of the relationships among platelet survival, platelet reactions during thrombosis, and platelet density in the 1970s. At that time we were investigating possible reasons for shortened platelet survival as a result of continuous vessel wall injury (Kinlough-Rathbone et al. 1983), and found that platelet survival was shortened by the removal of sialic acid residues with neuraminidase, or removal of membrane glycopeptides by treatment of the platelets with proteolytic enzymes such as plasmin, chymotrypsin or trypsin (Greenberg et al. 1975, 1979). However, platelet survival was not shortened by treatment with thrombin or ADP, although thrombin caused the release of a large proportion of the contents of platelet granules (Reimers et al. 1973, 1976; Packham et al. 1980). When the technique of separating platelets on the basis of differences in buoyant density by centrifugation through Stractan density gradients was introduced (Corash et al. 1977), we realized that it might be possible to detect platelets whose buoyant density had been altered by encounters with aggregating and release-inducing agents. Most of the experiments to be reviewed were done with rabbit platelets because the studies involved procedures that could be done only in experimental animals. For example, platelets were altered and labelled in vitro, and then returned to the circulation, or the effects of indwelling aortic catheters were investigated.

Our work will be reviewed under five main headings:

1. Evidence that, at least for the rabbit, the most dense platelets are enriched in young platelets and the least dense platelets are enriched in old platelets.
2. Comparison of results on discontinuous Stractan density gradients and continuous Percoll density gradients.
3. Review of the differences between most dense and least dense platelet subpopulations.
4. Description of the effects on platelet buoyant density of aggregating and release-inducing agents.
5. Results from in vivo experiments with rabbits and rats with indwelling aortic catheters.

Method of Separation of Platelets on Stractan Density Gradients

In most experiments, washed rabbit platelets suspended in a modified Tyrode–albumin solution (Ardlie et al. 1970; Rand et al. 1981) were layered over three layers of Stractan – 15%, 17% and 19% – and centrifuged for 45 minutes at 6460g. In many of the experiments, the platelets were isolated from 2.5-ml samples of blood so that a number of samples could be taken from the same rabbit on successive days (Rand et al. 1981). About 10% of the total platelet population was in the least dense platelet layer and about 20% was in the most dense platelet layer with these percentages of Stractan.

Types of Experiments

The question of the relation of platelet density to platelet age and platelet survival has been approached in four different types of experiments:

1. In vivo labelling.
2. Injection of a total labelled population of platelets, isolation of subpopulations of different densities at various times and determination of their relative specific radioactivity.
3. Injection of labelled most dense platelets or least dense platelets, followed by measurement of the amount of radioactivity in the circulation at various times.
4. Injection of labelled most dense platelets or least dense platelets, isolation of subpopulations of different densities at various times and determination of their relative specific radioactivity.

In Vivo Labelling

In our experiments, rabbits were given radioactive sulphate which labels the proteoglycans in the megakaryocytes so that the first labelled platelets that appear in the circulation are young platelets (Hirsh et al. 1968). This label is not re-utilized. Blood samples were taken at the times indicated in Fig. 3.1 for separation into density subpopulations (Rand et al. 1981). To calculate relative specific radioactivity, for each rabbit, the highest specific radioactivity attained by the total platelet population was assigned a value of 100%. This maximum occurred at 72 hours in all cases but one. The specific radioactivities of the platelet subpopulations on each day were expressed as percentages of this maximum specific radioactivity. By 24 hours labelled platelets began to appear in the circulation and the most dense platelet subpopulation was five times more heavily labelled than the least dense subpopulation. Since the label appeared in the most dense platelets more rapidly than in the least dense platelets, the most dense platelets must have the majority of the newly formed platelets, although some of the least dense platelets also must be young platelets. The relative specific radioactivity of the most dense platelets increased to a maximum between 48 and 72 hours and then decreased, whereas the specific radioactivity of the least dense platelets increased gradually over the 120 hours of observation. The relative specific radioactivity in the most dense platelets was higher than that of the least dense platelets throughout. These results are compatible with the concept that some of the most dense platelets are young platelets that become less dense as

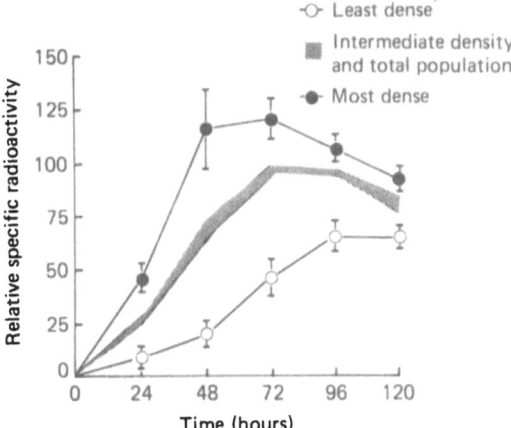

Fig. 3.1. Relative specific radioactivity curves of platelet subpopulations from rabbits injected with 2.5 mCi of $^{35}SO_4^{2-}$. The subpopulations were obtained by centrifugation on discontinuous Stractan density gradients. The relative specific radioactivity curve of the intermediate density platelet subpopulation was superimposable on that of the total population. Relative specific radioactivity was calculated as follows: for each rabbit, the highest specific radioactivity attained by the total platelet population, SA_{max} cpm/10^9 platelets, was assigned a value of 100%. (This maximum occurred in all cases but one at 72 hours.) The specific radioactivity of the platelet subpopulations on each day was then expressed as a percentage of SA_{max}. The percentages for each subpopulation on each day were meaned ($n=4$ for the 24, 48, and 72-hour time points and $n=5$ for the 96 and 120-hour time points; means ± SE). For all time points, the relative specific radioactivity values for the least dense and most dense subpopulations were significantly different ($p<0.001$). From Rand et al. (1981). Reproduced with permission from *Blood* 57:741–746.

they age in the circulation. One does not see the typical crossover of a precursor–product relationship, probably because old, least dense platelets are being removed from the circulation.

Listed in Table 3.1 are other investigators who used different types of density gradients and labelled platelets from several species in various ways. All of them except Boneu et al. (1973) obtained similar results, regardless of the type of gradient, species, or label. In every case but one, early labelling was greatest in the most dense platelets, although label did appear in all density subpopulations at early times. Nearly all investigators interpreted their data as indicating that most dense platelets are enriched in young platelets. In contrast, however, Boneu et al. (1973) and Penington and his colleagues (1976a, b) emphasized the appearance of label in all populations as indicative of the heterogeneity of platelets as they arise from megakaryocytes. Although Penington et al. (1976a) invoked increased protein synthetic activity in young, dense platelets to explain their observation of greater specific radioactivity of young, dense platelets, the validity of this explanation has been questioned by Corash et al. (1978), who suggested that contamination of the platelets with labelled leukocytes could account for the results of in vivo labelling with [^{75}Se]selenomethionine reported by Penington et al. (1976a).

Table 3.1. In vivo labelling of platelets by administration of a radioactive compound incorporated by megakaryocytes

Labelled compound administered	Species	Type of density gradient	Reference
[^{75}Se]Selenomethionine	Human	Silicone oils (discontinuous)	Amorosi et al. (1971)
[^{75}Se]Selenomethionine	Sheep	Sucrose (continuous)	Boneu et al. (1973)
[^{75}Se]Selenomethionine	Rabbit	Albumin (discontinuous)	Charmatz and Karpatkin (1974)
[^{75}Se]Selenomethionine	Rabbit	Differential centrifugation	Karpatkin (1978)
[^{75}Se]Selenomethionine	Rat	Ludox-PVP (continuous)	Penington et al. (1976a)
[^{3}H]Amino acids	Rabbit	Stractan (discontinuous)	Corash & Shafer (1982)
$^{35}SO_4$	Rabbit	Stractan (discontinuous)	Rand et al. (1981) Evans et al. (1985)

Total Population Label

The results from experiments in which *total* populations of rabbit platelets were labelled with ^{51}Cr and injected into rabbits are shown in Fig. 3.2 (Rand et al. 1983b). At the times indicated, platelets were separated into density subpopulations. When the 1-hour specific radioactivity of each subpopulation was expressed as 100% and the specific radioactivities at each time point as percentages of this, the relative specific radioactivity of the most dense platelets

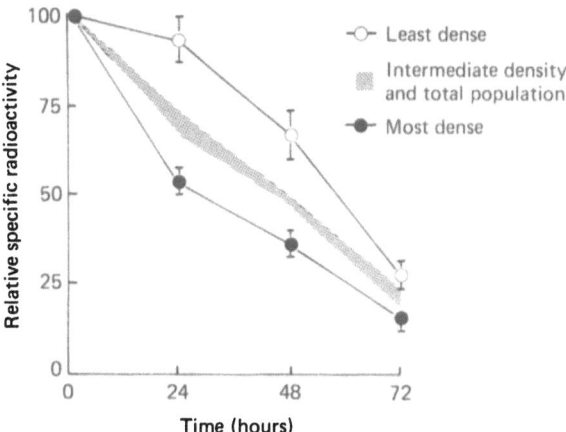

Fig. 3.2. Relative specific radioactivity curves of platelet density subpopulations from rabbits that had been injected with total populations of ^{51}Cr-labelled platelets. The subpopulations were obtained by centrifugation on discontinuous Stractan density gradients. The relative specific radioactivity of the intermediate density platelet subpopulation was superimposable on that of the total population. Relative specific radioactivity was calculated as described in Fig. 3.1. The specific radioactivity of each subpopulation 1 hour after injection of the labelled platelets was assigned a value 100%. The specific radioactivity of the platelet subpopulations on each day was then expressed as a percentage of the 1-hour value. Each point represents the mean ± SD of values from 3 animals. At 24, 48, and 72 hours, the relative specific radioactivity of the least dense platelet subpopulation was significantly greater than that of the most dense platelet subpopulation ($P<0.05$; paired t test). The least dense platelet subpopulation comprised 15%±7% (mean ± SD) of the total population, and the most dense, 37%±9%. From Rand et al. (1983b). Reproduced with permission from *Blood* 61:362–367.

decreased rapidly. In contrast, the relative specific radioactivity of the least dense platelets had not decreased significantly 24 hours after injection of the labelled *total* population. It then decreased gradually with time.

When the label remains in the least dense platelets longer, as it did in our experiments (Rand et al. 1983b) and those of Mezzano et al. (1984a) with dogs, two explanations are possible: either the most dense platelets become less dense, or the least dense platelets survive longer. Other investigators who did this type of experiment in humans, monkeys or baboons obtained the opposite result, finding that the low-density platelets survived for a shorter time than the high-density platelets. Consequently, they suggested the opposite possibilities that either the least dense platelets become more dense, or the most dense platelets survive longer (Mezzano et al. 1981, 1984b; Martin and Penington 1983; Watson and Ludlam 1986; Savage et al. 1986). One could reconcile the difference in the results by postulating that perhaps in the rabbit some of the most dense platelets do tend to become less dense, whereas in primates this change may not be so pronounced and the most dense platelets survive longer. In addition, as suggested by Watson and Ludlam (1986), sequestration of the most dense human platelets in the spleen could account for the longer survival of the most dense platelets, although the second study of Mezzano et al. (1984b) with splenectomized subjects would appear to rule out this possibility. Yet a third pattern of results was reported by Busch and Olson (1973), who found no difference over a 72-hour period in the distribution of ^{51}Cr in subpopulations of dog platelets of various densities. Boneu et al. (1973) also found no difference with ^{51}Cr-labelled human platelets.

Injection of Most Dense or Least Dense Platelets

In further experiments designed to distinguish between the survival of most dense and least dense subpopulations, we used two radioactive labels – [51]Cr and [111]In – and injected the labelled subpopulations into the same rabbits at the same time in order to reduce the effect of animal and experimental variability (Rand et al. 1983b). (In these experiments we first ensured that the survival in vivo of total populations labelled with one or other of these radioisotopes was identical under the conditions we were using.) Platelet suspensions were divided into two parts: half was labelled with ^{51}Cr and half with [111]In. The platelets were then separated into density subpopulations on Stractan gradients. For injection into rabbits 1–3, the least dense platelets labelled with ^{51}Cr were combined with the most dense platelets labelled with [111]In. For injection into rabbits 4–6, most dense platelets labelled with ^{51}Cr were combined with least dense platelets labelled with [111]In. Typical survival curves from one rabbit obtained with most dense and least dense platelet subpopulations labelled in this way are shown in Fig. 3.3. The curves for all six rabbits were similar to this, i.e. the least dense platelets disappeared more rapidly from the circulation. The platelet survival data are summarized in Table 3.2. There was a highly significant difference in the mean survival times of the subpopulations. Again, it seems likely that the most dense rabbit platelets are enriched in younger platelets which have a longer survival time than the older platelets in the least dense subpopulation.

These results that we obtained with rabbits are similar to those of Corash and his colleagues (1978) with rhesus monkeys and of Mezzano et al. (1984a) with

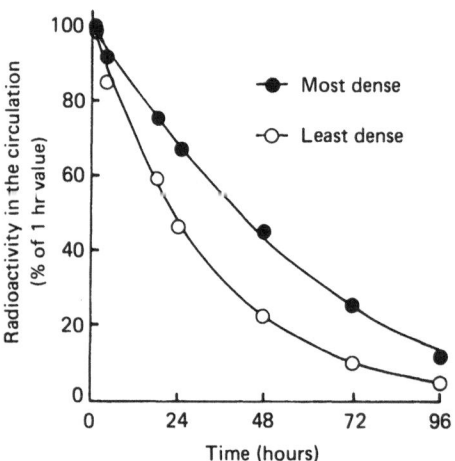

Fig. 3.3. Survival curves of platelet subpopulations obtained by centrifugation on discontinuous Stractan density gradients. In this experiment, the least dense platelets were labelled with ^{111}In, and the most dense with [51]Cr (see experiment 4 of Table 3.2 for mean platelet survival values). From Rand et al. (1983b). Reproduced with permission from *Blood* 61:363–367.

Table 3.2. Mean survival of least dense and most dense platelet subpopulations[a]

Experiment	Mean survival (h)	
	Least dense platelets[b]	Most dense platelets[b]
1	37.4	65.0
2	27.3	44.6
3	56.9	70.4
4	53.6	94.5
5	31.8	76.8
6	76.8	105.0
Mean±SD	47.3±18.7[c]	76.1±21.6[c]

[a] Survival experiments were performed concurrently in the same rabbits, and mean survival times were calculated using 1 hour as 100%.
[b] In the first three experiments, least dense platelet subpopulations were labelled with ^{51}Cr and most dense with ^{111}In. In the remaining experiments, the converse was the case. The least dense platelet subpopulation comprised 11%±3% (mean±SD) of the total population from which it was derived, and the most dense 28%±11% (mean±SD).
[c] A paired t test showed a significantly shorter survival of least dense platelets as compared to most dense platelets ($p < 0.0025$).
From Rand et al. (1983b). Reproduced with permission from *Blood* 61:362–367.

splenectomized dogs. However, our results differ from those of Mezzano et al. (1981) with humans in which the small platelets (presumably less dense) survived longer than the large, most dense platelets. An added complication in the interpretation of results from different groups is that Savage and his co-workers (1986) obtained still another pattern of observations. They reported that the different subpopulations of baboon platelets survived for similar times.

Injection and Re-isolation of Labelled Density Subpopulations

In the fourth type of experiment, labelled least dense platelets or most dense platelets were injected into rabbits, subpopulations were isolated at various times and their specific radioactivity was determined (Fig. 3.4) (Rand 1983). The label that was originally present in most dense platelets appeared in the least dense platelets, but the label that had originally been in least dense platelets did not appear in the most dense platelets. This result lends support to the view that, at least in rabbits, most dense platelets may decrease in density as they circulate. Corash and his colleagues (1978) obtained a similar pattern in the rhesus monkey and Mezzano et al. (1984a) in the one dog they studied. The data from similar experiments with human subjects reported by Mezzano et al. (1981) are difficult to interpret since the recovery of the labelled platelets after injection was less than 60%, and the possibility of sequestration in the spleen should be considered.

Recovery of Ability of Platelets to Synthesize Thromboxane After Aspirin Administration

Our findings with labelled platelets from rabbits were supported by the results of our studies of the synthesis of thromboxane by density subpopulations of rabbit

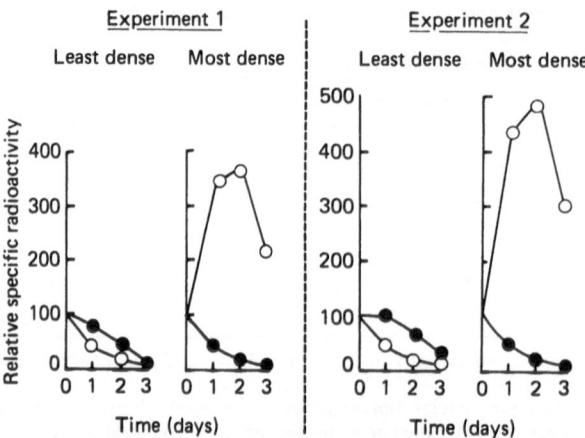

Fig. 3.4. Relative specific radioactivities of density subpopulations of platelets following injection of ^{51}Cr-labelled least dense and most dense subpopulations. The type of subpopulation injected is indicated at the top of each panel. The specific radioactivity of each re-isolated subpopulation at 1 hour was taken as 100% and the specific radioactivities of the platelet subpopulations on each day were expressed as percentages of the 1-hour values. Re-isolated least dense platelets (O), most dense platelets (●). Subpopulations were obtained by centrifugation on discontinuous Stractan density gradients (Rand 1983).

platelets after aspirin administration (Packham et al. 1985a). Aspirin irreversibly acetylates the cyclo-oxygenase of platelets and thus blocks the synthesis of thromboxane. As new platelets enter the circulation, the ability of platelets to synthesize thromboxane gradually returns. We took blood samples at times up to 72 hours, separated the platelets into density subpopulations, and determined the amount of thromboxane B_2 they formed in response to maximal stimulation with thrombin (Table 3.3). One hour after aspirin administration, residual cyclo-oxygenase activity was very low and similar in both subpopulations, but during the next three days the most dense subpopulation recovered its ability to

Table 3.3. Thrombin-induced TXB$_2$ production by least dense and most dense platelet subpopulations after aspirin administration to rabbits

Time after aspirin administration (h)	n	TXB$_2$ production[a] (percentage of pre-administration or 120-h value of corresponding subpopulation)		p[b]
		Least dense platelets (mean±SD)	Most dense platelets (mean±SD)	
Pre	6	100.0	100.0	
1	6	8.4±6.7	9.9±11.4	NS
24	6	16.1±8.6	26.4±21.7	NS
48	6	38.3±13.9	70.4±13.7	<0.005
72	4	85.1±10.5	100.7±14.6	<0.05

TXB$_2$, thromboxane B$_2$; NS, not significant.
[a] The platelets were stimulated with 0.75 U/ml of thrombin for 10 min.
[b] Paired difference analysis.
From Packham et al. (1985a). Reproduced with permission from *Blood* 66:287–290.

synthesize thromboxane B_2 more rapidly than did the least dense platelet subpopulation. The time required for the most dense platelets to recover completely corresponds to the mean survival time of rabbit platelets (65.7 ± 7.2 hours; Packham et al. 1980).

Our results are in sharp contrast to those of investigators who have studied human platelets in this way and reported that the least dense platelets recover the ability to synthesize thromboxane (or malondialdehyde) more rapidly than the most dense platelets (Boneu et al. 1980; Mezzano et al. 1981; McDonald and Ali 1983), although Leone et al. (1979) found the recovery times to be the same. In addition, an abstract by Chamberlain et al. (1984) from Penington's group, in which platelet monoamine oxidase (a mitochondrial enzyme) was irreversibly inhibited, showed more rapid recovery of the activity of this enzyme by the least dense human platelets. It is not clear whether the difference between our results and those of others is attributable to a species difference or to some other cause, such as activation of human platelets before or during density gradient centrifugation. In most of the experiments with human platelets, media with low concentrations of ionized calcium were used. Human platelets, but not rabbit platelets, are readily activated by close platelet-to-platelet contact in such media, with formation of thromboxanes (Packham et al. 1987). Activation at the interfaces of the discontinuous Stractan density gradients would be likely to occur with a resultant decrease in platelet density. Although Mezzano et al. (1981) added prostaglandin E_1 to prevent activation on the gradients, the other investigators who examined the recovery of cyclo-oxygenase activity do not appear to have taken precautions to prevent activation.

Conclusions About the Relation Between Density and Survival of Rabbit Platelets

From all these experimental approaches we have concluded that the least dense platelet subpopulations from rabbits have a shorter mean survival time than the most dense platelet subpopulation; that the least dense platelets are enriched in old platelets and the most dense platelets are enriched in young platelets; and that platelet senescence or ageing contributes to platelet density heterogeneity, although it is not the sole cause of it. Other investigators have agreed with our interpretation of the results with rabbit platelets, but have pointed out that there may be species differences (Penington 1984; Mezzano and Aster 1987).

Do Discontinuous Gradients Introduce Artefacts?

To investigate this possibility, we repeated some of our experiments using continuous Percoll gradients (3000 g, 75 minutes). Rabbits were given [^{35}S]sulphate, platelets were harvested at various times up to 120 hours, separated into density subpopulations by upward displacement of the Percoll gradient, and their

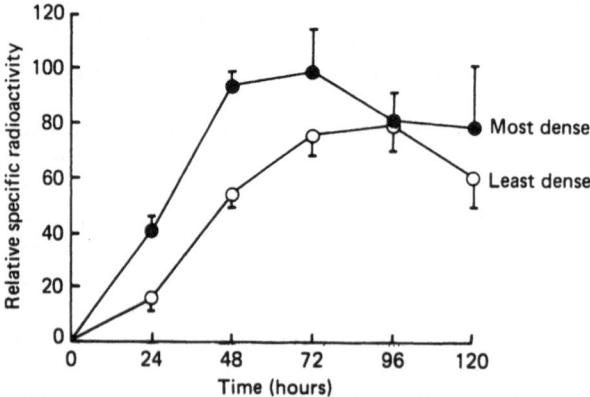

Fig. 3.5. Relative specific radioactivities of platelet subpopulations from rabbits injected with 2.5 mCi of $^{35}SO_4^{2-}$. The subpopulations were obtained by centrifugation on continuous Percoll gradients. See legend of Fig. 3.1 for details of methods of calculation, with the modification that the highest specific activity attained by the least dense platelet subpopulation was assigned the value of 100%.

relative specific radioactivity calculated (Fig. 3.5) (Evans et al. 1985). The relative specific radioactivity of the platelets that were most dense was at least twice that of the platelets that were least dense for at least 48 hours. The relative specific activity of the most dense platelets reached a maximum at 72 hours and then decreased gradually; the relative specific radioactivity of the least dense platelets reached a maximum 24 hours later. These results are very similar to those we obtained with the discontinuous Stractan gradients (Fig. 3.1). Thus the use of different types of density gradients may not explain the differences in results from different laboratories.

The various techniques of density gradient separation that had been used up to 1983 have been summarized by Martin et al. (1983).

Differences Between Most Dense and Least Dense Platelet Subpopulations

Some of the differences observed by many groups of investigators using various separation procedures and different species are listed in Table 3.4. The most dense platelets are larger, have more protein, more glycogen, more sialic acid, more α-granule contents and more dense granule contents. (Dog platelets seem to be the only exception to these generalities; Mezzano et al. 1986.) Platelet-associated IgG, Class I HLA antigen and HLA-A2 molecules are less with the most dense platelets, whereas the most dense platelets have more 1[A1] molecules and glycoprotein I. The amounts of the glycoprotein IIb/IIIa complex and Bak[a] antigen appear to be similar on platelets of different densities. Platelets of all densities seem to have the same lysosomal granule content. It is not clear whether the number of mitochondria is the same. The electrophoretic mobility of the most dense platelets has been reported to be less negative (Table 3.4).

Table 3.4. Differences in the characteristics of most dense and least dense platelets

Most dense platelets	Species	Reference
1. Larger size	Human	Karpatkin (1969), Karpatkin and Charmatz (1969), Penington et al. (1976a), Corash et al. (1977), Leone et al. (1979), Mezzano et al. (1981, 1986), Martin et al. (1983)
	Rabbit	Charmatz and Karpatkin (1974), Karpatkin (1978), Rand et al. (1981), Corash and Shafer (1982)
	Rat	Penington et al. (1976b)
	Dog	Minter and Ingram (1971)
Smaller size	Dog	Mezzano et al. (1986)
2. Greater protein content	Human	Friedhoff et al. (1978), Jung et al. (1985), Mezzano et al. (1986)
	Rabbit	Karpatkin (1978), Rand et al. (1981)
Same protein content	Dog	Mezzano et al. (1986)
3. More sialic acid per platelet	Human	Jung et al. (1985)
	Rabbit	Rand et al. (1981)
4. More glycogen	Human	Karpatkin and Charmatz (1969), Chamberlain et al. (1984)
5. More dense granule contents	Human	Karpatkin (1969), Corash et al. (1984), Mezzano et al. (1986)
(adenine nucleotides, 5-HT)	Rabbit	Cieslar et al. (1979)
Less 5-HT	Dog	Mezzano et al. (1986)
6. More α-granule contents (β-thromboglobulin, platelet factor 4, fibrinogen, von Willebrand factor, thrombospondin)	Human	Karpatkin (1969), Martin et al. (1983), Corash et al. (1984), Corash and Mok (1984), van Oost et al. (1984), Chamberlain et al. (1984), Jung et al. (1985), Illes et al. (1987), Parker et al. (1987)
	Rabbit	Cieslar et al. (1979)
7. Same lysosomal granule content	Human	Corash et al. (1984), Corash and Mok (1984), Chamberlain et al. (1984)
8. More mitochondria	Human	Penington et al. (1976b), Duyvené de Wit et al. (1987)
Same number of mitochondria	Human	Corash et al. (1977)
9. Less platelet-associated IgG	Human	Kelton and Denomme (1982), Khansari and Fudenberg (1983), Pfueller et al. (1986)
10. (a) More glycoprotein I	Human	Bolin et al. (1981), Jung et al. (1985)
(b) Same amount glycoprotein IIb/IIIa and Bak[a] antigen	Human	Bolin et al. (1981), Periera et al. (1988)
(c) More P1[A1] molecules		Periera et al. (1988)
(d) Less HLA-A$_2$ and Class I HLA antigens	Human	Periera et al. (1988)
11. Less negative electrophoretic mobility values	Human	Jung et al. (1985)

Nearly all investigators appear to agree that the most dense platelets are more functional than the least dense, although there are a few exceptions (Table 3.5). Corash et al. (1984) observed by electron microscopy that over a range of concentrations up to 0.5 U/ml, thrombin caused the same percentage loss of dense bodies from platelets of different densities. It was reported by van Oost et al. (1984) that lower concentrations of thrombin were required with less-dense platelets to induce the secretion of β-thromboglobulin, compared with concentrations of thrombin that caused the same percentage secretion of β-thromboglobulin from the most dense platelets.

Table 3.5. Functional differences between most dense and least dense platelets

Most dense platelets	Species	Reference
1. Greater rate of glycogenolysis, glycolysis and glycogen synthesis	Human	Karpatkin and Charmatz (1969), Karpatkin and Strick (1972)
2. Greater rate of aggregation and release of granule contents	Human	Karpatkin (1969)
β-Thromboglobulin secreted less readily in response to thrombin	Human	van Oost et al. (1984)
Same percentage loss of dense bodies in response to thrombin (electron microscopy)	Human	Corash et al. (1984)
3. More rapid 5-HT uptake	Human	Corash et al. (1984)
4.(a) More malondialdehyde formation in response to thrombin	Human	Leone et al. (1979)
Same malondialdehyde formation from arachidonic acid	Human	Boneu et al. (1980)
(b) Same TXB_2 formation in response to thrombin	Human	Martin et al. (1981)
More TXB_2 formation in response to thrombin	Rabbit	Packham et al. (1985a)
More TXB_2 formation from arachidonic acid	Human	Martin et al. (1981)
5. Higher mitochondrial enzyme activity	Human	Friedhoff et al. (1978), Corash et al. (1984), Chamberlain et al. (1984), Chamberlain and Penington (1988)

Effect of Aggregating and Release-Inducing Agents on Platelet Density

We have done a number of studies of the effect of aggregating and release-inducing agents on the density of rabbit platelets. The density distribution on discontinuous Stractan gradients of platelets that had been treated three times with 0.05 U/ml of thrombin was compared with the distribution of control platelets subjected to the same washing and resuspending procedures (Table 3.6) (Cieslar et al. 1979). Although the handling procedures decreased platelet density somewhat, the treatment with thrombin greatly increased the proportion of least dense platelets. Corash and Mok (1984) and van Oost and his co-workers (1983, 1984) have shown that thrombin also decreases the buoyant density of human platelets. Activation by ADP, adrenaline or collagen in citrated platelet-rich plasma, in which aggregation is accompanied by the release of granule contents, also decreases platelet density, according to van Oost et al. (1984).

Table 3.6. Effect of thrombin on density of rabbit platelets

Density	Percentage of platelets applied to gradient		
	Untreated	Control	Thrombin-treated
Least	5.6±1.1	9.6± 3.2	44.9±5.1
Intermediate	32.0±3.1	47.6± 8.0	43.3±5.4
Most	62.4±3.8	42.8±10.5	11.8±3.2

Mean±SE, $n=3$.
The control platelets were subjected to the same washing and centrifugation procedure as the thrombin-treated platelets.
From Cieslar et al. (1979). Data reproduced with permission from *Blood* 53:867–874.

The decrease in density caused by treatment of the platelets with thrombin persisted when the platelets were labelled with ^{51}Cr, returned to the circulation of rabbits and allowed to circulate for 18 hours (Table 3.7) (Cieslar et al. 1979). (We had shown previously that thrombin-treated platelets from rabbits survive for a normal length of time when they are returned to the circulation; Reimers et al. 1973, 1976.)

Table 3.7. Effect of thrombin on density of rabbit platelets (Labelled platelets injected, reharvested at 18 hours)

Density subpopulation	Percentage ^{51}Cr in each density fraction of reharvested platelets	
	Control platelets injected	Thrombin-treated platelets injected
Least	9.3	69.8
Intermediate	46.8	25.4
Most	43.9	4.8

Control platelets were subjected to the same labelling, washing, centrifugation, injection and reharvesting procedures as the thrombin-treated platelets.
From Cieslar et al. (1979). Data reproduced with permission from *Blood* 53:867–874.

Table 3.8 shows results of experiments in which rabbit platelets were treated with plasmin in different concentration ranges (Guccione et al. 1985). In these experiments, plasmin decreased the buoyant density of platelets, even at concentrations that did not cause release of the contents of the amine storage granules. These low concentrations of plasmin also increased the size of the platelets (from 4.44 fl to 5.62 fl). The increase in size, which could result from the uptake of water, could account for the decreased density caused by these low concentrations of plasmin, but loss of some α-granule contents may also be responsible since Vicic and Weiss (1983) and van Oost et al. (1984) have reported that a lack of α-granule contents, or release of α-granule contents from human platelets, decreases their density. In contrast to our findings with rabbit platelets, van Oost et al. (1983) reported that 0.15 CU/ml of plasmin did not cause a change in density, or the secretion of α-granule contents from human platelets.

Table 3.8. Effect of pretreatment of rabbit platelets with plasmin on their distribution after centrifugation in a discontinuous Stractan density gradient

	Concentration of plasmin (U/ml)	Percentage [¹⁴C]5-HT released in 30 min	Percentage of platelets in:		
			Most dense layer	Intermediate density layer	Least dense layer
Expt. 1	0	0	42	49	10
	0.1	0	21	55	22
	0.2	0	17	55	26
Expt. 2	0	0.1	34	53	13
	0.5	12	2	27	71
	1.0	54	2	17	80
Expt. 3	0	1.2	20	60	20
	1.5	94	2	16	82

Platelets were incubated with plasmin or buffer for 30 min at 37 °C before they were washed, resuspended and layered on the gradient.
From Guccione et al. 1985. Reproduced with permission from *Thromb Haemost* 53:8–14.

We have also shown that adenosine diphosphate (ADP) treatment of rabbit platelets decreases their density (Table 3.9) (Packham et al. 1985b). Although dense granule contents are not released from rabbit platelets upon stimulation with ADP, there is a slight loss of α-granule contents (Rand et al. 1983a; Harfenist et al. 1985). ADP treatment increases platelet size temporarily, but the platelets revert to normal within 1 hour, although the decrease in density persists. We repeated these experiments with ADP using albumin density gradients and again found that ADP treatment decreased platelet density (Packham et al. 1985b). Gear (1981) also reported an ADP-induced decrease in the density of human platelets without release of 5-HT; he suggested that uptake of water could account for the change he observed.

Table 3.9. Distribution of Stractan density gradients of control platelets and platelets aggregated with 10 μM ADP and allowed to deaggregate

Platelet subpopulations	Percentage in subpopulations			
	Control		ADP	
	15 min	4 h	15 min	4 h
Least dense	13± 4	13±5	26±4	27±5
Intermediate density	69±10	69±7	63±6	63±6
Most dense	18± 6	18±5	11±3	11±3

Mean values ± SE from 3 experiments. Rabbit platelets were incubated with ADP (10 μM) for 15 minutes or 4 hours at 37 °C with occasional gentle mixing. After these times they were recovered by centrifugation, resuspended and centrifuged through Stractan density gradients.
From Packham et al. (1985b). Reproduced with permission from *Blood* 65:564–570.

The agents to which platelets are likely to be exposed during thromboembolism include ADP, thrombin, thromboxane A_2 and plasmin. Probably all of them decrease platelet density, in most cases by causing the release of granule contents. van Oost and his co-workers (1982) have shown that some patients with thrombotic disease have a higher proportion of least dense platelets, and that the reactions that human platelets undergo during cardiopulmonary bypass decrease their density in vivo (van Oost et al. 1983). Boneu et al. (1983) detected an increased proportion of platelets of low density in blood from 9 of 11 patients hospitalized in an intensive care unit, most of whom were suffering from severe post-operative or post-traumatic infections or other conditions known to activate platelets.

Effect on Density of Raising the Concentration of Cyclic AMP in Rabbit Platelets

In experiments in which we were attempting to ensure that platelets were not activated, we added 10 μM prostaglandin E_1 (PGE$_1$) to the rabbit platelets before putting them on the Stractan density gradients and discovered a progressive decrease in density with time of incubation with PGE$_1$ (Table 3.10) (Packham et al. 1985b). Other agents such as forskolin, adenosine and papaverine that increase cyclic AMP had a similar effect (Table 3.11). During incubation with PGE$_1$, the decrease in density was paralleled by an increase in the median size of the platelets (Fig. 3.6). Since all these agents inhibit the release of granule contents, we believe that the decreased density is due to swelling (uptake of water). Concentrations of PGE$_1$ that markedly increased the size of rabbit platelets did not increase the size of human platelets under our experimental conditions. Mezzano et al. (1986) have reported that PGE$_1$ (1.1 μM) increases the size of human platelets, but not of dog platelets, in platelet-rich plasma; they

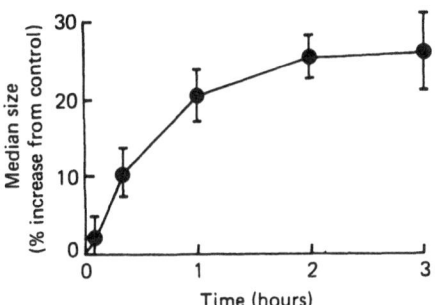

Fig. 3.6. Effect of time of incubation with 10 μM PGE$_1$ on the median size of platelets in Tyrode–albumin solution, expressed as a percentage increase from the median size of control platelets. The size of the control platelets did not change appreciably over the 3-hour period, although the median size of the platelets varied from rabbit to rabbit. Mean values±SE of 4 experiments are shown. From Packham et al. (1985b). Reproduced with permission from *Blood* 65:564–570.

found that there was no further increase in size when theophylline was added to the anticoagulant mixture that contained PGE_1. Other investigators have also used PGE_1, often in combination with theophylline, to inhibit activation of human or baboon platelets during density gradient centrifugation (Martin et al. 1983; van Oost et al. 1984; Watson and Ludlam 1986; Savage et al. 1986). It was reported by van Oost and his colleagues (1982) that PGE_1 had no additional effect on the density of human platelets when it was added to a suspending medium that already contained theophylline. However, it is not clear whether artefacts may have been introduced into the measurements of platelet size and density in some experiments in which these agents that increase the concentration of AMP in platelets were used.

Table 3.10. Distribution of Stractan density gradients of rabbit platelets incubated with PGE_1 for different times

Density subpopulation	Percentage in subpopulations (incubation, min)				
	0	15	60	105	150
Least	8.2	15.1	23.3	32.8	38.4
Intermediate	29.0	49.3	61.2	54.9	50.8
Most	62.7	35.6	15.5	12.3	10.8

Washed rabbit platelets were incubated with PGE_1 (10 μM) for 15, 60, 105 or 150 min at 37 °C before they were centrifuged through Stractan density gradients. The zero time sample was not exposed to PGE_1.
From Packham et al. (1985b). Reproduced with permission from *Blood* 65:564–570.

Table 3.11. Effects of agents that increase cyclic AMP in platelets on their distribution on Stractan density gradients

Agent	Percentage in subpopulations		
	Least dense	Intermediate density	Most dense
Control	7.9±2.3	46.3± 7.7	45.8± 9.7
PGE_1 (10 μM)	30.8±5.0	50.1± 1.9	19.1± 4.7
Control	7.0±4.0	35.3±12.9	57.3±17.2
Adenosine (100 μM)	18.4±8.8	55.9± 1.9	25.7± 7.5
Control	4.3±1.4	32.1± 2.0	57.8± 4.3
Forskolin (30 μM)	38.7±2.1	50.0± 4.4	11.5± 2.3
Control	2.9	24.8	72.3
Dibutyryl cAMP (5 μM)	12.7	51.1	36.2
Control	5.6	21.2	67.9
Papaverine (50 μM)	32.5	41.6	25.8

Mean values±SE of 7 experiments with PGE_1, 3 experiments with adenosine, 2 experiments with forskolin, 2 experiments with dibutyryl cAMP, and 1 experiment with papaverine. Suspensions of rabbit platelets in Tyrode–albumin, pH 7.35, were incubated with these agents for 30 min at 37 °C before centrifugation through the gradients.
From Packham et al. (1985b). Reproduced with permission from *Blood* 65:564–570.

Changes in Density In Vivo

In experiments with rabbits and rats, in which indwelling aortic catheters were inserted to cause continuous injury to the vessel wall, there were marked differences between the results in these two species.

In the rabbits, platelet density was decreased at 6–10 days while the catheters were in place, but returned toward pre-surgery values by 14 days (Table 3.12) (Somers et al. 1983; Somers 1984). The increased proportion of less-dense platelets and the decreased proportion of most dense platelets were associated with shortened platelet survival and the formation of thrombi around the catheters (sham operation: 61.1 ± 3.0 hours, $n=12$; aortic catheter: 44.2 ± 2.7 hours, $n=16$). It was also found that platelets harvested at 3 or 6 days from rabbits with indwelling catheters, labelled, and infused into normal rabbits survived significantly longer than platelets from sham-operated rabbits (Table 3.13), indicating that the platelets in the animals at 3 and 6 days were probably enriched with younger platelets (Somers 1984).

Table 3.12. Effect of indwelling aortic catheters on density distribution of rabbit platelets (percentage of platelets applied to the gradient)

Time of sample	Platelets in least dense fraction				Platelets in most dense fraction	
	n	Catheter	n	Sham	Catheter	Sham
Pre-surgery	11	33.8±2.3[a]	12	30.8±2.5	20.9±4.3	17.6±1.8
Post-surgery						
6 d	10	39.4±4.8	12	32.4±4.6	13.1±2.6	16.7±2.2
7 d	9	44.5±3.9	11	35.5±3.1	10.9±1.3	16.4±1.6
9 d	6	46.7±4.1	8	40.1±5.5	10.1±1.7	14.3±2.8
10 d	6	39.7±3.1	7	33.4±5.0	13.2±1.9	19.2±4.2
14 d	6	32.3±5.3	7	25.1±4.1	17.4±4.3	18.5±4.8
4 weeks	4	32.3±3.9	4	27.9±2.2	16.9±1.4	16.4±1.3
6 weeks	4	34.4±5.1	4	26.6±2.7	17.6±3.7	19.6±1.6

[a] Mean±SE.
Results of ANOVA:
   Platelets in least dense fraction, catheter v. sham, $p<0.05$; catheter v. time, $p<0.02$.
   Platelets in most dense fraction, catheter v. sham, $p>0.05$; catheter/sham v. time, $p>0.05$.
Platelets were isolated from whole blood obtained from rabbits before and at various times after the surgical procedure. The isolated platelets were separated into density subpopulations on discontinuous Stractan density gradients. The number of platelets in each density fraction was measured and expressed as a percentage of the platelets applied to the gradient.
From Somers 1984. Reproduced with permission.

In contrast, in rats with indwelling aortic catheters, the proportion of most dense platelets was increased at 4 days (Table 3.14) (Winocour et al. 1983). The increased proportion of most dense platelets was associated with shortened platelet survival (as in the rabbit), but no thrombi were observed around the catheters, although there was extensive vessel wall injury. Platelets harvested at 6 days from the rats with indwelling catheters, labelled, and infused into normal rats survived significantly longer than platelets from sham-operated rats (indwelling catheter: 113.3 ± 6.4 hours, $n = 8$; sham: 70.2 ± 4.8 hours, $n = 8$).

This difference between rats and rabbits was rationalized on the basis that thrombi form around the catheters in rabbits but not in rats. One could theorize

Table 3.13. Survival of platelets from rabbits with indwelling aortic catheters after injection into normal rabbits

Platelets from rabbits with	Number of rabbits	Platelet survival (h) (mean±SE)	p
3 days: catheter in situ	10	84.9±5.2	
			<0.01
3 days: sham operation	10	65.1±2.9	
6 days: catheter in situ	14	73.2±4.9	
			<0.05
6 days: sham operation	15	57.7±4.5	

From Somers 1984. Reproduced with permission.

Table 3.14. Effect of indwelling aortic catheters on density distribution of rat platelets (percentage of platelets applied to gradient)

Time of sample	n	Platelets in least dense fraction			Platelets in most dense fraction	
Pre-surgery	(4)	24.6±3.4[a]			55.1±2.8	
		Catheter		Sham	Catheter	Sham
Post-surgery 4 days	(9)	14.0±0.9 $p<0.05$	(8)	17.4±1.3	70.2±1.4 $p<0.001$	61.4±1.5

[a] Mean±SE.
Number of animals indicated in parentheses. Significance of difference: catheter v. sham.
From Winocour et al. 1983. Data reproduced with permission from *J Lab Clin Med* 101:175–182.

that some of the platelets that escape from thrombi in rabbits have had their density decreased by interactions with thrombin, ADP, thromboxane A_2 and plasmin, but that they have not been altered sufficiently to cause their rapid removal from the circulation, since only high concentrations of plasmin would shorten their survival (Guccione et al. 1985). In contrast, platelets that interact with the damaged wall in rats may not return to the circulation or, if they return, they may be sufficiently altered that they are immediately cleared. It seems reasonable to suggest that proteolytic degradation of platelet membrane glycoproteins may be necessary to free them from the subendothelial constituents to which they have adhered, and we have shown that proteolytic enzymes which remove glycopeptides from platelet membrane glycoproteins do shorten platelet survival (Greenberg et al. 1979). Regardless of whether they remain on the damaged wall or are freed from it in an altered state and immediately removed by the reticuloendothelial system, the rat platelets may be replaced by young platelets enriched in most dense platelets.

Conclusions

These are the overall conclusions with which most investigators seem to agree:

1. Some platelet heterogeneity is due to thrombopoiesis.
2. The most dense platelets tend to be larger, have more α- and dense granule contents, and are metabolically more active than the least dense platelets.

3. Platelets exposed to release-inducing agents or to ADP are decreased in density. This decrease persists in vivo.

4. Platelet density is decreased by cardiopulmonary bypass and in some patients with thromboembolic complications of atherosclerosis.

The conclusions we have drawn from our experiments and those of other investigators include the following points. In stable, healthy animals, the most dense platelets are enriched in younger platelets and least dense platelets are enriched in older platelets. Although there is a great deal of overlap, the most dense platelet subpopulations have a larger median size than the least dense subpopulations. Aggregating and release-inducing agents decrease platelet density and hence the characteristics of circulating platelets must be affected by the stimuli to which they are exposed. However, these effects can be complex, as is exemplified by the results with rabbits and rats with indwelling aortic catheters. Thus, studies of platelet density with humans with vascular disease may be difficult to interpret because the precise reactions in which platelets are taking part under various circumstances are incompletely understood.

References

Amorosi E, Garg SK, Karpatkin S (1971) Heterogeneity of human platelets. IV. Identification of a young platelet population with [^{75}Se]selenomethionine. Br J Haematol 21:227–232

Ardlie NG, Packham MA, Mustard JF (1970) Adenosine diphosphate-induced platelet aggregation in suspensions of washed rabbit platelets. Br J Haematol 19:7–17

Bolin RB, Medina F, Cheney BA (1981) Glycoprotein changes in fresh vs. room temperature-stored platelets and their buoyant density cohorts. J Lab Clin Med 98:500–510

Boneu B, Boneu A, Raisson C, Guiraud R, Biermé R (1973) Kinetics of platelet "populations" in the stationary state. Thromb Res 3:605–611

Boneu B, Sié P, Caranobe C, Nouvel C, Bierme R (1980) Malondialdehyde (MDA) re-appearance in human platelet density subpopulations after a single intake of aspirin. Thromb Res 19:609–620

Boneu B, Sié P, Eche N, Caranobe C, Hugo B, Nouvel C (1983) Platelet density analysis: a tool for the detection of acquired storage pool disease in man. Br J Haematol 55:523–532

Busch C, Olson PS (1973) Density distribution of ^{51}Cr-labelled platelets within the circulating dog platelet population. Thromb Res 3:1–11

Chamberlain KG, Chiu E, Penington DG (1984) Relationship of platelet density to ageing. Cohort studies using mono-amine oxidase activity. Pathology 16:355

Chamberlain KG, Penington DG (1988) Monoamine oxidase and other mitochondrial enzymes in density subpopulations of human platelets. Thromb Haemost 59:29–33

Charmatz A, Karpatkin S (1974) Heterogeneity of rabbit platelets. I. Employment of an albumin density gradient for separation of a young platelet population identified with Se^{75}-selenomethionine. Thromb Diath Haemorrh 31:485–492

Cieslar P, Greenberg JP, Rand ML, Packham MA, Kinlough-Rathbone RL, Mustard, JF (1979) Separation of thrombin-treated platelets from normal platelets by density-gradient centrifugation. Blood 53:867–874

Corash L, Mok Y (1984) Platelet heterogeneity: density distribution of alpha granule and lysosomal constituents in native and thrombin stimulated platelet density cohorts. Blood 64:245a

Corash L, Shafer B (1982) Use of asplenic rabbits to demonstrate that platelet age and density are related. Blood 60:166–171

Corash L, Tan H, Gralnick HR, Shafer B (1977) Heterogeneity of human whole blood platelet subpopulations. I. Relationship between buoyant density, cell volume, and ultrastructure. Blood 49:71–87

Corash L, Shafer B, Perlow M (1978) Heterogeneity of human whole blood platelet subpopulations. II. Use of a subhuman primate model to analyze the relationship between density and platelet age. Blood 52:726–734

Corash L, Costa JL, Shafer B, Donlon JA, Murphy D (1984) Heterogeneity of human whole blood platelet subpopulations. III. Density-dependent differences in subcellular constituents. Blood 64:185–193

Duyvené de Wit LJ, Badenhorst PN, Heyns AduP (1987) Ultrastructural morphometric observations on serial sectioned human blood platelet subpopulations. Eur J Cell Biol 43:408–411

Evans RM, Packham MA, Rand ML et al. (1985) Platelet buoyant density: similar results by centrifugation on discontinuous Stractan and continuous Percoll gradients. Thromb Haemost 54:243

Friedhoff AJ, Miller JC, Karpatkin S (1978) Heterogeneity of human platelets. VII. Platelet monoamine oxidase activity in normals and patients with autoimmune thrombocytopenic purpura and reactive thrombocytosis: its relationship to platelet protein density. Blood 51:317–323

Gear ARL (1981) Preaggregation reactions of platelets. Blood 58:477–490

Greenberg J, Packham MA, Cazenave J-P, Reimers HJ, Mustard JF (1975) Effects on platelet function of removal of platelet sialic acid by neuraminidase. Lab Invest 32:476–484

Greenberg JP, Packham MA, Guccione MA, Rand ML, Reimers H-J, Mustard JF (1979) Survival of rabbit platelets treated in vitro with chymotrypsin, plasmin, trypsin, or neuraminidase. Blood 53:916–927

Guccione MA, Kinlough-Rathbone RL, Packham MA et al. (1985) Effects of plasmin on rabbit platelets. Thromb Haemost 53:8–14

Harfenist EJ, Wrana JL, Packham MA, Mustard JF (1985) Measurement of fibrinogen concentrations in suspensions of washed rabbit and human platelets by radioimmunoassays. Thromb Haemost 53:110–115

Hirsh J, Glynn MF, Mustard JF (1968) The effect of platelet age on platelet adherence to collagen. J Clin Invest 47:466–473

Illes I, Pfueller SL, Hussein S, Chesterman CN, Martin JF (1987) Platelets in idiopathic thrombocytopenic purpura are increased in size but are of normal density. Br J Haematol 67:173–176

Jung SM, Tanoue K, Yamazaki H (1985) The electrophoretic mobility heterogeneity of human platelet subpopulations of different buoyant densities. Thromb Haemost 53:188–194

Karpatkin S (1969) Heterogeneity of human platelets. II. Functional evidence suggestive of young and old platelets. J Clin Invest 48:1083–1087

Karpatkin S (1978) Heterogeneity of rabbit platelets. VI. Further resolution of changes in platelet density, volume and radioactivity following cohort labelling with ^{75}Se-selenomethionine. Br J Haematol 39:459–469

Karpatkin S, Charmatz A (1969) Heterogeneity of human platelets. I. Metabolic and kinetic evidence suggestive of young and old platelets. J Clin Invest 48:1073–1082

Karpatkin S, Strick N (1972) Heterogeneity of human platelets. V. Differences in glycolytic and related enzymes with possible relation to platelet age. J Clin Invest 51:1235–1243

Kelton JG, Denomme G (1982) The quantitation of platelet-associated IgG on cohorts of platelets separated from healthy individuals by buoyant density centrifugation. Blood 60:136–139

Khansari N, Fudenberg HH (1983) Immune elimination of aging platelets by autologous monocytes: Role of membrane-specific autoantibody. Eur J Immunol 13:990–994

Kinlough-Rathbone RL, Packham MA, Mustard JF (1983) Vessel injury, platelet adherence, and platelet survival. Arteriosclerosis 3:529–546

Leone G, Agostini A, DeCrescenzo A, Bizzi B (1979) Platelet heterogeneity. Relationship between buoyant density, size, lipid peroxidation and platelet age. Scand J Haematol 23:204–210

Martin JF, Penington DG (1983) The relationship between the age and density of circulating ^{51}Cr-labelled platelets in the sub-human primate. Thromb Res 30:157–164

Martin JF, Shaw T, Jakubowski J, Penington DG, Martin TJ (1981) Production of thromboxane B_2 by platelets is related to their density. Thromb Haemost 46:198

Martin JF, Shaw T, Heggie J, Penington DG (1983) Measurement of the density of human platelets and its relationship to volume. Br J Haematol 54:337–352

McDonald JWD, Ali M (1983) Recovery of cyclooxygenase activity after aspirin in populations of platelets separated on Stractan density gradients. Prostaglandins Leukotrienes Med 12:245–252

Mezzano D, Aster RH (1987) Survival of platelet density subpopulations. Br J Haematol 65:505

Mezzano D, Hwang K-L, Catalano P, Aster RH (1981) Evidence that platelet buoyant density, but not size, correlates with platelet age in man. Am J Hematol 11:61–76

Mezzano D, Aranda E, Foradori A, Rodriguez S, Lira P (1984a) Kinetics of platelet density subpopulations in splenectomized mongrel dogs. Am J Hematol 17:373–382

Mezzano D, Aranda E, Rodriguez S, Foradori A, Lira P (1984b) Increase in density and accumulation of serotonin by human aging platelets. Am J Hematol 17:11–21

Mezzano D, Aranda E, Foradori A (1986) Comparative study of size, total protein, fibrinogen and 5-HT content of human and canine platelet density subpopulations. Thromb Haemost 56:288–292

Minter FM, Ingram M (1971) Platelet volume : density relationships in normal and acutely bled dogs. Br J Haematol 20:55–68

Packham MA, Guccione MA, Kinlough-Rathbone RL, Mustard JF (1980) Platelet sialic acid and platelet survival after aggregation by ADP. Blood 56:876–880

Packham MA, Guccione MA, O'Brien KM (1985a) Duration of the effect of aspirin on the synthesis of thromboxane by density subpopulations of rabbit platelets stimulated with thrombin. Blood 66:287–290

Packham MA, Perry DW, Kinlough-Rathbone RL et al. (1985b) Effects on the buoyant density of rabbit platelets of ADP and agents that increase the concentration of cyclic AMP. Blood 65:564–570

Packham MA, Kinlough-Rathbone RL, Mustard JF (1987) Thromboxane A_2 causes feedback amplification involving extensive thromboxane A_2 formation upon close contact of human platelets in media with a low concentration of ionized calcium. Blood 70:647–651

Parker RI, Shafer BC, Gralnick HR (1987) Platelet density-dependent partitioning of platelet-von Willebrand factor between alpha granule and non-alpha granule pools. Thromb Haemost 58:911–914

Penington DG (1984) Heterogeneity of platelets. Br J Haematol 56:351–352

Penington DG, Lee NLY, Roxburgh AE, McGready JR (1976a) Platelet density and size: The interpretation of heterogeneity. Br J Haematol 34:365–376

Penington DG, Streatfield K, Roxburgh AE (1976b) Megakaryocytes and the heterogeneity of circulating platelets. Br J Haematol 34:639–653

Pereira J, Cretney C, Aster RH (1988) Variation of class I HLA antigen expression among platelet density cohorts: a possible index of platelet age? Blood 71:516–519

Pfueller SL, Chesterman C, Illes I, Hussein S, Martin JF (1986) Relationship of platelet-associated immunoglobulin G and platelet protein to platelet size and density in normal individuals and patients with thrombocytopenia. J Lab Clin Med 107:299–305

Rand ML (1983) Studies of changes in rabbit platelets as they age in vivo. PhD thesis, University of Toronto, Toronto, Canada

Rand ML, Greenberg JP, Packham MA, Mustard JF (1981) Density subpopulations of rabbit platelets: size, protein, and sialic acid content, and specific radioactivity changes following labeling with ^{35}S-sulfate in vivo. Blood 57:741–746

Rand ML, Packham MA, Guccione MA, Mustard JF (1983a) Glycoproteins of rabbit platelets: Loss from granules during aging in vivo or as a result of the release reaction in vitro. Thromb Haemost 50:188

Rand ML, Packham MA, Mustard JF (1983b) Survival of density subpopulations of rabbit platelets: Use of [51]Cr- or ^{111}In-labeled platelets to measure survival of least dense and most dense platelets concurrently. Blood 61:362–367

Reimers HJ, Packham MA, Kinlough-Rathbone RL, Mustard JF (1973) Effect of repeated treatment of rabbit platelets with low concentrations of thrombin on their function, metabolism and survival. Br J Haematol 25:675–689

Reimers HJ, Kinlough-Rathbone RL, Cazenave J-P et al. (1976) In vitro and in vivo functions of thrombin-treated platelets. Thromb Haemost 35:151–166

Savage B, McFadden PR, Hanson SR, Harker LA (1986) The relation of platelet density to platelet age: survival of low- and high-density [111]Indium-labeled platelets in baboons. Blood 68:386–393

Somers DA (1984) The relation among vessel injury, thombus formation and platelet survival. PhD thesis, McMaster University, Hamilton, Ontario, Canada

Somers DA, Winocour PD, Kinlough-Rathbone RL, Mustard JF (1983) Relation among platelet survival, vessel injury, thrombosis and platelet density. Fed Proc 42:1027

van Oost BA, van Hien-Hagg IH, Veldhuyzen BFE, Timmermans APM, Sixma JJ (1982) Determination of the density distribution of human platelets: methodological aspects and comparison with other tests of platelet activation. Thromb Haemost 47:239–243

van Oost B, van Hien-Hagg IH, Timmermans APM, Sixma JJ (1983) The effect of thrombin on the density distribution of blood platelets: detection of activated platelets in the circulation. Blood 62:433–438

van Oost B, Timmermans APM, Sixma JJ (1984) Evidence that platelet density depends on the α-granule content in platelets. Blood 63:482–485

Vicic WJ, Weiss HJ (1983) Evidence that platelet α-granules are a major determinant of platelet density: studies in storage pool deficiency. Thromb Haemost 50:878–880

Watson HHK, Ludlam CA (1986) Survival of 111-indium platelet subpopulations of varying density in normal and post splenectomized subjects. Br J Haematol 62:117–124

Winocour PD, Kinlough-Rathbone RL, Perry DW, Rand ML, Packham MA, Mustard JF (1983) Changes in the properties of platelets from rats with experimentally induced shortened platelet survival. J Lab Clin Med 101:175–182

Technical Questions

Corash: I have one comment with respect to the in vivo incorporation data that you showed from David Penington's work in the *British Journal of Haematology* in 1976. I think that pair of papers had a considerable influence on the literature at the time of publication because of the controversy surrounding Karpatkin's work. One of the things a lot of people are not aware of and which we tumbled to in some subsequent work is that those experiments of Penington were contaminated with leukocytes. During the in vivo incorporation of selenomethionine, the specific activity of the leukocytes, particularly the lymphocytes, is very high. When you separate the cells on the gradients used by Penington, there is such significant contamination that interpretation of that data is extraordinarily difficult. I think John Martin appreciates this because subsequently he modified the techniques when doing the same sort of studies. I feel that is why Penington saw a lesser-fold enrichment than Karpatkin. However, Karpatkin had another artefact. He was working with platelet-rich plasma rather than a whole platelet population. Hence, it would appear to be a trade-off in two different directions. I feel that these points need to be emphasized and results treated with caution. Everybody must be made aware that leukocyte contamination is extraordinarily deleterious to interpreting the results of these experiments.

I would like to make another technical point. I do not believe that Percoll gradients can give isopycnic equilibrium. I think that this could be one cause for the difference in incorporation of specific activity. You still find a significant difference in incorporation between your most dense and least dense, but it is not as great as in your other experiments with arabino-galactan.

Packham: Yes, that is so.

Corash: It is pretty clear that there is a difference. Percoll is a large macromolecule. The *g* forces at which people have spun Percoll gradients are far less then the *g* forces that you use with the arabino-galactan gradients. If you spin Percoll for longer periods of times the macromolecules begin to separate themselves in the gradients, and the density gradient becomes unstable. That is why you cannot spin them over a long period of time. This became apparent to us when we did some red cell studies a number years ago. I think that this is another point we should be aware of in these systems.

Packham: I have a paper in my files entitled: Is Percoll innocuous to cells? [Wakefield JS, Gale JS, Berridge MV, Jordan TW, Ford HC (1982) Biochem J 202:795–797] Have you seen it?

Martin: I want to have a long discussion with Dr Corash about Percoll gradients and isopycnic centrifugation but I think we should leave that until we have answered the technical problems. Dr Packham, you say your two sulphur curves using the two different density gradients of arabino-galactan and Percoll are different. However, when you use the Percoll gradients they seem to be far closer together then they were with the arabino-galactan gradients, qualitatively at least. Is there a statistically significant difference between the two sets of curves, even though they are qualitatively similar?

Packham: I am sure you realize that all curves of this sort depend very much on the proportions of the total platelet population that one isolates in the least dense and most dense fractions. That, of course, accounts for some of the variability expressed by the standard deviation.

Martin: But if you use enough animals, then those errors should have a Gaussian distribution in both situations and you should be able to see differences. Just to my eye, it seems that there was less difference with the Percoll than there was with the arabino-galactan.

Packham: Well, I would agree, looking at the data that we have at present.

Thompson: I do not think you stated your hypothesis on the rabbits directly. However, I think the conclusion we all drew from hearing your lecture was that you felt the primary platelet heterogeneity, at least of density, was created by events that occurred in the circulation. You would say that those are submaximal stimulatory events that lead to granule release. Is that a fair reiteration of the hypothesis?

Packham: No. I would say that we think that heterogeneity arises both from the megakaryocytes and also from the encounters that platelets make in the circulation. It is a combination of the two.

Thompson: Let me restate that. It is a combination of the two but there is a significant percentage to account for the density distribution changes over age.

Packham: At least in rabbits.

Thompson: Have you done anything to test that hypothesis directly? If it is true then the obvious question would be: What happens to the density distribution with age if you shut off the partial release reactions, by inhibiting platelet release, in vivo? Could you do that physiologically? It seems to me that is the direct test of the hypothesis.

Born: This is a good point, but it sounds like general discussion.

Thompson: Can I ask just one further technical question quickly. Dr Packham, you made a point that the more dense platelets, you thought, had higher mitochondrial enzymatic activity. I wondered how that occurred? I think Dr Corash's lecture raised an important new point, which I have been thinking about a lot in the last couple of hours. The best proof that there has been a change during in vivo circulation is, in fact, that the mitochondrial content does not change while other things do change in the density gradients. How do you then explain that there is more mitochondrial enzymatic activity in the more dense platelets.

Packham: That is not my work. I was quoting Chamberlain and Penington. It is a recent paper in *Thrombosis and Haemostasis* 59:29–33, 1988.

Corash: You have raised two interesting points. With respect to the mitochondria, we measured MAO (monoamine oxidase) activity in the different density fractions with Dennis Murphy a number of years ago. If you express it as specific activity and you adjust for protein content then you find small but significant differences. The high-density platelets have more MAO activity than the low-density platelets. However, platelets have no real capacity for *de novo* synthesis. If you draw an analogy with some red cell systems, in which glycolytic enzymes fall in activity over a period of time, then this might account for the decline in MAO activity. It is not very significant and the half-life of that enzyme remains far greater than the life-span of the cell. I put forward this as a hypothesis but cannot prove it to you. With respect to the other question that Dr Thompson raised: if you inhibit the platelet release reaction do you see modification of platelet density? That experiment has been done, in fact, in a rather indirect way in a paper published in 1979 by Karen Kaplan in *Blood*. She looked at plasma levels, β-thromboglobulin and platelet factor 4 in people on aspirin and in people not taking any medication. She found that the plasma platelet factor 4 and β-thromboglobulin levels on aspirin went down significantly as if there was some decrease in the secretion process, but nobody has ever looked at density. That would be a fun experiment. The question is, would there be too much noise-to-signal for you to see anything? I think that might be hard.

Packham: In addition you could not do the experiment to shut down release completely because aspirin will not block release caused by thrombin.

Thompson: Right. I do not want to pursue that. I would just like to make one comment on mitochondria. I think Dr Corash's point is a good one, in that substrate from glycolytic enzymes is probably required by mitochondria for overall function, but the rest of their integrity has nothing to do with it. They maintain their own DNA content, they continue their ability to synthesize some RNAs, and they maintain their structural integrity. This is distinct from the rest of the platelet component, which does not have that self-renewing capability. I think that what Dr Corash suggested this morning, and this may turn out to be an important control for all of us, will be the mitochondria themselves. If we have a significant problem with mitochondrial enzymatic activity that is going to have to be addressed by all of us.

Discussion (Chapters 1–3)

The following is a discussion of the contributions forming Chapters 1, 2 and 3.

Rendu: Most of you have said that the α-granule content is the prime determinant of platelet density. I don't know what real evidence you have for that. I think dense bodies are also a determinant of platelet density. We have published that dense platelets contain more dense bodies [Lorez HP et al. (1977) J Lab Clin Med 89:200–206]. Platelets from patients with Hermansky–Pudlak syndrome that lack dense bodies are lighter than normal [Rendu F et al. (1979) Thrombos Haemostas 42:694–704]. Also we have shown that from a metabolic point of view the light platelets do not incorporate serotonin as much as dense platelets [Rendu F et al. (1972/1973) Haemostasis 1:161–168]. Hence, I think dense bodies are also an important determinant of platelet density. Finally, the Hermansky–Pudlak platelets do release less serotonin than normal platelets [Rendu F et al. (1987) Biochimie 69:305–313]. Can I make a further comment? It has been stated that in the release reaction the first components to appear were the α-granules. I think this is not the case. Since 1983 several groups have published different results [Ginsberg MH, Taylor L, Painter RG (1980) Blood 55:661–668; Skaer RJ (1981) Platelet degranulation, in: Gordon JL (ed) Platelets in biology and pathology, Vol. 2. Elsevier, Amsterdam, pp 321–348; Kawaguchi Y (1982) Acta Pathol Jpn 32:961–1002; Akkerman JWN, Gorter G, Kloprogge E (1982) Thrombos Res 27:59–64; Rendu F, Marche P, Maclouf J, Girard A, Levy-Toledano S (1983) Biochem Biophys Res Commun 116:513–519]. We demonstrated that the first granules to extrude their constituents were dense granules followed by α-granules and then lysosomes. This sequence in the release reaction has a physiological relevance since dense granules contain the pro-aggregating factors and α-granules contain adhesive proteins. So what could happen is that because the α-granules contain adhesive proteins they could be the first to stick the adhesive proteins onto the membrane. I think Mark Ginsberg has shown that [Ginsberg M, Plow EF (1981) J Supramol Struct 17:91–98]. But the first organelles which deliver their contents outside are the dense granules. This may be relevant to the release reaction in the different platelet densities.

    Corash: I think we might disagree. We have done some studies with very small doses of thrombin. Digressing slightly, that is another point I want to make. It tends to drive me a little crazy when I read papers and see thrombin doses given in units per millilitre. I always want to know the thrombin dose per number of platelets. Because thrombin binds to sites on the surface of the platelet, it seems to me that units of thrombin or molecules of thrombin per number of platelets is the most significant representation. When we use 0.01 units of thrombin per 10^8 platelets, probably α- or β-thrombin we get from John Fenton in the USA, we see α-granule secretion, and density modification, but we don't see very much happening to the dense bodies.

Your point about adhesive proteins is interesting. We have looked at GMP140 expression with very low doses of thrombin. I don't think of GMP140 as an adhesive protein. It is part of the internal membrane structure of the α-granule, according to the published studies of Paula Stenberg, who used immuno-gold microscopy. She has shown expression of GMP140 on the surface of the cell before movement of dense bodies. I would have to go back and look at your papers. It is interesting what you have to say and the point is well taken. I was relying, in part, on my impressions that have been formed, from the data of Karen Kaplan in 1979 who looked at that sequence. If I understand what you are saying, you have data that shows dense granules coming out before α-granules.

Rendu: There are several groups who describe that sequence [see earlier references].

Corash: I would like to get the references from you and explore it further.

Packham: Whether or not the contents of the dense granules are released before the contents of the α-granules might be different from whether or not they are released more easily. There is a time relationship and possibly a relationship to the concentration of stimulus. In all of the studies that have been reported here this morning, about change in density with stimulation by release-inducing agents, concentrations were used which would cause the release of a large proportion of both α- and dense granule contents.

Rendu: Yes.

Paulus: I would like to come back to the experiments describing selenomethionine, sulphate and amino acid incorporation into dense and light platelets. These experiments have been performed by several different groups. I submit that these experiments do not necessarily reflect changes in activity associated with platelet ageing, as is the general interpretation. They can be interpreted in a completely different way.

In Fig. D1.1, (a) shows the data obtained by Karpatkin, (b) by Rand et al., (c) by Corash and Shafer and (d) by Thompson et al. Only curve (c) shows the sequential appearance in platelets of radioactivity per unit weight, but from the values of platelet activity and volume or weight, the changes in specific activity can be determined in experiments (a), (b) and (d). Experiment (d) shows no change in specific activity in function of platelet volume: however, this is not so in experiments (a), (b) or (c) which all arrived at the same conclusion, namely that the initial specific activity is much greater in the large dense platelets than it is in the light small platelets. This is the basic point shown by several experiments. We have to address that question. I think the interpretation has not taken into account something fundamental which occurs at the end of thrombocytopoiesis. Consider the platelets that are labelled after 24 hours. These cells did not pick up the isotope themselves, it was incorporated by rather mature megakaryocytes. Again the platelets at 120 hours did not incorporate the isotope, whereas more immature megakaryocytes did. Compare these two kinds of megakaryocyte which incorporated the radioisotope at the two different times.

On the right of Fig. D1.2 is a mature megakaryocyte. This cell could have produced the platelets that are observed after 24 hours. In this megakaryocyte we

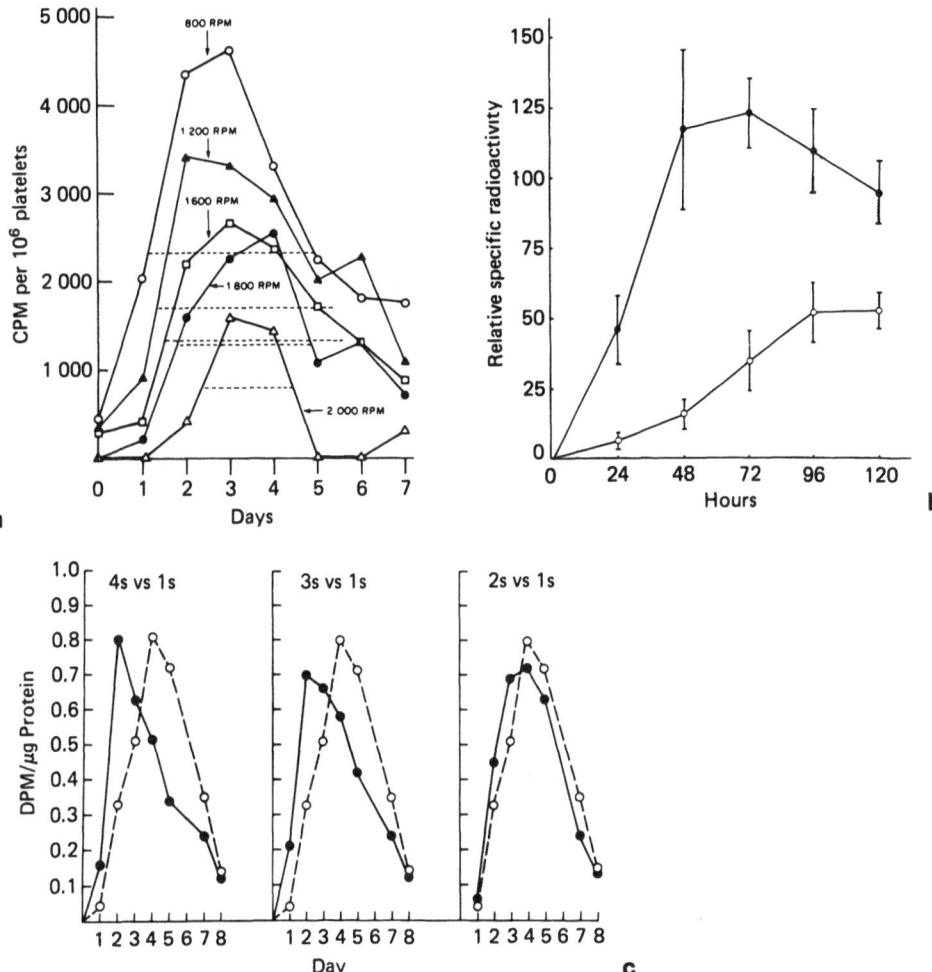

Fig. D1.1. A comparison of four experiments showing the sequential appearance of labelled platelets after administration of megakaryocyte labels to animals.

Platelet populations were separated as follows: **a** sequential centrifugation of rabbit PRP at increasing speed, yielding fractions labelled 800–2000 rev/min with mean platelet volumes of 3.33 fl (800 rev/min, 196 g), 3.10 fl (1200 rev/min, 420 g), 2.75 fl (1600 rev/min, 728 g), 2.56 fl (1800 rev/min, 924 g) and 2.26 fl (2000 rev/min, 1120 g); **b** isopycnic centrifugation of rabbit platelets in Stractan, yielding a least dense population, containing 1.39 mg protein per 10^9 platelets (O), a most dense population, containing 1.84 mg per 10^9 platelets (●), and a total population containing 1.48 mg per 10^9 platelets (shaded area); **c** isopycnic centrifugation of asplenic rabbit platelets in Stractan, yielding fractions labelled, from the least dense to the most dense, 1s (O – – – O in each case) to 4s; **d** size-dependent counterflow centrifugation of baboon platelets, yielding fractions with mean platelet volumes of 4.28 fl (1+2), 4.97 fl (3), 5.73 fl (4), 6.61 fl (5) and 7.2 fl (6+7).

Ordinates refer to **a** [^{75}Se]selenomethionine activity per 10^6 platelets; **b** [^{35}S]sulphate activity per 10^9 platelets in subpopulation sample divided by activity per 10^9 platelets in the total population sample having the highest activity (this maximum occurred in all cases but one at 72 hours); **c** [^{3}H]amino acid activity per microgram of protein; **d** [^{75}Se]selenomethionine activity per 10^9 platelets. Sequential changes in activity *per unit volume or weight* can be obtained by dividing the fraction's activity by the corresponding mean volume or protein content. With permission from **a** Karpatkin S (1978) *Br J Haematol* 39:459; **b** Rand ML et al. (1981) *Blood* 57:741; **c** Corash L, Shafer B (1983) *Blood* 60:166; **d** Thompson CB et al. (1983) *Blood* 62:487.

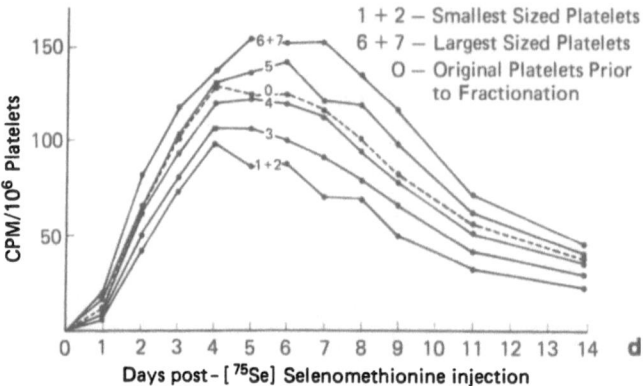

Fig. D1.1. (*continued*)

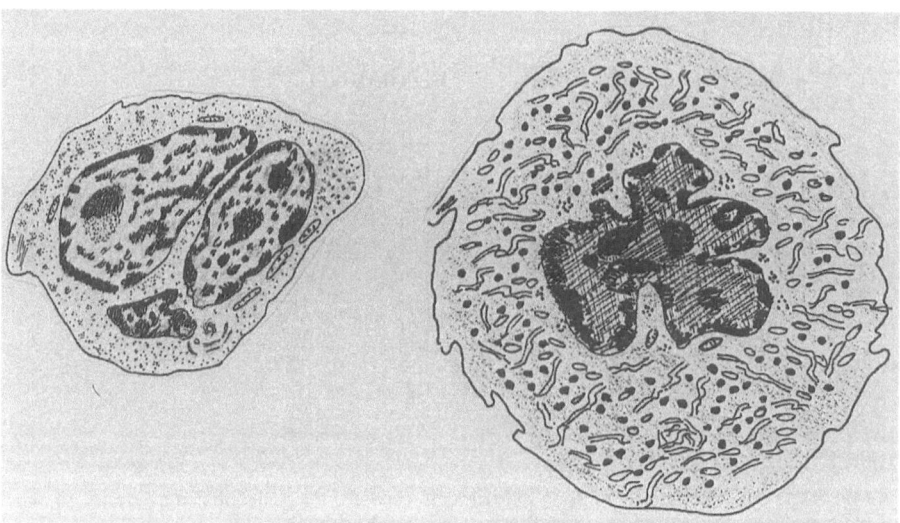

Fig. D1.2. Drawings of immature (*left*) and mature (*right*) megakaryocytes illustrating the concept that the more active, large dense fields are already individualized in mature megakaryocytes incorporating the radioisotope which will appear in 24-hour platelet samples. By contrast, platelet fields are not delineated in the immature cells which incorporate the bulk of the radioisotope to be measured in late (120-hour) samples.

have well-defined fields, some of which are large and some of which are small. The most logical explanation for what happens is that the large dense platelets which are seen at 24 hours come from the large dense fields which are present in mature megakaryocytes. If you remember radioisotope incorporation, knowing the greater activity per microgram of protein of the larger platelets, it must be that large fields incorporate more radioisotope per unit volume or weight than small light ones. Looking at the electron micrograph on the right you may very well imagine that large and small territories are produced together. The former are not necessarily younger than the other; they may be produced together, but the larger ones will have a greater specific activity than the smaller ones. That would explain all the points at 24 hours. On the contrary the megakaryocyte that incorporated the radioisotope, and produced platelets 120 hours later, would be much more immature and they would be like the megakaryocyte shown on the left half of the figure. In such a cell the radioisotope will be incorporated randomly in cytoplasmic zones that have still not grown and delineated platelet fields. Hence, after 120 hours the radioisotope would be dispersed randomly in large and small territories. The specific activities for the large dense platelets and the small light platelets would tend to become very similar. That is what is shown in experiments. You do not have to postulate that young platelets are large platelets.

Mustard: I think your point is an important one, but the critical aspect is really where you get the peak labelling. It is a difficult experiment to do, because you have to sample at least every 4 hours, in most animals. In the pig, the peak labelling is at about 72 hours. That labelling is much higher than at any other time. This peak indicates there is a bolus of platelets that come from the megakaryocytes. Although I cannot recall the actual experiments, people who have studied ^{35}S labelling of megakaryocytes find their results coincide. In those experiments you are getting a peak pouring out of labelled platelets. Your interpretation, I think, really should be geared to what actually takes place at that time. There is a very big difference. In all the curves you saw, the investigators were only sampling every 12 hours or 8 hours and they missed this peak.

Paulus: I agree. The peak essentially shows that the large dense platelets incorporate much more isotope per cubic micrometre or per milligram of protein. The situation is clearer at 24 hours, because then you know what kind of megakaryocyte has produced these platelets, and these are megakaryocytes which have already individualized their platelet territories. If you look at 72 hours, that is at 3 days, you might expect a mixture of megakaryocytes: those having individualized platelet territories, and those which have not. I think you have to consider both extremes to make the thing conceivable. The radioisotope which you measure at 24 hours was incorporated by megakaryocytes that were about to produce platelets, that is obvious. These megakaryocytes had individualized platelet territories, so the activity in the large dense platelets comes from the activity in these large territories. In the small platelets the activity comes from the small territories. The experiment indicates that the large territories have a greater growth capability, i.e. per milligram platelets protein or unit platelet volume, than the small territories. Later on this effect becomes diluted by the arrival of platelets derived from megakaryocytes that picked up the isotope before individualization of the platelet territories.

Corash: At the peak, the heights of the peak in the different density fractions should be equal if you are really considering specific activities. That, I think, is a very important point. That means the radioactivity per microgram of protein is the same eventually in those different populations. It is the temporal relationship which is different.

Mustard: There are problems associated with obtaining data about the peak labelling and also with sampling platelets after the peak and looking at their survival patterns. Your requirement, Dr Paulus, would be for a fairly homogeneous labelling over a period of time in which smaller platelets appear from the more immature megakaryocytes with a lower specific activity because theoretically they have had less isotope. The pattern of platelet disappearance from the peak is consistent with a bolus of platelets being produced. Subsequently, very few, if any, labelled platelets are derived from the megakaryocytes. The bulk of the platelet loss is from a group of mature platelets that have been produced from wherever they were labelled in the megakaryocytes at that peak time. The level of platelet radioactivity afterwards is almost entirely related to the platelet population produced at the time of the peak, not from another new supply of platelets that are produced from the megakaryocytes.

Jackson: The way I see this argument the two of you are not saying something that different. Dr Paulus is talking about the early part of the curve and I think you are talking about the peak, Dr Mustard. I would like to make a comment that agrees with what both of you said. In some unpublished studies of protein synthesis by different megakaryocyte populations, separated on the basis of their density, the most dense megakaryocytes tend to be the younger ones. We found that the highest incorporation of labelled methionine occurs in the youngest ones. So that protein synthesis, if you are using a protein synthesis label, is occurring primarily in the younger megakaryocytes. By the time you are getting to the mature megakaryocyte, like the one Dr Paulus has shown, protein synthesis is decreasing rapidly. Most of this label is incorporated in early megakaryocytes. I think Dr Paulus has an interesting point here.

Mustard: I think you are going to have to look at Fig. D1.3 This is one experiment showing the time when the peak occurs. That may not even be the true time or height of the peak because the sampling may not have been frequent enough. By 120 hours you are really dealing with a loss of radioactive platelets. If the platelets are harvested at the time of the peak and then put into another animal you get essentially the same pattern of disappearance of radioactivity. In other words there is very little influence of the megakaryocyte on the labelling pattern of that disappearance curve.

Thompson: Are you saying that a significant proportion of the platelets that are produced in the peak, it looks like that happens at about 52 hours, die within the next 24 hours?

Mustard: Yes, in the rabbit. The rabbit has a fairly short platelet half-life so

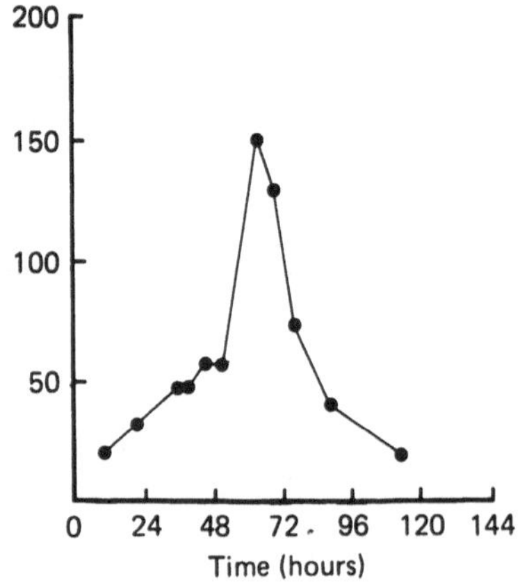

Fig. D1.3. The radioactivity of platelets isolated from the blood of a rabbit at intervals after the intravenous injection of $^{35}SO_4{}^{2-}$. The platelets were washed three times, and then their radioactivity was measured and expressed as counts per minute per milligram platelets on the ordinate.

that is not an unusual curve. I am more familiar with the pig, having used that animal in most of my experiments.

Thompson: So the platelet half-life is less than 24 hours?

Mustard: I don't think you can make a calculation of half-life specifically from just looking at the curve.

Thompson: That is not true. The half-life of any label can be estimated. You can argue that it might be shorter than what I am suggesting but you definitely cannot say that it is longer than that.

Mustard: I am saying that the pattern of labelling that you get with the peak is as shown. To calculate platelet survival from the curve is another issue. You would not calculate it from those data.

Thompson: You just look at the 52- or 56-hour point, or whatever it is, and then you look at the 72-hour point. That is at least 50% down, it looks to me to be 142 or 143 (at 52 hours) versus something around 68 (at 72 hours). Is that fair? Hence the half-life of those platelets . . .

Mustard: Look, let me come back to you in another way. If you do these experiments in pigs where your blood sampling and other things do not significantly change blood volume . . .

Thompson: But these are not pigs!

Mustard: Yes, but let me try to explain the nature of the problem. If you do the experiments in an animal where your sampling and other things do not change your blood volume hugely, such as in a pig, you will find the calculation of half-life, doing the ^{35}S experiment this way, is essentially the same as if you inject indium-labelled platelets and look at the disappearance.

You get the same calculation. The figure is from experiments with rabbits and is only shown to indicate the pattern of peak labelling.

Thompson: If you say this is peak labelling then either those platelets live a normal life-span or there is some artefact in the circulation. That might be blood volume, but it is hard to understand.

Mustard: I cannot explain it to you for the rabbit, but in the pig, where you get peak labelling which is very distinctive, and you study those platelets put into another pig's circulation the pattern of disppearance is the same as the pattern of disappearance of the ^{35}S radioactivity with this kind of labelling [Murphy EA, Robinson GA, Rowsell HC, Mustard JF (1967). The pattern of platelet disappearance. Blood 30:26–38].

Paulus: Dr Mustard, how do you interpret the first 24 hours?

Mustard: Well, I think you are quite right, that you have platelet heterogeneity which comes from the bone marrow. I think that there are labelled platelets being produced from megakaryocytes, some of which are going to be less dense and some more dense. I do not think that is a problem.

Bessman: From this curve does platelet production stop at 60 hours?

Mustard: I think you are dealing with a distributed function, which is really what Dr Paulus was getting at. A variety of megakaryocytes are incorporating the isotope and producing platelets. There is a core group of megakaryocytes which carry the label through as was shown by McDonald many years ago.

Bessman: I appreciate that. I would like an explanation of the rapid fall-off after the peak. Is it that post-core group megakaryocytes produce post-core group platelets, without isotope, that are being added to the circulation? Hence the calculation of the concentration of radioactivity in platelets is now being diluted as it were, rather rapidly, by post-core group megakaryocyte progeny.

Mustard: That could be an explanation. But as I tried to say, that experiment dealt with rabbits. In experiments with pigs the pattern of disappearance of ^{35}S-labelled platelets taken at the peak and put into another animal is exactly the same as the pattern of disappearance of the ^{35}S-labelled platelets in the animal that was given the radioactive sulphate initially. So your explanation does not hold for pig.

Bessman: Can I ask Dr Paulus one other question about his hypothesis? As I follow it, it suggests that in the megakaryocyte already there is not only a heterogeneity of size, indicated by the pre-demarcated megakaryocyte in which the platelet domains are reasonably well seen, but there is already an inexorable heterogeneity of platelet density that has been pre-formed. If that is the case could it be almost a geographic consideration. That is, are those domains of the megakaryocyte that are not only small but are light also lacking proportionately in cytoplasm? The megakaryocyte is not a nice cube or sphere from which can be cut equal equivalents. It contains bits of fins and narrowly opposed membranes, so that in fact it is mostly membrane. Therefore the big, dense, active, full-of-stuff portions are in fact those that disproportionately contain more cytoplasm rather than membrane.

Paulus: My main point is that, as far as size is concerned, the whole heterogeneity is present in the megakaryocyte. In each megakaryocyte there is enough to make a log normal distribution of platelet size, which is a very heterogeneous distribution by nature. In each megakaryocyte ploidy plays no part in heterogeneity. This characteristic is already present in each megakaryocyte. If you look at electron micrographs, either with demarcated territories, or with released processes of platelets, you can see that heterogeneity present at the end of megakaryocyte maturation. It is predetermined, in other words. Platelets are born heterogeneous as far as size is concerned. I do not comment on anything that apparently happens with density during the platelet life-span. I have not done those experiments myself, but as far as size is concerned everything can be explained by what happens in the late organization of megakaryocyte cytoplasm.

Martin: I do not accept all that Dr Paulus has said about pre-determination through demarcation membrane system, but I do agree with his point that there may be heterogeneity of uptake of isotope within those areas that are going to be platelets in the future.

Packham: Actually, it is not my figure of the rabbit data, it was Jack Hirsh's. It was when he was working with rabbit platelets in your laboratory, I think, Dr Mustard [laughter]. For the record it is in a paper with Jack Hirsh as first author [Hirsh J, Glynn MF, Mustard JF (1968) The effect of platelet age on platelet adherence to collagen J Clin Invest 47:466–473], and the fact that it is done as counts/min per milligram of platelets indicates to me that they must have been taking large volumes in order to be able to get enough platelets to weigh. I think this would answer your question, Dr Thompson, about the end of that curve not looking like a reasonable survival curve.

Thompson: Thank you.

Martin: Can I change the subject? We have considered heterogeneity as composed of volume, density and reactivity. Dr Packham and Dr Corash have spoken about density and Dr Thompson has spoken about volume. At breakfast this morning Dr Thompson was determined that he would have nothing to do with density. However, I think the two are linked. When Dr Thompson says that there is no change in survival of big platelets as opposed to small platelets we can interpret that as there is no change in survival of dense platelets as opposed to light platelets. Conversely when the other two speakers talk about density I also think about volume. I think we still have two opposed camps. Dr Corash said in the beginning that the mechanisms of thrombopoiesis and survival both determine overall heterogeneity. I do not think we have any concordance on that from what we have heard. As you know, I, when in Professor Penington's laboratory, measured the density of labelled platelets in 12 Japanese crab-eating monkeys, which is an exotic species. We found at 5 days that the label was still preserved within all density classes. We handled those platelets very carefully; we took them into prostacyclin when we harvested them from the monkey. The big difference between those results and the results of Dr Corash and Dr Packham is in the methodology used. Dr Corash and I can get similar results, I know, because at Sheffield with Drs Trowbridge and Warren we have just reproduced in the rat his very nice paper in the mouse that appeared in *Blood* on early changes in volume. This shows we can do similar experiments with similar results, but with density we have had radically different results in monkeys. You would agree Dr Corash? I see I get a nod of agreement from Dr Corash. The big difference I can see in the experiments is the use of discontinuous Stractan gradients and linear continuous Percoll gradients. That is the major difference. In addition, Dr Corash has always used slicing of the gradients, which he has argued is a very good way of taking the platelet population from the tube. He thinks that I might have some mixing when I pump the gradient up the tube [nod of assent from Dr Corash]. Those are the two differences, but, if you remember our paper from the *British Journal of Haematology*, we took interface sections from Stractan gradients and we put them down continuous linear Stractan gradients and continuous Percoll gradients. We found using the second methodology that within each interface there was a variety of populations of density that were greater than the ones to be found either side. Could this be the central difference between us; if not, Dr Corash, can you come up with any other explanation?

Corash: The reason we used discontinuous gradients arose from our experience of harvesting red cells which have very good markers in terms of glycolytic enzyme activities. If you look at hexokinase in a linear gradient of red cells spun to isopycnic equilibrium you find that by pumping-out methods you cannot extract these cells without mixing and get a good linear distribution of these activities. So we decided to slice the tubes. With a continuous linear gradient, where you slice the tube is made by an arbitrary decision, because without extracting the tube you do not know where the cells are in the tube, unless perhaps you could use some very sophisticated optical measurer of density or something like that to make decisions where to cut. So we went to a discontinuous gradient. If you slice and you do rebanding experiments with discontinuous gradients where you have prostaglandin E_1 (PGE_1) in the density medium you find good rebanding. So I do not agree with the results of your arabino-galactan rebanding experiments, Dr Martin. I have a lot of reservations about Percoll gradients and isopycnic equilibrium. I think that Percoll gradients respond at relatively low g forces so that you have a combination of velocity sedimentation and density separation going on. I think that is very hard to control.

Martin: When you say rebanding, did you reband into continuous, or reband again into discontinuous gradients?

Corash: Rebanding again into discontinuous gradients.

Martin: So you could be reproducing the same artefact that you were measuring in the first gradient?

Corash: Sure, except that those gradients are spun to isopycnic equilibrium and the total load of platelets put onto those gradients is relatively small. So you can spin them over a very long period of time.

Martin: That is right. As Dr Trowbridge and I pointed out in our theoretical paper on discontinuous gradients, isopycnic equilibrium in the discontinuous gradient is of a theoretically different quality to that in the continuous gradient. We stopped our Percoll gradients every 5 minutes until we found that time and that point in the gradient when the platelet mass went no further. In fact, when we spin them for a longer time we got secretion and the platelets started to go back up the gradient again. It was that time that we said was isopycnic.

Corash: I do not think that is right. I do not think you have reached isopycnic equilibrium. If you take a red cell which does not secrete and you put it into a Percoll gradient you cannot reach isopycnic equilibrium. The gradient deforms because you are dealing with a macromolecule. You cannot get the g force that you need.

Martin: The gradients did remain linear afterwards. Dr Corash, let us stop this because we are not going to agree. Answer my next question. If it is not a question of technique, if we both believe we have a reasonable technique, what is the explanation for the difference between our two monkey results, which are the most radical of all? I realize Dr Packham also has different results, but they are not as radical as those two sets of experiments.

Corash: First of all, let us go to Dr Thompson's data. If I remember those data correctly the survival is different between the small and large platelets.

Thompson: Let me comment on Dr Martin's statements and what Dr Corash is asking about the survival of different-sized platelets. I think we have very little useful information based on our separation technique for what the true relationship of density is to ageing. It is true that there is a positive correlation, as Dr Corash suggested earlier, between the size separation that we use and density, but I do not think we can make any inferences based on the small distribution in density difference in our data. It is true that consistently, by all the labelling techniques that we have used, it appears that the large platelets (with "large" being the primary determinant) seem to survive, by the best analyses we can do with a variety of different modelling systems, approximately, for a day longer in the circulation. Relative to total populations and observing total radioactivity being removed, relative to individual populations labelled by at least two independent mechanisms, we have five separate labelling techniques in which the data are consistently a day longer. But I do not think we can say a lot about the relationship of density from these data. Our opinion on the density is that it is very clear that in some animal systems, and that is why I pushed Dr Packham earlier and I think she stated very clearly what is true about density, from our observations of the density field there are two major components of heterogeneity: one is created during thrombopoiesis and the other is created during in vivo circulation. I think the simplest way for us to think about it is that the amount of contribution to heterogeneity, in terms of density, varies between species. Consistently in the rabbit model there has been a decrease in density; essentially every study has shown that. In other studies, we have come to the assumption that everybody is right, and all their data are correct, so it is just that all of our interpretations are wrong. So we have two opposed views in the primate, but that may simply reflect that, in fact, in this system the animal itself had some ongoing activation. Certainly we see this in our mice since we do much more immunology now. For example, for the next two months we cannot do a useful baseline resting lymphocyte assay because the mice are infected every year in the spring. So I think there are differences in terms of the ongoing activation that may occur even within a given animal model, depending upon the time at which the study is done and things like that. So I do not really have a problem, to be honest with you Dr Martin, between the fact that you and Dr Corash got opposing results. All the data simply say is there are two major mechanisms and in an individual animal or individual model you may see a balance shifted in one way or another, depending on a variety of conditions. I agree with you both that there are methodological differences, but I do not think that is why so many groups with so many different techniques come out with varying answers to the same question.

Corash: In response to your question to me, Dr Martin, what you are focusing on is the fact that in your primate experiment you did not find any difference between the survival of high-density and low-density platelets. Is that correct? I am concentrating on Dr Thompson's experiments, because I am trying to look for a theme of consistency in the literature, within the primate experiments that have been done. What I think I see in his experiments, and I believe this is what he has just said, is that although he has used primarily a size-dependent separation system he has enrichment of his large platelets with high-density cells. He does not have fantastic enrichment but he has enrichment to some extent and he has longer survival. If you consider that Dr Savage's data in his baboon experiments show prolonged survival of the high-density fraction, and if you take the Ludlam and Watson data they have prolonged survival of the high-density fraction and finally our own primate data show prolonged survival of the high-density fraction compared to the low-density fraction, so I see a theme of consistency there. I do not know how to explain the result that you got, Dr Martin, other than by the hypothetical questions I am raising about the problems with gradients, isopycnic equilibrium and extraction of gradients. I have fallen into some of those same pitfalls myself along the way and sometimes when you get negative data you do not like to publish it because nobody is too interested in it, but I know well the problems of extracting gradients and that is why I slice them. Slicing is difficult and a pain in the neck. I would much rather be able to pump them in or drip them out. I think there is a consistency in the literature. Therefore the experiments that I have described in primates do not stand as an isolated polarized result compared to your data, Dr Martin.

Martin: I accept that there may be two components to heterogeneity: one in the circulation and one from thrombopoiesis. The problem is what proportion of the component comes from thrombopoiesis in the normal physiological animal. I had always thought that by using young male monkeys we had a very small proportion of those platelets consumed in preserving endothelial integrity, for example. However, I do take Dr Thompson's point and your implied point, Dr Corash, that there may be animal differences as well that would increase that proportion, within various laboratories, of heterogeneity from circulating problems. But even if that is so it still means we are not dissecting out the problem. If we prescind from the fact that there may be changes in density due to thrombosis and preservation of vascular integrity, I still want to know in that pristine situation where there is no disease present what proportion of heterogeneity is determined by thrombopoiesis and what by ageing in the circulation. By ageing, I mean ageing independent of pathology. I still feel that my evidence points to the fact that there is approaching zero change in that pristine situation. Do you accept that statement or are we still saying that, disease apart, we have a component that is due to ageing in the circulation.

Corash: I do not think there is a pristine situation. We all have atherosclerosis, to some extent, even though we do not like to think about that. We all have a sort of continuing progression of non-fatal haemostatic events that involve platelets. I think the animals we use are subjected to some of those same considerations.

Martin: Let me put it another way. Do we all accept that the major component of density heterogeneity is thrombopoiesis? Would Dr Packham accept that?

Packham: I do not think I can put a percentage on the aspect that is due to thrombopoiesis and the aspect that is due to changes in the circulation. I would say that with rabbits there certainly are density changes as platelets circulate in these relatively young undiseased animals. They do not have atherosclerosis. I think we have to remember also that platelets have to be present to keep the endothelium intact, as I mentioned in my talk. We do not know how they do that and it is possible that they may be altered in doing so.

Born: It occurs to me that one should tackle the problem another way. We all have atherosclerosis, some of us worse than others. As you get older you have more and it is almost impossible to quantify. There has been all this work about shortened platelet survival in people with atherosclerosis. I do not know how well accepted this is, but could not one follow the changes in some way and relate them measurably, to changes in the circulation? Perhaps this has been done. Not these vastly obvious things which have been done, but is there some way in which one can get a better answer for the circulatory component and, as it were, extrapolate backwards? Is this possible? That is one thing; the other is a straight question. I do not know whether Dr Mustard knows the answer. Is the release reaction per platelet an all-or-none phenomenon, like a nerve impulse? Is that known? Once you start release of a platelet does it empty itself of all the dense granules that it has or all the α-granules that it has? I do not know the answer to that.

Packham: I do not think the answer is known. There has been an interesting paper from Elizabeth Simons' laboratory [Davies TA, Drotts D, Weil GJ, Simons ER (1988) Flow cytometric measurements of cytoplasmic calcium changes in human platelets. Cytometry 9:138–142] just recently. It shows that in a given population of platelets some of them respond to low concentrations of thrombin and others do not, which again is heterogeneity of response.

Born: But the ones that respond, do they respond totally, in other words with a nerve impulse it either fires or it does not, you reach the threshold and then the thing fires; is this true for platelets?

Jackson: We do not know the answer to that. I can make a comment from some unpublished data we have by flow cytometry, not on release; but it is related to what Dr Packham has said. If you study fibrinogen binding to platelets with increasing agonist concentration it is not an all-or-none phenomenon, you increase the amount of fibrinogen per platelet with increase in agonist concentration. That is not only from our data but this also has been observed by Johnston et al. [Blood 69:1401, 1987] for an α-granule protein that becomes exposed on the platelet surface during α-granule secretion.

Corash: I have a comment along the same lines, and I am interested to know whether or not your experiments confirm this. First to clarify the record, so to speak, the data we are talking about are the expression of unique activation antigens. We have been looking at the expression of GMP140 using McEver's S12 antibody. Also Shattil has an antibody called PAC 1 in which he is basically also looking at the fibrinogen-binding epitope on the surface of platelets. One of the things you find is a graded response with agonist for expression of this glycoprotein. So maybe that gets a little bit at your answer, but not completely. Also I have found that you cannot get expression on every single platelet, even if you use the maximal agonist dose. There is about 15–20% of platelets that will not express GMP140 on the surface. I do not know whether or not these are platelets which have already responded and GMP140 has been reinternalized or cleared off of the surface or handled by proteases in some way, or whether these cells are just duds. I asked Shattil that same question and he said that maybe there are some platelets that are made that are total duds and will never work. I do not know the answer to that, but I think that is the nature of the problem we are talking about.

Jackson: I might just make a couple more comments from our observations with this type of study. There is a relationship, as you would expect, between the amount of GPIIb/IIIa, the fibrinogen receptor, on platelets and their size, as determined by light scatter, in a flow cytometer. The platelets that do not respond to ADP, which is what we are using, this 20% or so that do not respond to ADP, tend to be those platelets that scatter light less. These tend to be the smaller platelets, but it is not an all-or-none type thing.

Trowbridge: I have listened very carefully. I did not want to say anything until I had listened to the experts [laughter]. It seems to me that we are talking about degrees of heterogeneity. Dr Paulus seems to be very dogmatic about the way that platelets are produced from megakaryocytes, that platelet territories are the particular aspects which determine both size and density. I think this afternoon we shall have some further argument about that, and therefore the discussion that is taking place now really is not taking place correctly, in the sense that we have not talked about platelet production in the way that we should if we are actually going to discuss the heterogeneity of density and volume. There appear to be two aspects. One is heterogeneity of volume and one is heterogeneity of density. The experiments that are done do not seem to tie up together in the sense that volume and density are not studied at the same time, not really. When density experiments are considered the heterogeneity studied seems to be either heavy platelets or light platelets; that is just two factors. That is what it appears to me. Whereas when we talk about volume heterogeneity, we are talking about a volume distribution. Now, I do not really understand, but I would like to know, is the density primarily determined by the granule content? If so those are integer quantities, aren't they, therefore we should be able to see if the platelets lose their granules in an integer way. Volume is not quite the same, it is a continuous smooth effect. Therefore, I do not really think the density and volume have been linked in a way which allows us to know what is going on with respect to ageing and thrombopoiesis. It may be that we need to go back again to this particular problem this afternoon.

Mustard: I think Dr Packham should answer that question about volume and density since Dr Trowbridge may have missed the point that you can have a change in platelet volume without the release reaction having occurred.

Packham: Actually this is something I took out of my talk because I did not have time to put it in. We did some experiments with PGE_1, which is a good inhibitor of the release reaction, and we showed that it will increase volume and decrease density if you leave rabbit platelets exposed to it [Packham MA, Perry DWS, Kinlough-Rathbone RL et al. (1985) Effects on the buoyant density of rabbit platelets of ADP and agents that increase the concentration of cyclic AMP. Blood 65:564–570]. ADP does this too, but there may be a slight release of α-granule contents with the ADP.

Trowbridge: Are you saying that if you incubate with PGE_1 the platelets increase in size?

Packham: Yes.

Trowbridge: I do not think that is what we found, is it Dr Martin?

Packham: I am talking about rabbit platelets. We tried the same thing with human platelets and at the same concentration we did not show much effect on human platelets, with just PGE_1.

Martin: We did a different experiment. We were showing that the artefactual increase in volume produced by activation with ADP was inhibited by PGE_1. We did not do your experiment, but I wonder what percentage of your experimental change is simply due to taking on water?

Packham: Yes, that is what I think is happening.

Martin: But then you are not answering Dr Trowbridge's question. He wants to see an integer loss of density as you lose the granule contents.

Packham: I was just asking Dr Corash how many α-granules there are per platelet. Does anyone know? [silence] Because if it is a large number then your distribution curve will be smoothed off and even though it is a Poisson distribution you will not see an integer change as granules discharge their contents.

Born: But, Dr Martin, one more point. I hope I am not too old-fashioned on this, but if you say that PGE_1 inhibits volume increase, here I would really like to have that volume increase controlled by an independent method. One must make quite sure it is not a shape change that happens, in a certain number of platelets. I think this would show up.

Martin: I think it is a shape change. In fact, we did the experiment because you had a personal observation in a paper that PGE_1 inhibited it, and we showed that this was in fact so. If you have an impedance method of measuring volume you can form what the physicists call a flock; whereby you start putting out fingers on your platelet and at some point there is a sudden jump from measuring the volume of the original surface to the external volume of all those fingers. That is what you can get if you have activated platelets. We showed PGE_1 can in fact, inhibit that activation.

4 Origins and Significance of Platelet Heterogeneity in a Non-human Primate Model

B. Savage, C. S. Hunter, L. A. Harker and S. R. Hanson

Introduction

Normal peripheral blood platelets are heterogeneous with respect to size, buoyant density, function, organelle content and metabolic capacity. Although it is now clear that normal thrombocytopoietic mechanisms produce a hetero-geneous platelet population, the extent to which platelets undergo modifications as they circulate in the bloodstream is not completely understood. Conflicting data from different laboratories over the past two decades have led to a variety of hypotheses concerning the mechanisms of platelet heterogeneity. Since the causes of platelet heterogeneity affect our interpretation of platelet kinetics and their clinical implications, it is important to resolve the current disparate views. Moreover, in addition to their obvious relevance to thrombotic disorders, mechanisms underlying platelet heterogeneity are also important for understanding other disease states characterized by alterations in platelet reactivity, destruction or production, including immune or thrombotic thrombocytopenias, myelodysplastic syndromes and myeloproliferative disorders.

The explanation for the variable results reported by different laboratories may relate to differences in experimental techniques and different interpretations of similar observations. The selection of appropriate animal models is an additional important consideration since there is significant variation in the size, volume, organelle content and survival of platelets among different animal species. For example, rodents have platelet counts greater than one million and a small mean platelet volume (MPV), in the range of 4.5 fl (Eason et al. 1986). Rabbits more closely approximate man in platelet count, but have a low MPV at 4.9 (Eason et al. 1986). The dense granule content of serotonin (5-hydroxytryptamine, 5-HT), ADP, ATP and divalent cations varies greatly among species, with the primate and dog bearing close resemblance to man (Meyers et al. 1982; Savage et al. 1988). The survival of normal platelets in the circulation reflects the balance between age-related removal and random platelet destruction. In certain animals, such as the rabbit, the exponential drop in labelled platelet radioactivity may indicate a substantial component of random destruction (Blajchman et al. 1981; Trowbridge and Martin 1983). Splenic haematopoiesis may complicate studies of platelet production in the mouse (Schalm et al. 1975). In this laboratory, we have elected to utilize a baboon model since we have shown that the haemostatic mechanism in the baboon closely resembles that of man in a number of respects, including platelet count, platelet volume, platelet morphology, platelet aggregation and release ex vivo, platelet density, platelet content of dense granule and α-granule constituents, and immunological cross-reactivity and concentrations of coagulation factors and fibrinolytic plasma proteins. We have also demonstrated cross-reactivity of several anti-human platelet monoclonal antibodies with epitopes expressed on baboon platelet membrane, including GPIa, GPIb, GPIIb/IIIa complex and with cryptic epitopes expressed after platelet activation.

To investigate the extent to which platelet properties are modified during their life-span in the peripheral circulation, platelets can be isolated according to a single property (e.g. density, size, function, electrophoretic mobility) to determine whether any correlations can be made with platelet age. Alternatively, platelets of uniform age may be examined with respect to their properties and compared with other platelet cohorts of known age or with control platelets of all ages. Both these approaches have been employed in this laboratory to investigate (a) the relation of platelet density to platelet age, and (b) the characteristics of young platelets with respect to kinetic properties, haemostatic function, organelle content, platelet volume, expression of platelet membrane glycoproteins and organ distribution.

It is also important to consider the extent to which intravascular events contribute towards platelet heterogeneity in health and disease. For example, it has been shown in human control subjects and in patients with thrombocytopenia that a fixed number of platelets are required to support vascular integrity (Hanson and Slichter 1985). In normal individuals, the fixed platelet requirement is modest: up to 18% of all platelets are destroyed in a random manner, while the remainder are probably removed through senescent mechanisms. It is not clear whether those platelets which participate in the maintenance of normal haemostasis and endothelial integrity are representative of the total circulating platelet population. It has been shown in both man and experimental animals that acute platelet destruction or elevated platelet turnover (due to cardiovascular prostheses or vascular disease) is associated with abnormalities in circulating platelets with respect to function (Buchanan et al. 1979; Clagett et al. 1981a), density (van Oost et al. 1982; Winocour et al. 1983), size (Volkmer et al. 1979; Yamazaki et al. 1980) and dense granule contents (Savage et al. 1983). Do platelets interact reversibly with thrombogenic surfaces and return to the circulation in a modified form? Alternatively, are certain platelet subpopulations selectively and irreversibly removed such that residual platelets remaining in the circulation display altered characteristics when compared with a control platelet population? The clinical significance of platelet heterogeneity and the diagnostic value of measuring quantitative platelet changes in vascular disease will remain uncertain until the underlying mechanisms have been clearly defined. In this chapter we review recent studies from this laboratory addressing some of these important issues.

Platelet Density

To determine the relationship between platelet density and platelet age in the baboon, we investigated changes in the density distribution of ^{111}In-labelled platelets following their maturation in the peripheral circulation (Savage et al. 1986). In these studies, baboons were transfused with ^{111}In-labelled autologous platelets (representing platelets of all densities). Blood was sampled at 1 hour following infusion of labelled platelets and at 24-hour intervals for 6 days. Platelets were isolated in high yield (>95%) from whole blood using the method developed by Martin et al. (1983), in which platelets are separated primarily on the basis of size on pre-formed Percoll density gradients. Platelets were then separated on the basis of density using linear Percoll density gradients under conditions producing true isopycnic separation of platelets. Following fractionation of the gradients, platelet number and platelet-associated ^{111}In activity were measured in each density fraction.

At 1 hour following infusion of ^{111}In-labelled autologous baboon platelets, the density distribution of ^{111}In-labelled platelets coincided closely with the distribution of total platelets, indicating that the labelling procedure did not affect platelet density and that platelets of all densities were labelled in an equivalent manner (Fig. 4.1). The platelet density distribution profile remained constant for a period of five days, as would be expected under basal physiological conditions. However, there was a small but detectable transition in the distribution of ^{111}In-labelled platelets towards platelets of higher densities (the peak density shifted from 1.061 to 1.063 g/ml; $p<0.001$, χ^2 test). This shift was most apparent after 5 days (Fig. 4.1), when the labelled platelets remaining in the circulation represented a relatively old platelet population, i.e. approaching the average platelet life-span in baboons of 5–6 days.

These data are compatible with either of the following interpretations: (a)

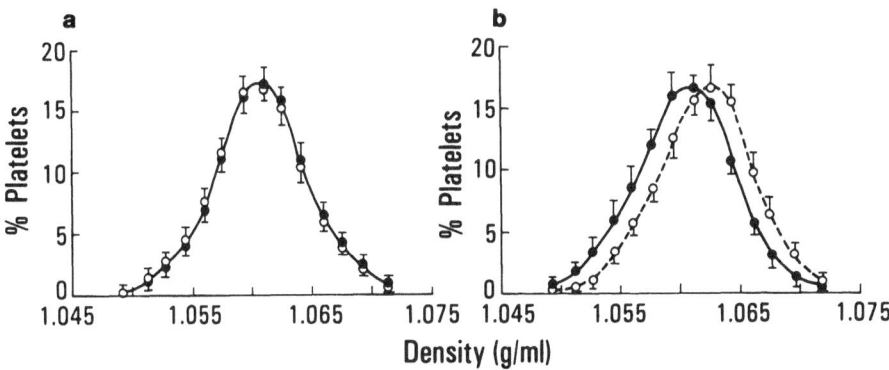

Fig. 4.1. Comparison of total platelet (●) and ^{111}In-labelled platelet (○) density distributions. Platelets were separated in linear continuous Percoll density gradients at 1 hour (a) and at 5 days (b) following infusion of ^{111}In-labelled autologous platelets in baboons. Error bars represent ±1 SD ($n=6$). Reproduced with permission from Grune & Stratton, Inc.

platelets of all densities increase in density on ageing in the circulation, producing a symmetrical shift in the total platelet population towards higher densities; or (b) low-density platelets have a shorter survival time and are therefore cleared from the circulation at a faster rate than the more dense platelets. To distinguish between these two possibilities, the survival characteristics of low-density (1.052–1.056 g/ml) and high-density (1.064–1.068 g/ml) ^{111}In-labelled platelets were investigated. There were no significant differences between the mean survival times of low-density platelets (5.0±0.49 days), high-density platelets (4.9±0.56 days) or control platelets representing platelets of all densities (4.9±0.38 days) (Fig. 4.2). Therefore, although these studies show a slight increase in the density of all platelets upon ageing, the principal finding is that platelet preparations with different mean densities have similar survival times. Thus, these data support the concept that thrombocytopoiesis, not platelet ageing, is the major determinant of platelet density heterogeneity in primates. The slight increase in the density of all platelets occurring during their subsequent life-span in the circulation contributes little to the density heterogeneity of platelets in normal physiology. Whereas several groups of investigators have proposed that platelet maturation in the peripheral circulation is associated with a concomitant decrease in platelet density (Karpatkin 1978; Corash et al. 1978; Rand et al. 1983), other groups have concluded either that platelet density increases with platelet age (Mezzano et al. 1981; Boneu et al. 1982) or that platelet density heterogeneity is determined during megakaryocyte maturation (Penington et al. 1976). This long-standing controversy probably reflects, in part, the different methodologies adopted by

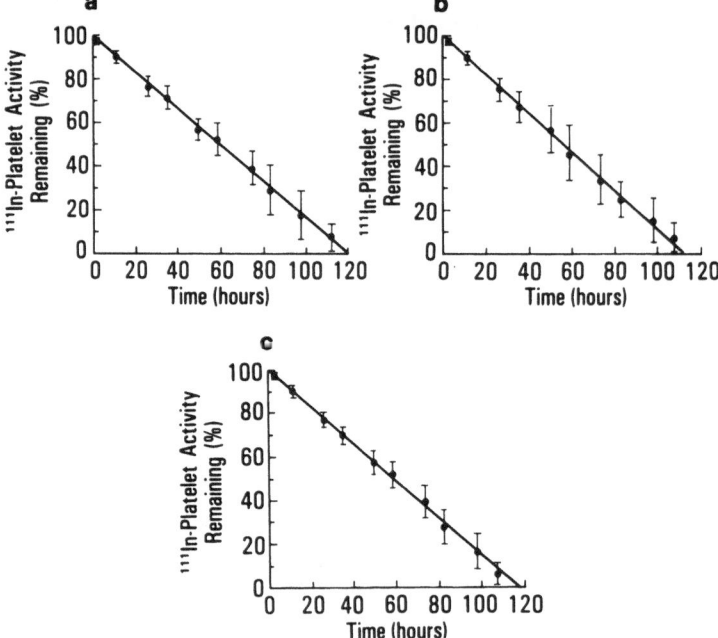

Fig. 4.2. In vivo ^{111}In platelet disappearance patterns. ^{111}In-labelled low-density platelets (**a**), high-density platelets (**b**), and control platelets representing platelets of all densities (**c**) are compared. Error bars represent ±1 SD (*n*=6). Reproduced with permission from Grune & Stratton, Inc.

various laboratories for the density separation of platelets. Previous studies have used sucrose (Booyse et al. 1968; Rendu et al. 1979a), inert silicone oils (Karpatkin 1969), albumin (Charmatz and Karpatkin 1974; Boneu et al. 1982), arabino-galactan polysaccharide (Stractan) (Corash et al. 1978; Rand et al. 1983; Vicic and Weiss. 1983) and Percoll (Martin et al. 1983; Martin and Penington. 1983) gradient systems. The physical characteristics (viscosity, osmolality) of the gradient medium often impose important limitations on its application to the density separation of platelets. Furthermore, theoretical considerations, expounded by Martin and Trowbridge (1982), suggest that major constraints are imposed by discontinuous gradient techniques, since platelets of variable density may be trapped at multiple-step interfaces resulting in stress-induced platelet activation. Platelet activation may cause organelle secretion, leading to decreased platelet density (van Oost et al. 1982) without necessarily affecting platelet survival (Reimers et al. 1973). The necessity for a valid isopycnic centrifugation technique should also be emphasized. Since the principal factors that determine the separation of platelets in density gradients are platelet volume and density, the viscosity of the medium and the speed of centrifugation, the use of high-viscosity gradients (e.g. Stractan) will necessitate longer centrifugation times if true platelet density separation is to be achieved. If centrifugation is stopped before equilibrium conditions have been reached, platelet volume will affect the distribution.

Martin and Penington (1983) have also demonstrated a slight increase (5%) in the mean density of platelets in monkeys 5 days after infusion of ^{51}Cr-labelled autologous platelets, using continuous linear Percoll density gradients and isopycnic equilibrium conditions. These results and their interpretation are in agreement with the work reported by Boneu and co-workers (1982) and Mezzano and co-workers (1981) in humans, but contrast with the observations reported by Corash and co-workers (1978) using rhesus monkeys and by Rand and co-workers (1983) using similar methods and rabbits. Meaningful comparisons of data from different laboratories can only be made when similar methodologies and animal models are used. It is well documented that platelets from different species display considerable variation with respect to structural, kinetic, functional and biochemical properties. For example, Mezzano and co-workers (1984) have presented evidence suggesting that the direction of the change in platelet density with age is dependent on the species studied. Thus, these workers reported that mongrel dog platelets decrease in density with age, in contrast with their observation that human platelets increase in density with age, despite the use of similar techniques and experimental designs.

Characterization of Young Platelets

The relationship of platelet age to platelet heterogeneity can be directly assessed by isolating a platelet population of uniform age and defining its properties. This has generally been done by harvesting platelets during recovery from acute thrombocytopenia induced by anti-platelet antibodies (Ginsburg and Aster 1972; Tong et al. 1987), drugs (Shulman et al. 1968; Packham et al. 1985), or radiation

(Blajchman et al. 1981). Unfortunately, the characteristics of young platelets produced following such manipulations may not be representative of the properties of young platelets produced under conditions of steady-state thrombocytopoiesis. Many investigators have demonstrated that within a few hours of the infusion of anti-platelet sera, a burst of large platelets is released, which we shall refer to as "proplatelets" (Trowbridge et al. 1986; Tong et al. 1987). Because several days are required before the emergence of "stress" or "shift" platelets through an increase in the rate of megakaryocyte production and maturation (Penington and Olsen 1970; Odell et al. 1976; Corash et al. 1987), proplatelets must result from a direct effect on the mature megakaryocyte. Whether this is due to binding of anti-platelet antibodies to the megakaryocyte (Rolovic et al. 1970; McMillan et al. 1978), or as a result of the release of humoral intermediates which affect mature megakaryocyte fragmentation (Leven and Yee 1987), is unclear. In any event, the earliest platelets produced may not be representative of normal young platelets. In addition, the survival of newly released platelets in the circulation may be shortened as a consequence of antibody binding to circulating platelets in states of antibody excess, or the binding of antibody to the platelet while it is still a component of the megakaryocyte. Both these events could lead to accelerated platelet clearance by Fc receptor-mediated mechanisms.

To avoid these limitations, we developed a non-immune, rapid method of depleting circulating platelets through the use of a series of glass bead columns which retain $\geqslant 90\%$ of all circulating platelets during a 1-hour exposure period. The platelets harvested during recovery from acute thrombocytopenia survive normally, are removed from the circulation by predominantly senescent mechanisms, and are not increased in size. Therefore, their properties may more accurately reflect those of normal young platelets than do platelets produced by other methods.

The Baboon Model of Acute Thrombocytopenia

The baboon is uniquely suited for studies of the haemostatic system. Work from this laboratory and others has confirmed the baboon's similarity to man with respect to coagulation factors, platelet kinetics and granular contents, and platelet and plasma proteins as measured by human radioimmunoassays (Hampton and Mathews 1966; Todd et al. 1972; Hanson et al. 1985a, b). The baboon vascular anatomy and accessibility allow for the placement of femoral arteriovenous shunts which will remain patent for at least several weeks. These Teflon–silastic shunts do not detectably shorten platelet survival or produce measurable platelet activation (Hanson et al. 1985b; Savage et al. 1986). Animals remain awake for the duration of each experiment, thereby avoiding the possible effects of anaesthetic agents. All of our experiments were performed on juvenile male baboons (*Papio cynocephalus/anubis*) weighing 8–13.5 kg. All animals were observed to be disease-free for at least 6 weeks prior to use. Procedures were approved by the institutional Animal Care and Use Committee in accordance with federal guidelines (*Guide for the Care and Use of Laboratory Animals*).

After systemic heparinization, platelets were removed from the circulation by perfusion of blood over a series of glass bead columns and distally placed 20-μm pore size paediatric transfusion filters interposed between the arterial and venous limbs of the shunt (Fig. 4.3). Columns were made from the filter chambers of two

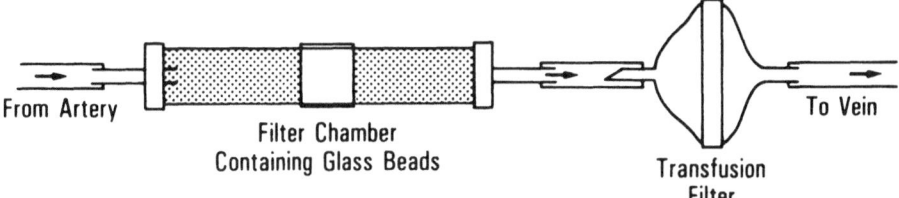

Fig. 4.3. Glass bead column and blood transfusion filter. The filter chamber (200-μm filter, 20-ml capacity) was filled with spherical glass microbeads (0.5–0.6 mm diameter). The column, blood filter (20 μm pore size) and connecting Silastic tubing (4.0 mm i.d.) were primed with sterile isotonic saline before connecting to the arterial and venous shunt sites and establishing blood flow. Mean blood flow rates through the column and filter were measured continuously using a Doppler ultrasonic flowmeter fitted around the Silastic tubing connected to the arterial shunt site.

blood component recipient sets and filled with 18 ml of spherical glass micro-beads, 0.5–0.6 mm in diameter. The distal filter prevented the recirculation of platelet aggregates dislodged from the column which might otherwise accumulate in the pulmonary vasculature. Mean blood flow rates through the circuit ranged from 100 to 150 ml/min at the start of each experiment. Eight columns and four filters placed sequentially over a period of 1 hour removed ≥90% of circulating platelets. Platelet counts then recovered in a linear fashion over the next week (Fig. 4.4). The platelet population present at 20 hours post-depletion was enriched in young platelets and was harvested for further study as described in subsequent sections of this report.

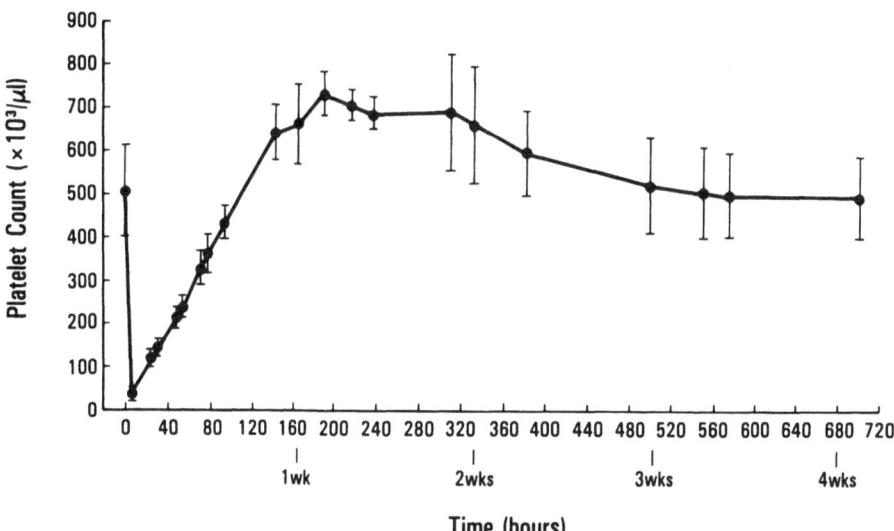

Fig. 4.4. Recovery from acute thrombocytopenia induced by the exposure of flowing blood to glass microbeads. The average circulating platelet count is shown at various time intervals after the onset of acute thrombocytopenia. Error bars represent ±1 SD ($n=4$). Reproduced with permission from Blackwell Scientific Publications Ltd.

Platelet Kinetics

The fate of platelets in animals and man has been an issue of some controversy. In previous studies, mathematical modelling of the survival curves of radioisotopically labelled platelets in normal individuals has suggested that up to half of all circulating platelets may be removed through random processes (Davey 1966; Trowbridge and Martin 1983). However, it is clear that such estimates may be influenced strongly by both the slight curvature of normal platelet disappearance patterns in man, and the reported variability in normal platelet life-span, e.g. 7–10 days. In addition, platelet survival could be influenced by platelet injury during collection and labelling, non-random sequestration of platelets by the spleen, the labelling of homologous versus autologous cells, non-random cell labelling and the quality of the data. Although measurements of platelet survival may be useful for documenting increased platelet destruction, in general we agree with the view of earlier investigators that analysis of the shape of platelet survival curves may not provide insight into the mechanisms normally responsible for the removal of platelets from the circulation (Aster 1971; Mustard et al. 1966).

In a previous report we performed platelet kinetic studies in normal subjects and in patients with moderate and severe thrombocytopenia secondary to decreased platelet production (Hanson and Slichter 1985). The data were subsequently analysed to determine whether the decrease in platelet survival observed in these patients could be explained on the basis of a fixed platelet requirement. The analysis indicated that in normal individuals no more than about 20% of all platelets would be utilized by random haemostatic processes during their life-span, with the remainder being removed through senescent mechanisms. This prediction was consistent with the observations in patients showing that platelet survival was only reduced when the circulating platelet count fell below approximately 100 000 platelets/μl. While this study concluded that platelet removal is predominantly age-related in man, the demonstration was indirect (being based on the relationship between platelet survival and platelet count) and subject to the variabilities of clinical patient studies. A more direct demonstration of senescent platelet removal could be achieved by following the survival of platelet subpopulations of fixed age.

A population of normal young platelets removed from the circulation on the basis of age alone should exhibit a survival curve which is concave downwards, a characteristic of a cohort of newly produced cells (Aster 1971). Attempts to demonstrate this survival pattern in the past have met with only partial success. Harker (1977) studied a patient recovering from quinidine-induced thrombocytopenia and observed a disappearance pattern consistent with the age-dependent clearance of a young platelet cohort, but it is difficult to draw firm conclusions from the study of a single patient. In rats, Ginsburg and Aster (1969) observed a prolonged survival of younger platelets, but the anti-platelet serum and exchange transfusions used to produce young platelets may have caused some ill-effects on the hosts.

In our study, 11 animals were rendered acutely thrombocytopenic using the glass bead filter approach described previously. Autologous baboon platelets were labelled with [^{51}Cr]sodium chromate prior to the procedure to determine the number of residual platelets remaining in the circulation after platelet depletion and during recovery from acute thrombocytopenia. Twenty hours post-depletion, residual platelet-associated ^{51}Cr radioactivity and platelet counts were measured to determine the relative proportion of young platelets present. A mean of 72% young platelets were present at 20 hours post-depletion (by subtraction of residual ^{51}Cr-labelled platelets from the total platelet population). These platelets were then harvested and relabelled with [^{111}In]indium oxine. The kinetics of the total (residual + young) platelet population were determined by serial sampling and survival analysis. Following platelet depletion, baboons displayed the composite platelet survival pattern shown in solid symbols (Fig. 4.5). Also shown are the ^{51}Cr disappearance patterns of platelets labelled prior to the acute depletion procedure (open symbols in Fig. 4.5). Subtraction of the survival pattern of the residual platelets from the composite survival pattern yielded the platelet disappearance curve shown in Fig. 4.6. To rule out any adverse effects of the procedure on the host, a second group of recipient animals also received labelled platelets harvested from the depleted animals 20 hours post-depletion. We have previously shown that homologous platelets do not exhibit shortened survival in normal baboons. In the present study the disappearance pattern of the young platelets in normal recipients was indistinguishable from that seen in the donors. These data convincingly demonstrated that a population of young platelets had been isolated, and that their removal from the circulation was predominantly dependent on normal senescent mechanisms.

The average half-life of the labelled platelet cohorts was greater than 5 days, as compared to a normal half-life of 2.5–3.0 days as determined from control studies. Curve-fitting analysis of these data indicated that the young platelets were initially cleared at a rate of approximately 2% per day, a value comparable to the rate of random platelet destruction in normal humans (Hanson and Slichter

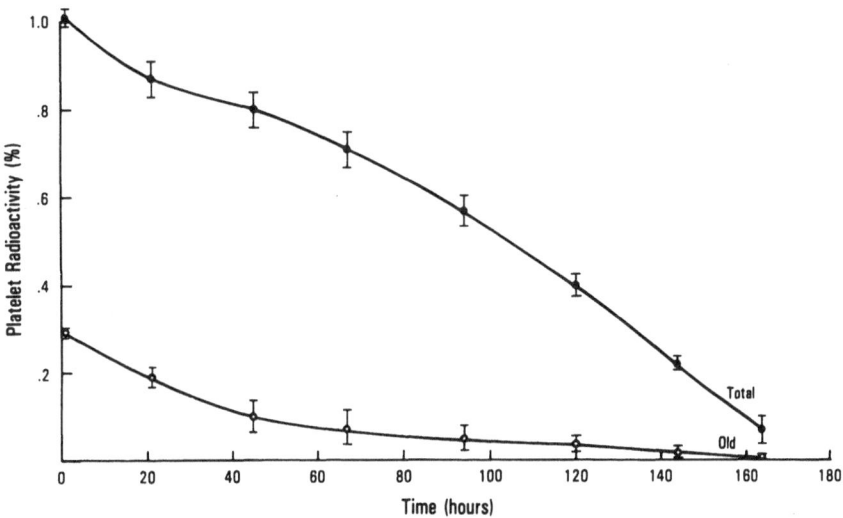

Fig. 4.5.   Platelet kinetics during recovery from acute platelet depletion induced by glass bead filters. Circulating platelets were labelled with ^{51}Cr prior to inducing acute thrombocytopenia (O) and with ^{111}In one day following platelet depletion (●). The ^{51}Cr-labelled residual ("old") platelets comprised approximately 30% of the total platelet population initially, and were rapidly cleared over subsequent days. The total cell population comprised of "old" and newly produced platelets exhibited a prolonged and non-linear disappearance pattern. Values are mean ±1 SEM of observations in 4 animals. Reproduced with permission from Grune & Stratton Inc.

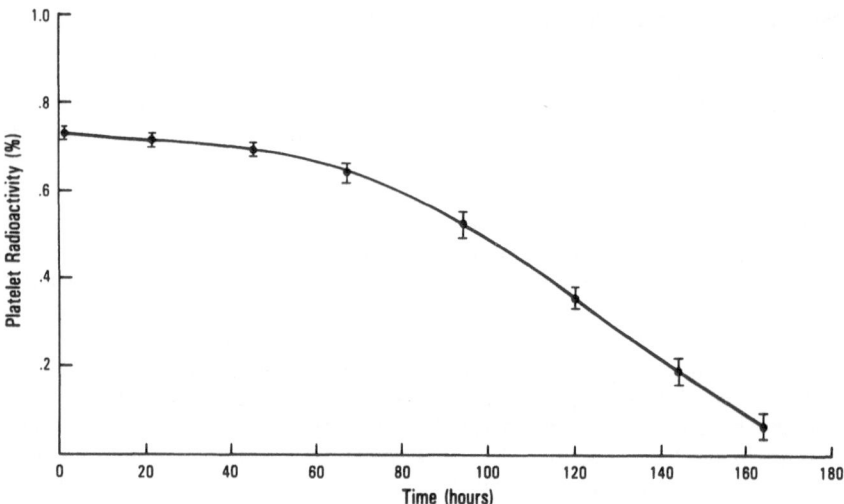

Fig. 4.6. ^{111}In-platelet kinetics of a cohort of newly produced cells. The survival curve of "young" platelets produced following induction of non-immune-mediated acute thrombocytopenia was determined from the data shown in Fig. 4.5 by subtracting the disappearance pattern of "old" platelets (labelled pre-depletion) from that of the "total" ("young" plus "old") platelet population (labelled post-depletion). The shallow slope of the curve over 0–2 days indicated that approximately 90% of the cells were cleared by age-related (senescent) mechanisms. Values are mean ± 1 SEM of observations in 4 animals. Reproduced with permission from Grune & Stratton, Inc.

1985). In addition, these results were consistant with a process of random platelet destruction involving approximately 10% of all platelets during their life-span, with the remaining 90% of cells being removed through age-related mechanisms.

Organ Localization

It has been well documented that the spleen retains a portion of the circulating platelet pool (Kotze et al. 1986), but it is not known whether this sequestration affects all platelets equally or whether a select population of platelets has greater affinity for the spleen. In 1968, Shulman harvested platelets from human volunteers with intact spleens and healthy donors who had previously undergone splenectomy. Upon transfusion of these platelets into thrombocytopenic recipients, a longer survival for the platelets from asplenic donors was reported. He concluded that young platelets were preferentially sequestered by the spleen and therefore could only be harvested from the asplenic individuals. This led to the theory that the spleen may participate in the process of platelet maturation. In support of this concept, Freedman and Karpatkin (1975) presented evidence that the rabbit spleen preferentially sequesters megathrombocytes, and Watson and Ludlam (1986) concluded that platelets of higher density were preferentially retained by the spleen. In both cases the platelet population under study was presumed to be younger than average. Finally, Wichmann and Gerhardts (1981) developed a mathematical model which suggested that the spleen's storage of young platelets could explain the sagging commonly observed in normal platelet survival curves.

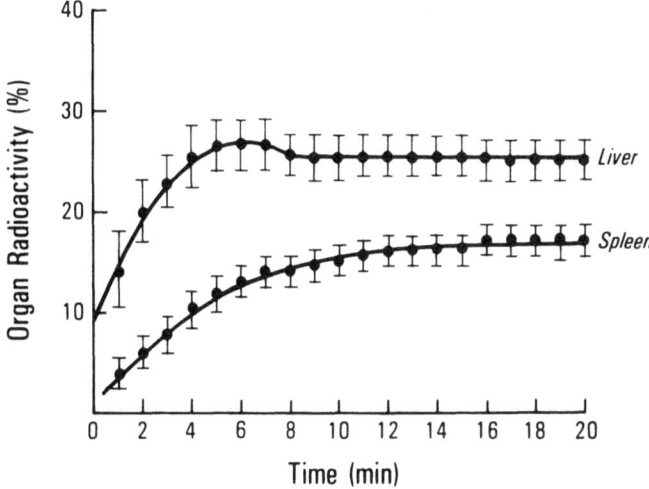

Fig. 4.7. The attainment of equilibrium after injection of ^{111}In-labelled young platelets. Organ radioactivity was determined at 1-minute intervals and expressed as a percentage of whole body activity. Error bars represent ±1 SEM ($n=10$).

Our model provided an opportunity for direct assessment of the role of the spleen in sequestering young platelets. Platelets were harvested 20 hours post-depletion and labelled with quantities of [111]indium oxine sufficient to provide high-quality scans with standard gamma camera imaging techniques. Twenty minutes after injection, equilibrium was attained (Fig. 4.7), and organ counts were computed from the geometric mean of 1-minute anterior and posterior regions of interest. Whole body counts were calculated from the geometric mean of the sums of four anterior and four posterior sections (head, thorax, abdomen/pelvis and lower extremities), each acquired for 1 minute. Statistical comparisons were made using Student's t test after organ radioactivity was expressed as a percentage of whole body radioactivity.

Six depleted animals, four normal animals serving as recipients of labelled young platelets, and six controls receiving labelled autologous platelets were imaged. Recipients were evaluated to rule out any influence of the depletion procedure on the reticuloendothelial system of the host. Results are shown in Table 4.1. There were no significant differences in the distribution of organ

Table 4.1. Comparison of the organ distribution of ^{111}In-labelled young platelets and ^{111}In-labelled control platelets

Group	n	Mean organ activity at equilibrium (% of whole body ^{111}In activity)	
		Liver	Spleen
Donors	6	27.0±5.9 ($p=0.29$, NS)[a]	19.5±1.6 ($p=0.45$, NS)
Recipients	4	17.2±4.4 ($p=0.11$, NS)	16.7±8.7 ($p=0.98$, NS)
Controls	6	23.1±6.4	16.8±7.9

All values are expressed as mean ± 1 SD
[a] p value for comparison with the control group. NS, not significant.

radioactivity between any of the groups. It is also important to note that our controls were comparable to previously published normal values for baboons (Kotze et al. 1985). The animals in our study had a rapid and predictable rise in platelet counts after depletion, with no lag period which might suggest the retention of a select group of young platelets in the spleen, making them unavailable for relabelling. All baboons were healthy at the time of the experiment and had received no prior platelet transfusions, in distinct contrast to the group of patients studied by Shulman (1968), many of whom were seriously ill and had presumably received numerous prior platelet transfusions. These data do not support the long-held concept that young platelets are preferentially sequestered by the spleen, but rather suggests that such sequestration is a random process.

Platelet Size

The baboon model described above has also been utilized to examine the size characteristics of young platelets harvested during immediate recovery (23 hours) from acute experimental thrombocytopenia, and at daily intervals during rebound thrombocytosis and normalization of platelet count (Savage et al. 1988). Whole blood platelet counts and platelet volume measurements were performed on blood sampled into EDTA (4 mg/ml) and measured within 1 hour of sampling, using a Model 810 Platelet Analyzer (Baker Instruments Corp., Allentown, Pennsylvania). Baseline platelet volume distributions (measured at time $t=0$, Table 4.2) were log-Gaussian with an MPV of 7.3 ± 0.3 fl. The MPV measured at 23 hours after the onset of acute thrombocytopenia, and at subsequent time points, was not significantly different from the baseline value (Table 4.2). No changes were observed in the dispersion about the mean platelet volume.

These data contrast with previous studies in which immune-mediated acute experimental thrombocytopenia was associated with an increase in MPV during the immediate recovery phase. Odell and co-workers (1969) observed "giant" platelets at 12 hours after the injection of anti-platelet serum (APS) in rats. Similarly, Trowbridge and co-workers (1986) reported an increase in the MPV within a few hours of APS injection in rats. These studies documented changes in platelet volume heterogeneity caused by the immediate stress of acute thrombocytopenia, before an increase in the rate of platelet production could be effected. More recent studies by Corash and co-workers (1987) utilized a murine model to study thrombocytopoiesis serially after the induction of experimental thrombocytopenia of variable severity and duration using APS. These workers observed an increase in platelet volume which preceded, and was therefore independent of, major changes in the megakaryocyte ploidy distribution. The peak increment in MPV occurred at 24 hours after the induction of acute thrombocytopenia and slowly declined to basal values at 96 hours. However, when interpreting these data it is important to consider the effects that anti-platelet antibodies may exert on platelets released into the circulation subsequent to the infusion of APS. It is possible that smaller platelets, being more readily saturated by anti-platelet antibodies, are removed from the circulation at a faster rate than larger platelets, resulting in an increased MPV. In the studies by Trowbridge and colleagues

Table 4.2. Platelet volume, α-granule contents and aggregation ex vivo during recovery from non-immune-mediated acute thrombocytopenia in baboons

Time (h)	Platelet count ($\times 10^9$/l)	Mean platelet volume (fl)	Platelet β-TG (μg/10^9 platelets)	Platelet PF-4 (μg/10^9 platelets)	Platelet aggregation ex vivo EC$_{50}$ ADP (μM)	EC$_{50}$ collagen (μg/ml)
0	509±107	7.3±0.3	9.6±1.5	9.7±2.4	7.6±2.3	13.1±7.0
23	119± 21	7.3±0.6	14.2±2.4	10.1±1.6	n.d.[a]	n.d.
47	214± 24	6.8±0.3	14.5±0.8	9.1±1.4	3.6±1.7	6.0±3.4
71	326± 37	6.8±0.4	11.6±0.4	9.2±1.1	3.7±0.7	4.6±1.3
143	645± 59	6.6±0.4	8.9±1.0	8.5±1.2	5.2±1.5	6.8±1.9
167	665± 94	6.9±0.4	9.5±0.9	8.8±1.8	5.0±0.9	7.0±1.9
191	736± 48	6.7±0.5	11.0±0.7	10.5±3.2	5.6±1.3	6.5±1.0
216	711± 36	6.8±0.4	10.6±0.8	9.2±1.2	5.7±1.2	8.3±2.0
310	697±144	6.8±0.7	9.6±0.9	7.1±1.2	6.3±2.3	6.7±2.2
383	599± 98	6.9±0.6	9.3±1.3	8.7±0.8	7.0±2.8	10.2±6.6
500	525±109	6.7±0.5	10.5±1.5	10.5±1.1	7.8±2.6	10.9±4.0
575	500± 98	6.9±0.5	12.8±1.2	9.8±1.3	8.0±2.1	10.9±5.5
695	494± 89	6.8±0.4	10.7±0.9	9.9±1.8	7.9±1.9	11.4±4.5

All values are expressed as mean ± 1 SD.
[a] Not determined due to inadequate platelet counts for the standardized aggregation platelet concentration of 200×10^9/l.

(1986), the rate of platelet production did not exceed the rate of platelet destruction until 12 hours after the infusion of APS in rats. Thus, the nadir in the circulating platelet count was prolonged over several hours before a measurable increase in platelet count was seen. This platelet recovery profile is in contrast with our observations (Fig. 4.4) in which non-immune mediated acute thrombocytopenia was associated with an immediate increase in the circulating platelet count.

It has recently been suggested by Tong and co-workers (1987) that large circulating megakaryocyte fragments or proplatelets may contribute significantly to the immediate increase in platelet volume observed during recovery from APS-induced acute thrombocytopenia, before significant increases in megakaryocyte size and ploidy can be demonstrated. Whereas changes in megakaryocyte maturation rate, size, number and ploidy occur over several days and affect immature megakaryocyte and precursor cells, large platelets released during the immediate recovery phase of acute thrombocytopenia may derive from mature megakaryocytes directly affected by the thrombocytopenic state. It has been shown that plasma obtained from rabbits with immune thrombocytopenia contains a factor that stimulates cytoplasmic fragmentation of isolated megakaryocytes (Leven and Yee 1987). This effect was not seen when anti-rabbit platelet serum alone was used. The fact that we failed to show any significant changes in the MPV of circulating platelets throughout the entire period of altered thrombocytopoiesis suggests that APS may affect megakaryocytes directly, possibly influencing the extent of proplatelet formation and the rate of their release into the circulation. Alternatively, mature megakaryocytes may respond to a humoral factor(s) associated only with APS-induced thrombocytopenia.

Platelet Function

It has been demonstrated that large platelets are metabolically and enzymatically more active and are functionally more competent, as assessed by ex vivo aggregometry, than small platelets (Karpatkin 1969, 1978; Thompson et al. 1982; Thompson et al. 1983). It therefore seems likely that larger platelets may be more active haemostatically (Van der Lelie and Van dem Borne 1985). In this context, it has been shown that the MPV is an important indicator of haemorrhagic risk in thrombocytopenic patients (Eldor et al. 1982). The property of increased haemostatic effectiveness has been attributed to young platelets (Harker and Slichter 1972), and it has been widely accepted that young platelets may be larger with an enhanced functional capacity as compared with the total platelet population. In view of these observations it was of interest to evaluate platelets following recovery from non-immune mediated acute thrombocytopenia to determine whether young platelets were intrinsically more functional or whether previous observations of increased function could be explained on the basis of an increased MPV. Since we did not observe significant changes in the MPV during recovery from acute thrombocytopenia, the baboon model afforded the opportunity to investigate any changes in platelet function that were independent of changes in platelet size.

Ex vivo platelet aggregation induced by ADP and collagen was measured (Savage et al. 1988; Harker 1974). Data were plotted as per cent aggregation against log (concentration of agonist) and the concentration of agonist required to produce 50% of the maximal achievable amplitude (EC_{50}) was compared with the concentration required to produce the same change at serial times after the onset of acute thrombocytopenia. Platelet aggregation induced by ADP or collagen became more pronounced when measured on the second day after acute thrombocytopenia (Table 4.2), i.e. the concentration of agonist required to induce 50% aggregation decreased from basal values of 7.6 ± 2.3 μM and 13.1 ± 7.0 $\mu g/ml$ to 3.6 ± 1.7 μM and 6.0 ± 3.4 $\mu g/ml$ after 47 hours for ADP and collagen, respectively (Table 4.2). A gradual normalization of these values occurred in concert with a return to basal steady-state platelet counts. These findings are consistent with the clinical evidence that the functional capacity of platelets produced during thrombocytopenia may be enhanced (Harker and Slichter 1972). Moreover, the present findings support the concept that young platelets are functionally more responsive and that this is an intrinsic platelet property, not attributable to an increase in the MPV.

Membrane Glycoproteins

Membrane glycoproteins are critical for the maintenance of platelet functional integrity. They serve as cytoadhesins to mediate both platelet interactions with the subendothelium and platelet aggregation. Analysis of normal platelets reveals significant variability in the number of glycoprotein (GP) molecules detected per platelet (Johnston et al. 1984), as well as in the distribution of glycoproteins within the membrane. It has been shown that GPIIb/IIIa is initially arranged uniformly over the platelet surface, but becomes redistributed upon exposure to physiological agonists (Loftus and Albrecht 1984). Likewise, GPIb, which normally forms small clusters on the unstimulated platelet, redistributes into large patches upon thrombin stimulation (Polley et al. 1981). Stimulation of platelets in vivo may also lead to the expression of functional receptors, new membrane glycoproteins, such as GMP140 (Stenberg et al. 1985) or increased expression of pre-existing epitopes, as with GPIIb/IIIa (Niiya et al. 1987). Finally, the addition of certain drugs or proteolytic enzymes such as plasmin may alter the number or distribution of glycoproteins detected on the platelet surface, contributing further to heterogeneity (Coller 1982; Adelman et al. 1985).

A relationship between membrane glycoproteins and platelet age has been proposed. George and co-workers (1976) have suggested that fragments of platelet membrane are lost in the process of reversible haemostatic interactions. They presented evidence that the more dense platelets (presumed to be younger) expressed more membrane glycoproteins than older, less-dense platelets (George et al. 1976; Blajchman et al. 1981). Haver and Gear (1982) separated platelets on the basis of function and analysed membrane glycoproteins to conclude that more reactive (presumed younger) platelets expressed more membrane glycoprotein. Further study by this group suggested that the difference between the "more reactive" and "less reactive" groups was that membrane glycoproteins were not lost, but became inaccessible, most likely as a result of conformational changes.

A final line of evidence linking membrane protein heterogeneity to platelet age comes from the study of megakaryocytes. Some platelet antigenic determinants are not expressed on the megakaryocyte surface at all, while others are expressed only on fully mature megakaryocytes (Hyde and Zucker-Franklin 1987). If platelet release is accelerated under conditions of thrombocytopoietic stress, the antigenic profile of the platelets so produced may be altered. Taken together, this work suggests that the membrane glycoprotein profile of young platelets may differ substantially from that of platelets of normal age distribution and may contribute to enhanced function. We therefore evaluated membrane glycoproteins on young platelet populations harvested 20 hours after platelet depletion and compared the number of molecules bound per platelet and dissociation constants with normal controls (total population platelets obtained prior to platelet depletion).

Murine monoclonal antibodies (all IgG) to human platelet glycoproteins were purified from ascites by DEAE Affigel blue (Bruck et al. 1982) or protein A Sepharose (Duhamel et al. 1979) column chromatography. Purity was assessed by polyacrylamide gel electrophoresis. Radiolabelling with ^{125}I was performed according to the Iodogen method (Fraker and Speck 1978). These monoclonal antibodies displayed cross-reactivity with epitopes expressed on baboon platelets. Binding assays were performed by incubating gel-filtered platelets with various concentrations of labelled antibody in modified Tyrode's buffer. Bound label was separated from free label by centrifugation through a 20% sucrose, 2% bovine serum albumin solution. Saturable binding isotherms were analysed according to the Ligand program (Munson and Rodbard 1980) to determine the number of molecules bound per platelet and the dissociation constants.

Monoclonal antibodies studied included CP8 for GPIIb/IIIa (Niiya et al. 1987), 12F1 for GPIa (Pischel et al. 1987) and S12 for GMP140 (Stenberg et al. 1985). CP8 and S12 binding were measured on resting platelets in the presence of EDTA (5 mM) and PGE$_1$ (1 μM), and on platelets stimulated by α-thrombin in the presence of EDTA (5 mM) alone to a degree sufficient to produce >60% 5-HT release. In control experiments, binding of these monoclonal antibodies to baboon platelets in the presence of EDTA (5 mM) or Ca^{2+} (2 mM) was unchanged. 12F1 binding was assessed on resting platelets only, since no differences were observed in the binding of 12F1 to resting and stimulated platelets. A comparison of membrane glycoproteins on control and young platelets is shown in Table 4.3. S12 binding to resting platelets was negligible for both control and young platelets. No differences were seen between the dissociation constants of control and young platelets.

Table 4.3. Comparison of platelet membrane glycoprotein epitopes expressed on control platelets and on young platelets obtained during recovery from non-immune-mediated acute thrombocytopenia in baboons

Antibody (IgG)	Epitope	Molecules bound per platelet at saturation		P value[a]	kD (M)
		Control	Young		
CP8 bound to resting platelets	GP IIb/IIIa	28 700 ±4419	32 079 ±10 334	0.430 NS	10^{-7}
CP8 bound to stimulated platelets	GP IIb/IIIa	38 735 ±6105	34 920 ±8290	0.173 NS	10^{-7}
12F1 bound to resting platelets	GP Ia	3076 ±244	2980 ±553	0.793 NS	10^{-10}
S12 bound to stimulated platelets	GMP-140	7476 ±553	6014 ±1852	0.275 NS	10^{-10}

All values are expressed as mean ± 1 SD.
[a] t test for comparison between means for control platelets and young platelets.
NS, not significant.

Of note is that when CP8 binding to resting and α-thrombin-stimulated platelets are compared at baseline (prior to depletion), there was a significant difference between the two: the number of molecules bound to stimulated platelets increased by 35%, with a p value of 0.005 (t test for paired comparisons). This difference was not seen with young platelets, in which there was only a 5% difference between resting and stimulated platelets ($p=0.45$). There is controversy whether the increased number of GPIIb/IIIa epitopes expressed on stimulated human platelets is related to the presence of GPIIb/IIIa within the superficial canalicular membrane system which becomes accessible upon stimulation, or to the presence of GPIIb/IIIa on α-granule membranes which are fused with the surface membrane upon release (Gogstad et al. 1981; Zucker-Franklin 1981; Stenberg 1984; Wencel-Dranke et al. 1986; Niiya et al. 1987). One interpretation of our data is that the number of GPIIb/IIIa molecules per platelet is constant and is determined at the time of platelet formation, with some reorganization of platelet membranes during maturation in the circulation (specifically, further invagination of the canalicular system). In support of this, measurement of CP8 binding at 48 hours after depletion, when the mean platelet age is slightly older, reveals an increased difference in the binding of CP8 to resting and thrombin-stimulated platelets, but not a complete return to the difference seen with baseline platelets. Overall, these data do not support a relationship between epitopes expressed on membrane glycoproteins and platelet age, at least with respect to GPIIb/IIIa, GPIa and GMP140. Heterogeneity of GPIIb/IIIa, GPIa and possibly other cytoadhesins is most likely determined at the level of the megakaryocyte, although there may be some reorganization which takes place after release of platelets from the marrow.

Platelet Organelle Content

Platelets are heterogeneous with respect to the number of subcellular cytoplasmic organelles, including mitochondria, lysosomes, dense bodies and α-granules. It has been shown by morphometric analysis (Duyvené de Wit et al. 1987) and by analysis of platelet subcellular organelle constituents (Corash et al. 1984) that both α-granule and dense granule numbers are increased, per platelet, with increasing platelet density and size. Large platelets are also enriched in surface sialic acid and sulphydryl groups and in internal glycogen, ATP, ADP, and Ca^{2+} when compared to small platelets, even when normalized per unit volume (Carty and Gear 1986). It has been proposed that platelets may undergo secretion of subcellular granules, particularly α-granules and dense bodies, as they age in the circulation (Corash et al. 1984). Reimers and co-workers (1976) have shown in rabbits that thrombin-induced platelet aggregation in vitro with extensive release of granule constituents is not irreversible and that thrombin treatment does not result in more rapid elimination of damaged platelets from the circulation following re-infusion. Furthermore, it has been proposed that such platelets can still be haemostatically effective. It is therefore important to distinguish between heterogeneity in subcellular granules due to processes occurring in vivo during the platelet life-span and the intrinsic heterogeneity imparted during thrombocytopoiesis.

Using the baboon model of acute thrombocytopenia to investigate platelet properties as a function of platelet age, the relationship between platelet age and platelet content of dense granule and α-granule constituents was examined. Total platelet and thrombin-induced releasable ATP and ADP levels were measured by high-performance liquid chromatography (HPLC) analysis of neutralized perchloric acid extracts (Savage et al. 1988). Total platelet content of ADP and platelet dense granule ADP were significantly reduced at 23 hours after the onset of thrombocytopenia (3.7 ± 0.9 and 2.8 ± 0.4 $\mu mol/10^{11}$ platelets respectively, compared with baseline values of 4.7 ± 0.6 and 3.9 ± 0.3 $\mu mol/10^{11}$ platelets respectively; $p<0.01$; Fig. 4.8). In contrast, total platelet content of ATP did not change significantly, but varied randomly about the mean basal value of 5.2 ± 0.7 $\mu mol/10^{11}$ platelets ($p>0.1$) (Fig. 4.9). Although a significant reduction in dense granule ATP was observed at all time points up to 21 days after the onset of thrombocytopenia (Fig. 4.9), the magnitude of the decrease was less than that seen for dense granule ADP, as reflected by an increase in the dense granule ATP/ADP ratio from 0.60 ± 0.04 to 0.86 ± 0.14 ($p<0.01$). Furthermore, the platelet content of βTG and PF4 did not change significantly throughout the period of observation (Table 4.2).

Although the mechanism underlying the selective reduction in dense granule ADP has not been clearly defined, it is unlikely that secretion of dense granule constituents can account for this observation since the content of α-granule constituents (which are secreted at a lower threshold in response to a variety of platelet agonists compared with dense granule contents) did not change significantly throughout the study. Further evidence that platelet α-granules were unchanged in the young platelet population was obtained from binding studies

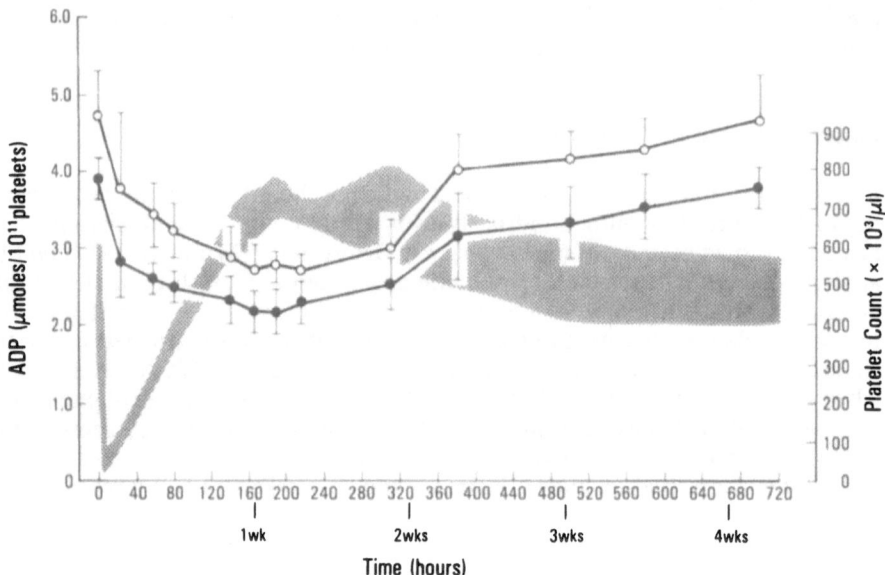

Fig. 4.8. Effect of non-immune mediated acute thrombocytopenia on platelet ADP levels. Total platelet ADP (○) and thrombin-releasable ADP (●) were measured in platelets isolated from blood sampled at the times indicated. The *shaded area* represents the range in the circulating platelet count during recovery from acute thrombocytopenia. Error bars represent ±1 SD ($n=4$). Reproduced with permission from Blackwell Scientific Publications Ltd.

with the monoclonal antibody S12. As outlined previously in this chapter, S12 binds to GMP140, an α-granule membrane glycoprotein that becomes exposed on the platelet surface following secretion (Stenberg et al. 1985). There was no significant difference in the number of S12 molecules bound per platelet between baseline-stimulated platelets and young stimulated platelets obtained at 23 hours post-depletion, despite stimulation by γ-thrombin to a degree sufficient to produce >60% 5-HT release (a prerequisite for maximal expression of GMP-140).

Although the mechanism for uptake of nucleotides and their storage within the platelet dense granule is poorly understood, evidence has been presented suggesting that dense granule precursors are formed in the megakaryocyte (Robblee et al. 1973). Furthermore, it has been shown that ATP can be transferred from the cytoplasmic pool across the storage organelle membrane, where it is partially hydrolysed to yield ADP (Reimers et al. 1977). Since the young platelet populations obtained in our studies were characterized by a selective depletion in dense granule ADP, with normal total platelet ATP levels, it seems plausible that maturation of platelets in the circulation is associated with an interconversion of adenine nucleotides within the granule, resulting in changes in the granular ATP/ADP ratio. We therefore propose that newly released platelets from mature megakaryocytes in normal thrombocytopoiesis have an adenine nucleotide profile different from that seen in the total platelet population. This consideration should therefore evoke a re-evaluation of previous studies of reduced ADP levels in experimental and clinical reports. In the past, many investigators have interpreted reduced levels of dense granule ADP to

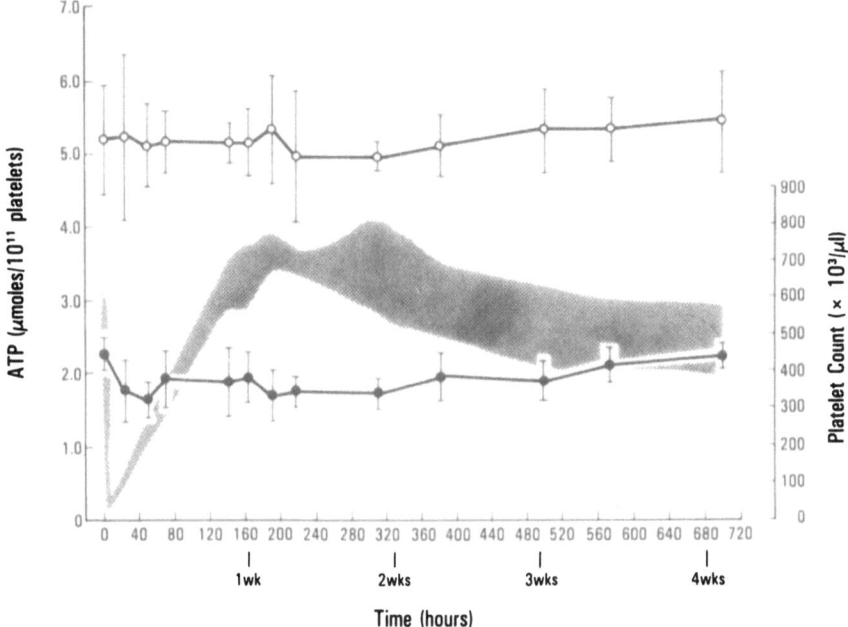

Fig. 4.9. Effect of non-immune mediated acute thrombocytopenia on platelet ATP levels. Total platelet ATP (○) and thrombin-releasable ATP (●) were measured in platelets isolated from blood sampled at the times indicated. The *shaded area* represents the range in the circulating platelet count during recovery from acute thrombocytopenia. Error bars represent ±1 SD ($n=4$). Reproduced with permission from Blackwell Scientific Publications Ltd.

reflect a loss of ADP from circulating platelets in vivo. While that interpretation may be correct for myelodysplastic patients (Malpass et al. 1984; Elias et al. 1987), most reports have failed to document an actual loss of dense granule contents in vivo (Holmsen and Weiss 1972; Rendu et al. 1979b; Hourdille et al. 1980; Yamazaki et al. 1980; Broughton et al. 1977). Although the selective consumption of dense-enriched platelets or altered megakaryocytopoiesis may contribute towards decreased platelet ADP levels, a shift in the age distribution of circulating platelets towards a younger mean age platelet population should also be considered.

Platelet Enzymes

The enzymes of the Embden–Myerhoff and related pathways yield ATP used by the platelet as an energy source. The activities of these enzymes have been extensively studied in red blood cells. There it can be demonstrated that the activities of hexokinase, glucose phosphate isomerase, aldolase, triose phosphate isomerase, glyceraldehyde phosphate dehydrogenase and glucose-6-phosphate dehydrogenase decline with advancing red cell age (Beutler 1983). Platelet glycolytic enzymes have been shown to decline after storage at room temperature for 3 days. The most significant changes were seen in the activities of enolase, triose phosphate isomerase and lactate dehydrogenase (LDH; Tegos and Beutler

1979). Thompson and co-workers (1982) demonstrated that large platelets (previously suggested to be younger) contained higher concentrations of LDH per unit of platelet volume than small platelets, indicating a possible correlation between platelet enzyme activity and platelet age.

To investigate directly the relationship between platelet enzyme activity and platelet age, we assayed the enzymes listed in Table 4.4 in young platelets, harvested on the day following depletion, according to the method of Beutler (1984). No differences were found between the enzyme activity levels in young platelets and a control group of baseline platelets. This result is consistent with the hypothesis that platelet heterogeneity with respect to metabolic capacity is not a process of progressive ageing in the circulation. It does not exclude the possibility that subtle changes might occur which do not become significant over the relatively short life-span of the platelet since changes in red cell enzyme levels are observed over a considerably longer period of time.

Table 4.4. Comparison of platelet glycolytic enzymes in control platelets and in young platelets obtained during recovery from non-immune-mediated acute thrombocytopenia in baboons

Enzyme	Mean enzyme activity (mU/mg protein)	
	Control platelets	Young platelets
Hexokinase	167	182
Glucose phosphate isomerase	1407	1478
Glucose-6-phosphate dehydrogenase	75	85
6-Phosphogluconate dehydrogenase	19	18
Phosphofructokinase	112	96
Aldolase	64	56
Triose phosphate isomerase	13 262	9856
Glyceraldehyde phosphate dehydrogenase	1381	1682
Phosphoglycerate kinase	1345	1846
Pyruvate kinase	542	498
Lactate dehydrogenase	1862	1836
Glutathione reductase	54	65
Glutathione peroxidase	146	202
Glutathione S-transferase	96	106
Glutamate-oxaloacetate transaminase	49	40

Chronic Thrombocytopenia

As an extension of our studies on the properties of young platelets, we elected to explore further the possibility that platelets produced under an intense or prolonged thrombocytopoietic stimulus may have unique properties, different from platelets produced at thrombocytopoietic equilibrium. The baboon model of acute thrombocytopenia produced young platelets that were not substantially different from the total platelet population, suggesting that platelet heterogeneity, with respect to the measured parameters, is largely independent of platelet age.

If platelet heterogeneity is essentially a consequence of megakaryocyte production factors, it should be possible to produce an altered platelet by influencing conditions at the megakaryocyte level. Studies performed with repeated infusions of anti-platelet sera in rodents demonstrated augmentation of megakaryocyte numbers, accelerated megakaryocyte maturation, and an upward shift of the model megakaryocyte ploidy class several days after the onset of chronic thrombocytopenia (Penington and Olsen 1970; Corash et al. 1987). There is evidence to suggest that megakaryocytes of higher ploidy may produce larger and more heterogeneous platelets (Bessman 1984). In addition to changes in size, these "stress" platelets may have other unique attributes. To evaluate this phenomenon using a non-immunological method, we have extended out model to simulate chronic thrombocytopenia by a process of repeated platelet depletions.

In a pilot experiment, serial platelet depletions were performed for 7 days. Glass bead columns were inserted into the shunt circuit to reduce the daily post-depletion platelet count to a mean of $78\,000/\mu l$. The mean platelet volume, initially 6.1 fl, increased gradually to 7.95 fl at 24 hours after the final platelet depletion process. Platelet distribution histogram analyses revealed that an actual shift of the mean had occurred, rather than a skewing of the distribution curve due to the presence of red blood cell fragments or platelet aggregates. Platelet production rates increased from approximately 115 000 platelets per microlitre per day for the first three days of the experiment to 155 000 platelets per microlitre per day for the last 3 days of platelet depletion, but returned to baseline values within 2 days following cessation of the platelet depletion process.

The number of GPIIb/IIIa epitopes expressed, as assessed by CP8 antibody binding at 19 hours after the final depletion, decreased by 30% from baseline for both resting and stimulating platelets. This difference was still apparent at 163 hours after the final depletion. The number of GMP140 molecules recognized by S12 binding to stimulated platelets and the number of GPIa molecules demonstrated by 12F1 binding remained constant throughout the experiment and for 7 days thereafter. There were no detectable changes in the dissociation constants of any of the antibodies compared with baseline values. From these preliminary observations, we have demonstrated that it is technically possible to perform daily platelet depletions without adverse effects on the animal. The platelet population so produced is larger and displays some altered membrane characteristics. Additional studies of "stress" platelets in this setting are warranted.

Acquired Platelet Alterations

Changes in the average properties of the circulating platelet pool with respect to physical, functional and biochemical characteristics have been reported in humans with disorders involving both acute platelet destruction and chronic elevations of platelet turnover. Acute platelet alterations, which are unlikely to be due to mechanisms related to platelet ageing, have been most extensively studied in patients undergoing cardiopulmonary bypass. These changes include reductions in platelet density (Van Oost et al. 1983), platelet count (Martin et al. 1987), levels of surface membrane glycoproteins (George et al. 1986), α-granule platelet factor 4 and β-thromboglobulin (Harker et al. 1980; Mezzano et al. 1986), and the dense granule constituents ADP and 5-HT (Beurling-Harbury and Galvan 1978; Mezzano et al. 1986). A reduction in dense granule components has also been reported in a patient with acute disseminated intravascular coagulation (DIC) (Pareti et al. 1976). Such platelet alterations were usually associated with inhibition of platelet haemostatic function, characterized by a marked bleeding tendency. In general, these results have been interpreted to support the concept that platelets may undergo activation and granular release with continued circulation in vivo (O'Brien 1978; Pareti et al. 1979). This hypothesis has been based in part on the demonstration in rabbits that platelets having undergone dense granule release in vitro exhibited a normal disappearance pattern following reinfusion in vivo (Reimers et al. 1973, 1976). While these observations are intriguing, the continued survival of platelets following granular release in vivo has not been directly demonstrated in man or any other species. Indeed, an equally compelling, but also untested, hypothesis could be based on the observed functional heterogeneity of normal platelets. In this model, acute platelet destruction (e.g. during bypass) would result in the selective removal of cells having the greatest functional capacity as determined by factors related to density, granular contents, membrane components or other characteristics. Thus the average properties of the circulating platelet pool might change due to the irreversible (fatal) activation of particular platelet subpopulations, but with no measurable effects on those platelets remaining in the circulation. This hypothesis is supported by recent observations using flow cytometry showing that individual platelets may vary markedly with respect to their capacity to undergo α-granule secretion (Johnston et al. 1987).

Chronic disorders associated with increased platelet destruction in man are also characterized by platelet alterations. For example, reduced platelet α-granule contents in peripheral artery disease (O'Brien et al. 1984), and reduced dense granule contents in patients with artificial heart valves (Beurling-Harbury and Galvan, 1978), prosthetic vascular grafts (Savage et al. 1983) and chronic DIC (Yamazaki et al. 1980) have been reported. While these observations are also consistent with a process involving the selective utilization of particular platelet subpopulations, platelet changes in chronic disease may also reflect altered megakaryocytopoiesis or an increased proportion of younger cells in the general circulation (as described earlier).

Attempts, using various animal models, to define changes in platelet proportions following the exposure of thrombogenic surfaces in vivo have produced variable results. Rabbits with indwelling aortic cannulae in place for 20 hours exhibited prolonged bleeding and a diminished capacity to form thrombus at a second injury site in the carotid arteries (Buchanan et al. 1979). In baboons, the deposition of ^{111}In-labelled platelet thrombus was equivalent on vascular grafts (exposed to flowing blood for 1 hour) placed at 1, 24, 48 and 72 hours after injection of the labelled cells, despite ageing of the labelled platelets in the circulation and their repeated exposure to the thrombogenic grafts (Hanson et al. 1985b). Platelets from these animals also showed no reduction at intraplatelet α-granule proteins or dense granule ADP. In other studies, placement of chronic aortic cannulae in rats caused no changes in platelet size, or the sensitivity of platelets to aggregating and release-inducing agents (Winocour et al. 1983). In addition, the survival of platelets from rats with aortic cannulae, or from baboons with vascular grafts or chronic arteriovenous shunts, was not reduced following removal of the thrombogenic surface or cross-transfusion of donor platelets into normal recipient animals (Winocour et al. 1983; Meuleman et al. 1980; Harker and Hanson 1979; Hanson et al. 1985b). In contrast, the placement of chronic aortic grafts in dogs impaired the functional capacity of circulating platelets, diminished the level of platelet dense granule 5-HT, and caused a shortening in platelet survival following the transfusion of donor cells into normal recipient animals (Clagett et al. 1981a, b).

To examine these differences and to assess the capacity of platelets to undergo acute granular release and other changes in vivo, we have employed a baboon model of platelet activation and thrombus formation. Autologous baboon platelets were labelled with both $[^{51}Cr]$sodium chromate (a cytoplasmic label) and $[^{14}C]5$-HT (a dense granule label). Platelet release was induced in vivo by intravenous injection or infusion of several agents known to activate platelets. These agents included Type I rat skin and bovine fibrillar collagen (bolus injection of 1–40 mg), purified human thrombin (a gift from Dr A. Thompson) infused continuously (up to 6 units/kg per minute for 4 hours), bacterial endotoxin (0.01–0.5 mg/kg bolus, E. coli LPS, Sigma), purified bovine von Willebrand factor (a gift from Dr R. Counts, 10–60 units/kg bolus) and antibody against baboon platelets (0.08 ml/kg bolus, rabbit anti-platelet serum). As illustrated in Fig. 4.10, the disappearance patterns of platelets doubly labelled with ^{51}Cr and $[^{14}C]5$-HT were measured throughout the platelet life-span as well as during the experimental interval. We consistently observed parallel disappearance patterns for the two isotopes with no evidence of a preferential loss of $[^{14}C]5$-HT relative to the ^{51}Cr-platelet label. The disappearance of $[^{14}C]5$-HT was slightly prolonged relative to ^{51}Cr due to modest re-uptake of 5-HT, which in baboons averages only about 10% of the exogenous amine (this laboratory, unpublished observations). It is unlikely that the limited re-utilization of this label in vivo could have prevented detection of a significant dense granule release reaction, since 60–80% of the platelet $[^{14}C]5$-HT was releasable in vitro. In addition, the use of imipramine to block 5-HT re-utilization failed to enhance any difference between $[^{14}C]5$-HT and ^{51}Cr-platelet disappearance patterns (Fig. 4.10).

The relative loss of $[^{14}C]5$-HT and ^{51}Cr radioactivities from the circulating platelets due to the administration of various agents is shown in Fig. 4.11. The percentage reductions in both ^{51}Cr-platelet and $[^{14}C]5$-HT activities were calculated by comparing pre-infusion values with measurements taken 4 hours after agonist injection, by which time all changes in platelet numbers and radioactivities appeared irreversible. The agonists and doses used were chosen to cause reductions in platelet numbers in vivo ranging from 0 to 100%. A direct one-to-one relationship was found between the loss of platelet cytoplasmic ^{51}Cr and dense granule $[^{14}C]5$-HT, implying no selective or preferential loss of the releasable platelet label. While these results do not preclude the possibility of significant release in other settings or in non-primate species, they suggest that dense granule release in vivo is associated with the rapid clearance of platelets from the circulation.

We subsequently investigated the effects of acute thrombus formation on platelet chracteristics in vivo. We have previously shown that short Dacron vascular grafts (10 cm × 4 mm i.d.) exposed in an arteriovenous system for 1 hour

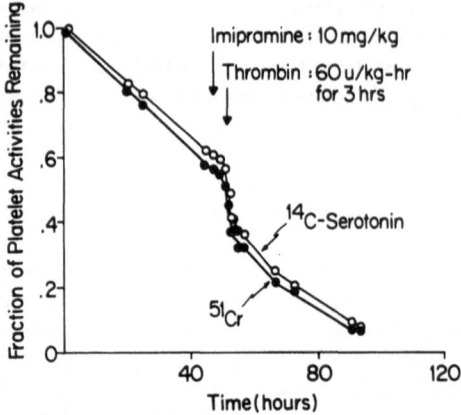

Fig. 4.10. Disappearance patterns for baboon platelets doubly labelled with ^{51}Cr (a cytoplasmic label) and [^{14}C]5-HT (a dense granule label). Thrombin infusion caused significant platelet destruction, but did not induce a preferential loss of [^{14}C]5-HT relative to ^{51}Cr from platelets which continued to circulate. Imipramine was given to inhibit the re-uptake of released 5-HT.

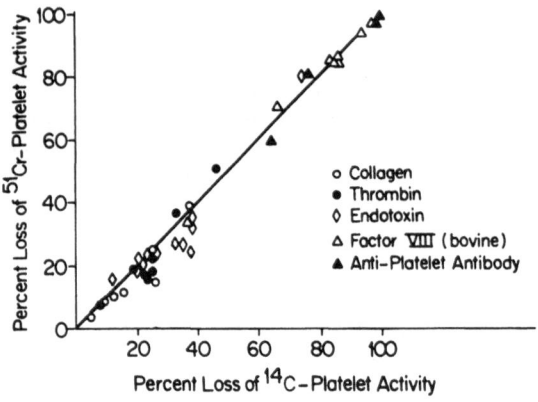

Fig. 4.11. Loss of ^{51}Cr and [^{14}C]5-HT platelet radioactivity following infusion of activating and release-inducing substances in vivo. In response to the agents shown there was an equivalent irreversible reduction in baboons of cytoplasmic ^{51}Cr and granular [^{14}C]5-HT, with no evidence of continued circulation of platelets depleted of dense granule components.

caused no detectable platelet changes (Hanson et al. 1985b). In the present series of experiments a substantially greater challenge to the haemostatic system was provided by increasing the graft surface area (80 cm × 4 mm i.d.). In eight animals, graft exposure for 1 hour caused a reduction in mean platelet counts from 528 000±28 000/μl to 216 000±27 000/μl (Table 4.5). Platelet deposition was irreversible and the survival of the remaining circulating platelets was unaffected as demonstrated by the normal disappearance pattern of the residual ^{111}In-labelled platelets. Whereas the plasma levels of platelet factor 4 increased

Table 4.5.   Effect of Dacron grafts on circulating platelet properties

	Pre-	Post-	Significance
Platelet count (per μl)	528 000±28 000	216 000±27 000	$p<0.01$
Mean platelet volume (fl)	6.7±0.6	6.5±0.7	$p>0.2$
Mean platelet density (g/ml)	1.062±0.003	1.061±0.003	$p>0.5$
Thromboxane B$_2$ (μg/10^9 platelets)	1.8±0.9	1.2±0.4	$p>0.05$

All values are expressed as mean ± SD.

approximately tenfold, the mean platelet volume, density and the platelet content of PF4 did not change significantly (Table 4.5 and Fig. 4.12). In spite of a significant reduction in platelet dense granule ADP (from 2.6±0.5 to 1.8±0.5 μmol/10^{11} platelets, $p<0.01$), the net reductions in [^{14}C]5-HT and ^{111}In were equivalent, averaging 57% and 60% respectively, and indicating that platelets remaining in the circulation had not undergone dense granule release. Since our previous results argue against a sublethal dense granule release reaction in vivo, and since dense granule release in the absence of α-granule release seems unlikely, these results suggest that as a consequence of platelet granular heterogeneity the irreversible removal of platelet subpopulations which are rich in granular ADP may have little effect on the contents in residual platelets of endogenous α-granule proteins or newly absorbed 5-HT. We believe these hypotheses merit further attention for the interpretation of both animal and clinical studies of mechanisms of platelet utilization in vivo.

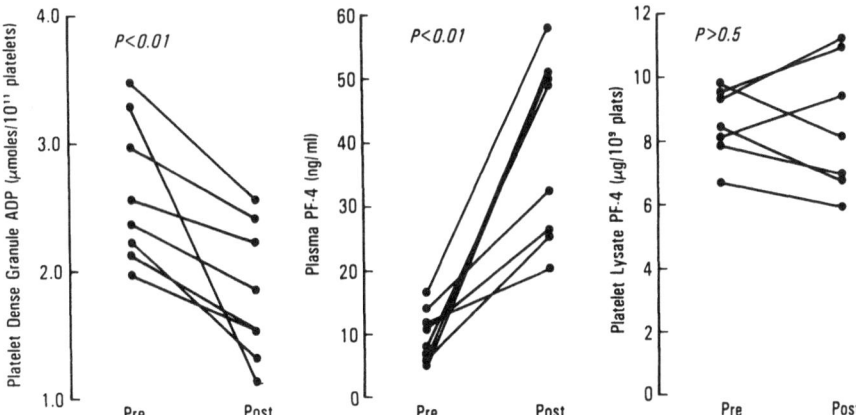

Fig. 4.12.   Platelet changes associated with acute thrombus formation. Exposure in 8 baboons for 1 hour of Dacron vascular grafts caused a consistent reduction in dense granule ADP, increased plasma levels of PF-4, but no change in the intraplatelet level of PF-4. The results are consistent with the selective removal of platelets which are rich in dense granule contents (ADP) but not α-granule contents (PF-4).

Conclusions

Data from this laboratory support the concept that platelet density heterogeneity is primarily determined during the thrombocytopoietic process. The slight increase in the density of all platelets occurring during their life-span in the circulation contributes little to the density heterogeneity of platelets. One of the primary difficulties with investigating platelet density heterogeneity has been the failure to establish standardized methodologies and appropriate animal models so that definitive data can be obtained and a consensus reached regarding the relation of platelet density to platelet age.

Our studies of young platelets, produced after non-immune-mediated acute thrombocytopenia, suggest that in health platelets are not substantially modified as they circulate, but rather undergo subtle changes with respect to the redistribution of dense granule adenine nucleotides and the re-orientation of functional membrane glycoproteins. New platelets released into the circulation were not significantly altered in size, and were removed from the circulation by predominantly senescent mechanisms.

Acquired changes in the platelet heterogeneity profile in acute thrombosis may reflect a process of platelet activation, reversible platelet interactions with thrombogenic surfaces, or selective platelet consumption. In studies of acute thrombosis in the baboon, we have demonstrated a process of selective platelet consumption, with the irreversible removal of dense granule-enriched platelets. Residual circulating platelets, while having reduced dense granule ADP levels, had not undergone dense granule release in response to the thrombogenic stimulus, were unaffected in their content of α-granule constituents and did not have compromised viability.

As more information emerges about how altered megakaryocytopoiesis affects platelet heterogeneity, the interpretation of changes in the platelet heterogeneity profile will become more clinically relevant. Continued investigations of acquired platelet alterations may provide additional insight into the underlying physiological disorder and may be relevant to a further understanding of diseases such as disseminated intravascular coagulation, thrombotic thrombocytopenic purpura, and other consumptive thrombocytopenias. Efforts to define markers of platelet senescence in the circulation should prove fruitful. Such studies could improve the efficacy of therapeutic platelet transfusions and further our understanding of the mechanisms of platelet removal. With the increasingly common measurement of platelet size distribution, and the availability of flow cytometric techniques for assessing cell to cell variability, the description of platelet heterogeneity in disease states should receive greater attention. Through these types of studies we can understand more fully the complex relationships between platelet heterogeneity, health, and disease.

This research was supported in part by research grants HL 31950, HL 31469, HL 36602 and RR 00833 from the National Institutes of Health, US Public Health Service. This is publication number 5439 BCR from the Research Institute of Scripps Clinic, La Jolla, California.

References

Adelman B, Michelson AD, Loscalzo J, Greenberg J, Handin RI (1985) Plasmin effect on platelet glycoprotein 1B–von Willebrand factor interactions. Blood 65:32–40

Aster RH (1971) Factors affecting the kinetics of isotopically labelled platelets. In: Paulus JM (ed) Platelet kinetics: radioisotopic, cytological, mathematical and clinical aspects. Elsevier/North Holland, Amsterdam, pp 3–23

Bessman JD (1984) The relation of megakaryocyte ploidy to platelet volume. Am J Hematol 16:161–170

Beurling-Harbury C, Galvan C (1978) Acquired decrease in platelet secretory ADP associated with increased postoperative bleeding in post-cardiopulmonary bypass patients and in patients with severe valvular heart disease. Blood 52:13–23

Beutler E (1983) Energy metabolism and maintenance of erythrocytes. In: Williams WJ, Beutler E, Erslev AJ, Lichtman MA (eds) Hematology, 3rd edn. McGraw Hill, New York, pp 331–345

Beutler E (1984) Red cell metabolism, 3rd edn. Grune & Stratton, Orlando

Blajchman MA, Senyi AF, Hirsh J, Genton E, George JN (1981) Hemostatic function, survival, and membrane glycoprotein changes in young vs old rabbit platelets. J Clin Invest 68:1289–1294

Boneu B, Vigoni F, Boneu C, Caranobe C, Sie P (1982) Further studies on the relationship between platelet buoyant density and platelet age. Am J Hematol 13:239–246

Booyse EM, Hoveke TP, Rafelson ME, Jr (1968) Studies on human platelets. II. Protein synthetic activity of various platelet populations. Biochim Biophys Acta 157:660–663

Broughton BJ, Corbett WEN, Ginsburg AD (1977) Myeloproliferative disorders: A paradox of in vivo and in vitro platelet function. J Clin Pathol 30:228–234

Bruck C, Portetelle D, Glineur C, Bollen A (1982) One-step purification of mouse monoclonal antibodies from ascitic fluid by DEAE affi-gel blue chromatography. J Immunol Methods 53:313–319

Buchanan MR, Carter CJ, Hirsh J (1979) Decreased platelet thrombogenicity in association with increased platelet turnover and vascular damage. Blood 54:1369–1375

Carty DJ, Gear ARL (1986) Fractionation of platelets according to size: functional and biochemical characteristics. Am J Hematol 21:1–14

Charmatz A, Karpatkin S (1974) Heterogeneity of rabbit platelets. 1. Employment of an albumin density gradient for separation of a young platelet population identified with ^{75}Se-selenomethionine. Thromb Diath Haemorrh 31:485–492

Clagett GP, Russo M, Hufnagel H (1981a) Platelet changes after placement of aortic prostheses in dogs. I. Biochemical and functional alterations. J Lab Clin Med 97:345–359

Clagett GP, Russo M, Hufnagel H (1981b) Platelet changes after placement of aortic prostheses in dogs. II. Impaired surface-induced thrombosis. J Lab Clin Med 97:360–368

Coller BS (1982) Effects of tertiary amine local anesthetics on von Willebrand factor dependent platelet function: alteration of membrane reactivity and degradation of GPIB by a calcium dependent protease. Blood 60:731–743

Corash L, Shafer B, Perlow M (1978) Heterogeneity of human whole blood platelet subpopulations. II. Use of a subhuman primate model to analyze the relationship between density and platelet age. Blood 52:726–734

Corash L, Costa JL, Shafer B, Donlon JA, Murphy D (1984) Heterogeneity of human whole blood platelet subpopulations. III. Density dependent differences in subcellular constituents. Blood 64:185–193

Corash L, Chen HY, Levin J, Baker G, Lu H, Mok Y (1987) Regulation of thrombopoiesis: effects of the degree of thrombocytopenia on megakaryocyte ploidy and platelet volume. Blood 70:177–185

Davey MG (1966) The survival and destruction of human platelets. Karger, New York, pp 64–70

Duhamel RC, Schur PH, Brendel K, Meczan E (1979) pH gradient elution of human IgG1, IgG2, and IgG4 from protein A-sepharose. J Immunol Methods 31:211–217

Duyvené de Wit LJ, Badenhorst PN, Heyns A du P (1987) Ultrastructural morphometric observations on serial sectioned human blood platelet subpopulations. Eur J Cell Biol 43:408–411

Eason CT, Pattison A, Howells DD, Mitcheson J, Bonner FW (1986) Platelet population profiles: significance of species variation and drug-induced changes. J Appl Toxicol 6:437–441

Eldor A, Avitzour M, Or R, Hanna R, Penchas S (1982) Prediction of heamorrhagic diathesis in thrombocytopenia by mean platelet volume. Br Med J 285:397–400

Elias L, Van Epps DE, Smith K, Savage B (1987) A trial of recombinant alpha 2 interferon in the myelodysplastic syndrome. II. Characterization and response of granulocyte and platelet dysfunction. Leukemia 1:111–115

Fraker PJ, Speck JC (1978) Protein and cell membrane iodinations with a sparingly soluble chloroamide, 1,3,4,6-tetrachloro-3α,6αdiphenyl glycoluril. Biochem Biophys Res Commun 80:849–857

Freedman ML, Karpatkin S (1975) Heterogeneity of rabbit platelets. V. Preferential sequestration of megathrombocytes. Br J Haematol 31:255–262

George JN, Lewis PC, Sears DA (1976) Studies on platelet plasma membranes. II. Chracterization of surface proteins of rabbit platelets in vitro and during circulation in vivo using diazotized ^{125}I-diiodosulfanilic acid as a label. J Lab Clin Med 88:247–260

George JN, Pickett EB, Saucerman S et al. (1986) Platelet surface glycoproteins. Studies on resting and activated platelets and platelet membrane microparticles in normal subjects, and observations in patients during adult respiratory distress syndrome and cardiac surgery. J Clin Invest 78:340–348

Ginsburg AD, Aster RH (1969) Kinetic studies with [51]Chromium labelled platelet cohorts in rats. J Lab Clin Med 74:138–144

Ginsburg AD, Aster RH (1972) Changes associated with platelet aging. Thromb Diath Haemorrh 27:407–415

Gogstad GO, Hagen I, Korsmo R, Solum NO (1981) Characterization of the proteins of isolated human platelet alpha granules: evidence for a separate alpha granule pool of the glycoproteins IIb and IIIa. Biochim Biophys Acta 670:150–162

Hampton JW, Mathews C (1966) Similarities between baboon and human blood clotting. J Appl Physiol 21:1713–1716

Hanson SR, Slichter SJ (1985) Platelet kinetics in patients with bone marrow hypoplasia: evidence for a fixed platelet requirement. Blood 66:1105–1109

Hanson SR, Harker LA, Bjornsson TD (1985a) Effects of platelet modifying drugs on arterial thromboembolism in baboons: aspirin potentiates the antithrombotic action of dipyridamole and sulfinpyrazone by mechanisms independent of platelet cyclooxygenase inhibition. J Clin Invest 75:1591–1599

Hanson SR, Kotze HF, Savage B, Harker LA (1985b) Platelet interactions with Dacron vascular grafts: a model of acute thrombosis in baboons. Arteriosclerosis 5:595–603

Harker LA (1974) Control of platelet production. Ann Rev Med 25:383–400

Harker LA (1977) The kinetics of platelet production and destruction in man. Clin Haematol 6:671–693

Harker LA, Hanson SR (1979) Experimental arterial thromboembolism in baboons: mechanisms, quantitation and pharmacologic prevention. J. Clin Invest 64:559–569

Harker LA, Slichter SJ (1972) The bleeding time as a screening test for evaluation of platelet function. N Engl J Med 287:155–159

Harker LA, Malpass TW, Branson HE, Hessel II EA, Slichter SJ (1980) Mechanism of abnormal bleeding in patients undergoing cardiopulmonary bypass: acquired transient platelet dysfunction associated with selective alpha-granule release. Blood 56:824–834

Haver VM, Gear ARL (1982) Functional fractionation of platelets: aggregation kinetics and glycoprotein labeling of differing platelet populations. Thromb Haemost 48:211–216

Holmsen H, Weiss HJ (1972) Further evidence for a deficient storage pool of adenine nucleotides in platelets from some patients with thrombocytopathia – "storage pool disease". Blood 39:197–209

Hourdille P, Bernard P, Reiffero J, Broustet A, Boisseau MR (1980) Platelet dense bodies loaded with mepacrine: study in chronic idiopathic thrombocytopenic purpura (ITP).Thromb Haemost 43:208–210

Hyde P, Zucker-Franklin D (1987) Antigenic differences between human platelets and megakaryocytes. Am J Pathol 127:349–357

Johnston GI, Heptinstall S, Robins RA, Price MR (1984) The expression of glycoproteins on single blood platelets from healthy individuals and from patients with congenital bleeding disorders. Biochem Biophys Res Commun 123:1091–1098

Johnston GI, Pickett EB, McEver RP, George JN (1987) Heterogeneity of platelet secretion in response to thrombin demonstrated by fluorescence flow cytometry. Blood 69:1401–1403

Karpatkin S (1969) Heterogeneity of human platelets. I. Metabolic and kinetic evidence suggestive of young and old platelets. J Clin Invest 48:1073–1082

Karpatkin S (1978) Heterogeneity of rabbit platelets. VI. Further resolution of changes in platelet density, volume and radioactivity following cohort labeling with ^{75}Se-selenomethionine. Br J Haematol 39:459–469

Kotze HF, Lotter MG, Badenhorst PN, Heyns A du P (1985) Kinetics of In-111-platelets in the baboon. II. In vivo distribution and sites of sequestration. Thromb Haemost 53:408–410

Kotze HF, Heyns A du P, Wessels P, Pieters H, Badenhorst PN, Lotter MG (1986) Evidence that ^{111}In labeled platelets pool in the spleen, but not in the liver of normal humans and baboons. Scand J Haematol 37:259–264

Leven RM, Yee MK (1987) Megakaryocyte morphogenesis stimulated in vitro by whole and partially fractionated thrombocytopenic plasma: a model system for the study of platelet formation. Blood 69:1046–1052

Loftus JC, Albrecht RM (1984) Redistribution of the fibrinogen receptor of human platelets after surface activation. J Cell Biol 99:822–829

Malpass TW, Savage B, Hanson SR, Slichter SJ, Harker LA (1984) Correlation between prolonged bleeding time and depletion of platelet dense granule ADP in patients with myelodysplastic and myeloproliferative disorders. J Lab Clin Med 103:894–904

Martin JF, Penington DG (1983) Relationship between the age and density of circulating chromium-51 labeled platelets in the subhuman primate. Thromb Res 30:157–164

Martin JF, Trowbridge EA (1982) Theoretical requirements for the density separation of platelets with comparison of continuous and discontinuous gradients. Thromb Res 27:513–522

Martin JF, Shaw T, Heggie J, Penington DG (1983) Measurement of the density of human platelets and its relationship to volume. Br J Haematol 54:337–352

Martin JF, Daniel TD, Trowbridge EA (1987) Acute and chronic changes in platelet volume and count after cardiopulmonary bypass induced thrombocytopenia in man. Thromb Haemost 57:55–58

McMillan R, Luiken GA, Levy R, Yelonosky R, Longmire RL (1978) Antibody against megakaryocyte in idiopathic thrombocytopenic purpura. J Am Med Assoc 239:2460–2462

Meuleman DG, Vogel GMT, van Delft AML (1980) Effects of intra-arterial cannulation on blood platelet consumption in rats. Thromb Res 20:45–55

Meyers KM, Holmsen H, Seachord CL (1982) Comparative study of platelet dense granule constituents. Am J Physiol 243:R454–R461

Mezzano D, Hwang K-I, Catalano P, Aster RH (1981) Evidence that platelet buoyant density but not size, correlates with platelet age in man. Am J Hematol 11:61–76

Mezzano D, Aranda E, Faradori A, Rodriguez S, Lina P (1984) Kinetics of platelet density subpopulations in splenectomized mongrel dogs. Am J Hematol 17:373–382

Mezzano D, Aranda E, Urzua J et al. (1986) Changes in platelet β-thromboglobulin, fibrinogen, albumin, 5-hydroxytryptamine, ATP, and ADP during and after surgery with extracorporeal circulation in man. Am J Hematol 22:133–142

Munson PJ, Rodbard D (1980) Ligand: a versatile computerized approach for characterization of ligand-binding systems. Anal Biochem 107:220–239

Mustard JF, Rowsell HC, Murphy EA (1966) Platelet economy (platelet survival and turnover). Br J Haematol 12:1–24

Niiya K, Hodson E, Bader R et al (1987) Increased surface expression of the membrane glycoprotein IIb/IIIa complex induced by platelet activation: relationship to the binding of fibrinogen and platelet aggregation. Blood 70:475–483

O'Brien JR (1978) "Exhausted" platelets continue to circulate. Lancet ii:1316–1317

O'Brien JR, Etherington MD, Pashley M (1984) Intra-platelet platelet factor 4 (IP.PF4) and the heparin-mobilisable pool of PF4 in health and atherosclerosis. Thromb Haemost 51:354–357

Odell TT Jr, Jackson CW, Friday TJ, Charsha DE (1969) Effects of thrombocytopenia on megakaryocytopoiesis. Br J Haematol 17:91–101

Odell TT Jr, Murphy JR, Jackson CW (1976) Stimulation of megakaryocytopoiesis by acute thrombocytopenia in rats. Blood 48:765–775

Packham MA, Guccione MA, O'Brien KM (1985) Duration of the effect of aspirin on the synthesis of thromboxane by density subpopulations of rabbit platelets stimulated with thrombin. Blood 66:287–290

Pareti FI, Capitanio A, Mannucci PM (1976) Acquired storage pool disease in platelets during disseminated intravascular coagulation. Blood 48:511–515

Pareti FI, Capitanio A, Mannucci L, Ponticelli C, Mannucci PM (1979) Acquired dysfunction due to the circulation of "exhausted" platelets. Am J Med 69:235–241

Penington DG, Olsen TE (1970) Megakaryocytes in states of altered platelet production: cell numbers, size and DNA content. Br J Haematol 18:447–463

Penington DG, Lee NLY, Roxburgh AE, McGready JR (1976) Platelet density and size: the interpretation of heterogeneity. Br J Haematol 34:365–376

Pischel KD, Hemler ME, Huang C, Bluestein HG, Woods VL Jr (1987) Use of the monoclonal antibody 12F1 to characterize the differentiation antigen VLA-2. J Immunol 138:226–233

Polley MJ, Leung LLK, Clark FY, Nachman RL (1981) Thrombin induced platelet membrane glycoprotein IIb and IIIa complex formation: an electron microscope study. J Exp Med 154:1058–1068

Rand ML, Packham MA, Mustard JF (1983) Survival of density subpopulations of rabbit platelets: use of ^{51}Cr- or ^{111}In-labeled platelets to measure survival of least dense and most dense platelets concurrently. Blood 61:362–367

Reimers HJ, Packham MA, Kinlough-Rathbone RL, Mustard JF (1973) Effect of repeated treatment of rabbit platelets with low concentrations of thrombin on their function, metabolism and survival. Br J Haematol 25:675–686

Reimers HJ, Kinlough-Rathbone RL, Cazenave JP et al (1976) In vitro and in vivo functions of thrombin-treated platelets. Thromb Haemost 35:151–166

Reimers HJ, Packham MA, Mustard JF (1977) Labeling of the releasable adenine nucleotides of washed human platelets. Blood 49:89–99

Rendu F, Nurden AT, Lebret M, Caen JP (1979a) Relationship between mepacrine-labeled dense body number, platelet capacity to accumulate ^{14}C-5-HT and platelet density in the Bernard–Soulier and Hermansky–Pudlak syndromes. Thromb Haemost 42:694–704

Rendu F, Lebret M, Nurden A, Caen JP (1979b) Detection of an acquired platelet storage pool disease in three patients with a myeloproliferative disorder. Thromb Haemost 42:794–796

Robblee LS, Shepro D, Belamarich FA, Towle C (1973) Platelet calcium flux and the release reaction. Ser Haematol 6:311–316

Rolovic Z, Baldini M, Dameshek W (1970) Megakaryocytopoiesis in experimentally induced immune thrombocytopenia. Blood 35:175–188

Savage B, Malpass TW, Stratton JR, Harker LA (1983) Platelet adenine nucleotide levels in patients with Dacron vascular prostheses. Thromb Res 32:365–372

Savage B, McFadden PR, Hanson SR, Harker LA (1986) The relation of platelet density to platelet age: survival of low and high density ^{111}In labeled platelets in baboons. Blood 68:386–393

Savage B, Hanson SR, Harker LA (1988) Selective decrease in platelet dense granule adenine nucleotides during recovery from acute experimental thrombocytopenia and ensuing thrombocytosis in baboons. Br J Haematol 68:75–82

Schalm OW, Jain NC, Carrol EJ (1975) Veterinary hematology, 3rd edn. Lea & Febiger, Philadelphia

Shulman NR, Watkins SP Jr, Itscoitz SB, Students AB (1968) Evidence that the spleen retains the youngest and haemostatically most effective platelets. Trans Assoc Am Phys 81:302–313

Stenberg PE (1984) Redistribution of alpha granules and their contents in thrombin-stimulated platelets. J Cell Biol 98:748–760

Stenberg P, McEver RP, Shuman MA, Jacques YV, Bainton DF (1985) A platelet alpha-granule membrane protein (GMP-140) is expressed on the plasma membrane after activation. J Cell Biol 10:880–886

Tegos C, Beutler E (1979) Platelet glycolysis in platelet storage. I. The glycolytic enzymes. Transfusion 19:203–205

Thompson CB, Eaton KA, Princiotta SM, Rushin CA, Valeri CR (1982) Size dependent platelet subpopulations: relationship of platelet volume to ultrastructure, enzymatic activity and function. Br J Haematol 50:509–520

Thompson CB, Jakubowski JA, Quinn PG, Deykin D, Valeri CR (1983) Platelet size as a determinant of platelet function. J Lab Clin Med 101:205–213

Todd ME, McDevitt E, Goldsmith EI (1972) Blood clotting mechanism of nonhuman primates: choice of the baboon model to simulate man. J Med Primatol 1:132–141

Tong M, Seth P, Penington DG (1987) Proplatelets and stress platelets. Blood 69:522–528

Trowbridge EA, Martin JF (1983) A biological approach to the platelet survival curve with criticism of previous interpretations. Phys Med Biol 28:1349–1377

Trowbridge EA, Warren CW, Martin JF (1986) Platelet volume heterogeneity in acute thrombocytopenia. Clin Phys Physiol Meas 7:203–210

Van der Lelie J, Von dem Borne AEGKR (1985) The clinical significance of platelet volume analysis. Neth J Med 28:457–461

Van Oost BA, van Hien-Hagg IH, Veldhuyzen BFE, Timmermans APM, Sixma JJ (1982) Determination of the density distribution of human platelets: methodological aspects and comparison with other tests for platelet activation. Thromb Haemost 47:239–243

Van Oost B, van Hien-Hagg IH, Timmermans APM, Sixma JJ (1983) The effect of thrombin on the density distribution of blood platelets: detection of activated platelets in the circulation. Blood 62:433–438

Vicic WJ, Weiss HJ (1983) Evidence that platelet alpha granules are a major determinant of platelet density: studies in storage pool deficiency. Thromb Haemost 50:878–880

Volkmer I, Nienhaus K, Wenzel E et al. (1979) Anti-thrombin III and platelet volume in correlation with hemolysis after valve replacements using xenografts. Thromb Haemost 42:73 (abstract)

Watson HHK, Ludlam CA (1986) Survival of 111-Indium platelet subpopulations of varying density in normal and post-splenectomized subjects. Br Haematol 62:117–124

Wencel-Drake JD, Plow EF, Kunicki TJ, Woods VL, Keller DM, Ginsberg MH (1986) Localization of internal pools of membrane glycoproteins involved in platelet adhesive responses. Am J Pathol 124:324–334

Wichmann HE, Gerhardts MD (1981) Platelet survival curves in man considering the splenic pool. J Theor Biol 88:83–101

Winocour PD, Kinlough-Rathbone RL, Perry DW, Rand ML, Packham MA, Mustard JF (1983) Changes in the properties of platelets from rats with experimentally induced shortened platelet survival. J Lab Clin Med 101:175–182

Yamazaki H, Motomiya T, Watanabe C et al. (1980) Consumption of larger platelets with decrease in adenine nucleotide content in thrombosis, disseminated intravascular coagulation and post-operative state. Thromb Res 18:77–88

Zucker-Franklin D (1981) Endocytosis by human platelets: metabolic and freeze fracture studies. J Cell Biol 91:706–715

5 Platelet Formation, Platelet Density and Platelet Ageing

K. G. Chamberlain, M. Tong and D. G. Penington

Introduction

Microscopic examination of both platelets and megakaryocytes shows them to vary widely in size and ultrastructure. This structural diversity was noted by early investigators (Bunting 1909) and interest in its origin and significance has continued to the present day. While haemostasis is undoubtedly the major life-preserving function of platelets, several other functions have been attributed to them, such as phagocytosis, promotion of wound healing and IgE-dependent killing of schistosomes (Joseph et al. 1983). Platelets have also been implicated in inflammatory disease (Ginsberg 1981), atherosclerosis and thrombosis. There is little evidence at present that any of these functions are exclusively performed by distinct subsets of platelets analogous to the well-characterized subsets of the lymphocyte population. In general, platelet populations show continuous variation in structural or functional properties, although they are often divided up into arbitrary "subpopulations" for the purpose of analysis. While we must remain open to the possibility that categorically different types of platelets may exist, our main effort will continue to be directed towards understanding how this continuously variable platelet population arises and how it achieves its known functions.

The first section of this chapter will focus on the "proplatelet" theory of platelet formation which was first advanced by Wright (1906) but then suffered a partial eclipse until its recent revival by Radley and other workers. A correct understanding of the mechanism of platelet formation is essential if we are to explain the origin of the platelet volume distribution. This section will include a description of some of our own studies on the morphology and frequency of circulating proplatelets. The following section of the chapter will deal with our studies on platelet density heterogeneity and its relationship to platelet ageing in normal human subjects.

The Proplatelet Theory of Platelet Formation

The process of thrombopoiesis involves many stages from the initial commitment of megakaryocyte precursors to the emergence of discoid platelets. In this section we wish to focus on the final stage of platelet formation, which has often been poorly understood but is likely to play a vital role in the determination of platelet heterogeneity.

Wright (1906, 1910) was the first to establish clearly that blood platelets arose from the largest haemopoietic cells in the bone marrow. He also described the process by which the cytoplasm of the megakaryocytes appeared to be packaged out to form individual platelets. He observed that mature megakaryocytes were motile cells which inserted long pseudopods in the marrow sinusoids. These processes developed constrictions which demarcated nascent platelets and were possible sites of detachment from the parent megakaryocyte. Wright suggested that single platelets could be released from the terminus of a pseudopod or, alternatively, longer segments could become detached and fragment into individual platelets in other parts of the circulation. Although Wright's observations were rapidly confirmed and extended by Bunting (1909), other mechanisms of platelet formation were suggested by later investigators and these later suggestions have often overshadowed Wright's original concept and created considerable confusion in this field. The following review will adhere strongly to Wright's concept but include some discussion of alternative views.

Proplatelet Formation in Bone Marrow

Most of the stages in platelet formation suggested by Wright on the basis of his light microscope observations were amply confirmed by subsequent studies of bone marrow using scanning and transmission electron microscopy (Behnke 1969; Muto 1976; Becker & De Bruyn 1976; Lichman et al. 1978). These studies have shown that megakaryocytes are preferentially located close to the walls of marrow sinuses and are capable of inserting long pseudopodal processes through the endothelial lining cells into the vascular sinuses. Becker and De Bruyn (1976) named these processes "proplatelets" and reported that their width varied from 1.5 to 3.5 μm and their length varied up to 120 μm. The proplatelet processes often occurred in clusters, suggesting a common origin from a single megakaryocyte, and they frequently showed beading with constrictions separating platelet-sized segments. Residual platelets in the sinusoids sometimes showed a teardrop shape which may have indicated recent separation from one of these constriction sites. Scurfield and Radley (1981) showed that megakaryocytes situated some distance from a marrow sinusoid were capable of extending pseudopodia a considerable distance through the extravascular compartment in order to contact and penetrate the sinus endothelium. Handagama et al. (1986) described proplatelet processes up to 500 μm in length extending into the marrow sinusoids of both dogs and rats but found no evidence of platelet release within the haemopoietic spaces of the marrow.

Proplatelet Formation In Vitro

Fixed marrow preparations can only give a snapshot view of the dynamic process of platelet formation and so other investigators have obtained valuable insights by studying living megakaryocytes in short-term cultures. Thiery and Bessis (1956) showed that a proportion of freshly prepared megakaryocytes from rat bone marrow maintained in sealed chambers at 37°C were capable of transforming themselves from globular cells to squid-like forms with long pseudopodal extensions. After about 4 hours in culture these pseudopods had lengthened enormously and developed the typical beaded appearance of the proplatelets later described in fixed marrow preparations. Following this, Pulvertaft (1958) observed similar dramatic transformations in preparations of human bone marrow. After a gap of about 25 years, the same process was described by Radley and Haller (1982, 1983) in explants of mouse bone marrow, and subsequently by Handagama et al. (1987b–d) in enriched megakaryocyte preparations from dogs and rats and by Leven and Yee (1987) in purified preparations of guinea-pig megakaryocytes.

Fig. 5.1 shows two megakaryocytes from one of our own preparations in different stages of proplatelet formation. The cells were flushed from a rat femur using "CATCH" medium (citrate–adenosine–theophylline in Hank's balanced salt solution; Levine and Fedorko 1976) and allowed to settle on a glass slide in a humidified chamber for 1 hour. The first megakaryocyte has just begun to form two major processes at opposite ends of the cell, while the second megakaryocyte shows one process which has become greatly elongated and is beginning to show the typical beaded appearance of proplatelets.

Factors Controlling Proplatelet Formation

In vitro preparations have allowed detailed investigation of the factors controlling the process of proplatelet formation. Although Pulvertaft and Humble (1956) examined hundreds of bone marrow cultures from human and animals, they saw only one megakaryocyte in these preparations undergo the transformation described by Thiery and Bessis (1956). Pulvertaft (1958) then discovered that the condition required to cause megakaryocyte motility and proplatelet formation was a reduction in oxygen tension. When the culture medium was saturated with 95% N_2/5% CO_2 instead of air, the mature megakaryocytes began to move and extend processes within 5 hours. This surprising result makes sense given that the marrow itself may be relatively hypoxic, since most of its arterial supply has already passed through capillaries in the surrounding bone (De Bruyn 1981). Pulvertaft (1958) pointed out that thrombopoiesis is also stimulated by haemorrhage and travel to high altitudes – both conditions associated with hypoxia.

Radley and Haller (1982, 1983) reported marked retraction of pseudopodal processes from mouse megakaryocytes in response to cold (4 °C for 2 hours) or the microtubule-disrupting agent vincristine. Handagama et al. (1987c) reported that CATCH medium, containing the platelet inhibitors adenosine and theophylline, decreased proplatelet formation in culture. Using a modified RPMI-1640 medium they found that about 9% of isolated rat megakaryocytes were producing proplatelets after 24 hours. They also reported that proplatelet formation was inhibited by the microtubule-disrupting agents vincristine and colchicine but

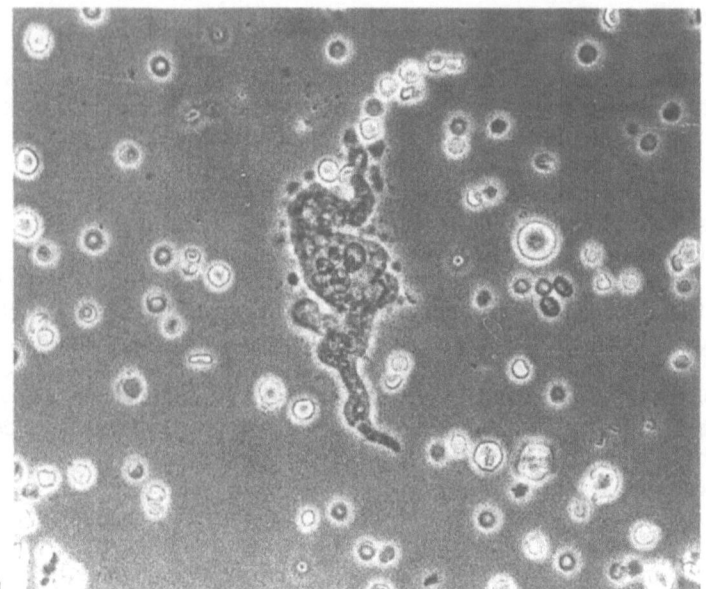

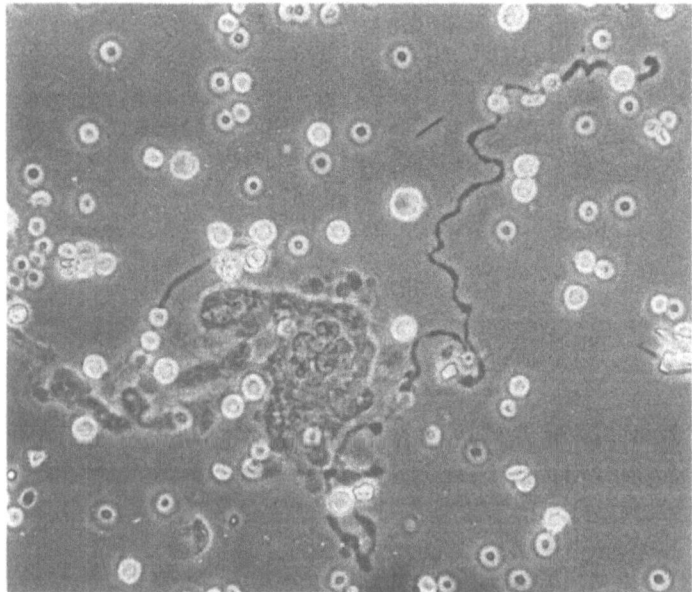

Fig. 5.1. Phase microscope images of megakaryocytes flushed from rat femoral marrow and allowed to settle under a coverslip on a glass slide for 1 hour in a humidified chamber. The other cells present are mainly erythrocytes. **a** The development of the thick pseudopodia signals an early stage in proplatelet formation. **b** Proplatelet formation has developed further in this cell, which shows one very long attenuated process with alternate swellings and constrictions. Reprinted from Penington (1987).

found that cytochalasin B (which interferes with microfilament extension) was less inhibitory. Proplatelet formation was inhibited by the glycolytic inhibitor NaF but hardly affected by the respiratory inhibitor NaCN. This reliance on glycolysis as an energy source is not surprising given the effect of hypoxia on proplatelet formation. Handagama et al. (1987d) reported that anti-platelet serum inhibited proplatelet formation and related this to the deficient platelet production which has been reported in some cases of idiopathic thrombocytopenic purpura (ITP) (Ballem et al. 1987), in which circulating antibody may bind to intravascular proplatelets and possibly also penetrate the extravascular space of the marrow.

Eldor et al. (1986) studied guinea-pig megakaryocytes which had adhered to an extracellular matrix secreted by bovine endothelial cells. These cells remained quiescent under static conditions, but up to 60% of them fragmented into a proplatelet network if exposed to flow conditions caused by rocking the culture dishes for 24 hours. Under these conditions the incipient platelets still remained attached to each other by thin cytoplasmic threads. Leven and Yee (1987) incubated guinea-pig megakaryocytes in open culture dishes for 18 hours and reported little spontaneous proplatelet formation. These authors then isolated thrombocytopenic plasma from rabbits injected 4 hours previously with guinea-pig anti-rabbit platelet serum. Addition of normal rabbit plasma to the 18-hour megakaryocyte cultures resulted in proplatelet extension by only 0.1% of the megakaryocytes after 3 hours, but addition of thrombocytopenic plasma induced 5.3% of the megakaryocytes to produce proplatelets. A 60%–80% ammonium sulphate cut of the thrombocytopenic plasma was even more potent, inducing proplatelet formation in 18% of the megakaryocytes.

These results demonstrate that a factor rapidly produced in response to thrombocytopenia (thrombopoietin?) is capable of accelerating the formation of proplatelet extensions by existing megakaryocytes. This goes a long way towards explaining the rapid appearance of large platelet forms after the induction of acute thrombocytopenia, despite possible injury to some megakaryocytes by the anti-platelet serum and prior to the changes in megakaryocyte number, size and ploidy which subsequently occur.

Leven and Yee (1987) also demonstrated that vincristine and colchicine inhibited proplatelet formation but, in contrast to the results of Handagama et al. (1987c), they found that cytochalasins B and D were able to initiate proplatelet formation in a high proportion of megakaryocytes. The resultant proplatelets seemed to lack the irregular beading observed normally, although this was observed when cytochalasins were added together with thrombocytopenic plasma. These results seem to indicate a major role for microtubules in proplatelet formation and perhaps a role for microfilament reorganization in the formation of the proplatelet constriction sites.

Proplatelet Structure

Behnke (1969) described the alignment of microtubules with the long axis of megakaryocyte pseudopodia which were penetrating the sinusoidal endothelium. Leven and Yee (1987) used indirect immunofluorescence to demonstrate that proplatelet extensions from cultured megakaryocytes contained many microtubules parallel to the long axis. Scurfield and Radley (1981) found that the parallel microtubules which traversed the constrictions between cytoplasmic segments often occupied nearly all of the available space in these sites and they pointed out the similarity of these constrictions to the narrow cytoplasmic bridges joining mitotic cells near the completion of cytokinesis.

Centrioles are frequently associated with microtubule organizing centres. The number of centrioles in megakaryocytes is determined by ploidy and may exceed eight, while the number of pseudopod extensions per megakaryocytes varies from one to nine (Haller and Radley, 1983; Handagama et al. 1987b). Radley and Scurfield (1980) suggested that ploidy may determine the maximum number of pseudopodia extended by each megakaryocyte. They found that centrioles were located near the nucleus in immature megakaryocytes but near the cell periphery in mature megakaryocytes, and a single centriole was found in each of eight proplatelet extensions examined by serial sectioning. Radley (1986) has recently expressed some doubts about the concept that the microtubules of each pseudopod originate from separate centrioles in the light of a study on processes in neuroblastoma cells (Sharp et al. 1982). He now suggests that all microtubules in megakaryocytes may originate at a common pericentriolar zone, while the centrioles found within processes may be non-functional.

The linear extended shape of most proplatelet segments contrasts with the smooth discoid shape of mature platelets which indicates the presence of a marginal microtubule coil. Leven and Nachmias (1988) reported the existence of occasional microtubule coils in the cytoplasm of guinea-pig megakaryocytes induced to spread by the action of ADP, and Leven and Yee (1987) reported that microtubule rings were sometimes seen in proplatelet processes in addition to longitudinal microtubules. Radley and Hartshorn (1987) also reported that detached proplatelet fragments occasionally showed a terminal putative platelet with a rounded profile containing a microtubule coil in addition to longitudinal microtubules. More frequently, however, the proplatelet fragments showed tapered ends with longitudinally arranged microtubules. A few free platelets in these preparations were atypical in appearance – showing teardrop or spindle shapes, suggesting recent separation from proplatelet chains. These observations suggest that the marginal microtubule coil usually arises after proplatelet fragmentation. A similar structural rearrangement is known to occur when platelets are rewarmed after cooling to 4 °C.

Cooling of discoid platelets leads to sphering and disappearance of the microtubule coil. On rewarming to 37 °C most platelets reassemble their mcrotubulc coil and rcsumo their lentiform shape, but a minority adopt an elongated form with a microtubule bundle parallel to the long axis (Behnke 1970). Zucker and Borrelli (1954) reported that although 24% of platelets had adopted this shape 20 minutes after rewarming, the proportion decreased to 12% after 50 minutes, suggesting that there was a natural tendency to revert to the discoid conformation at 37 °C. Larrimer et al. (1970) reported a low frequency of elongated forms in all their preparations, including those fixed immediately after blood sampling. These may be the young platelets which have just separated from proplatelet chains and have not yet organized a marginal microtubule bundle. Examples of elongated forms are shown in Fig. 5.3(a).

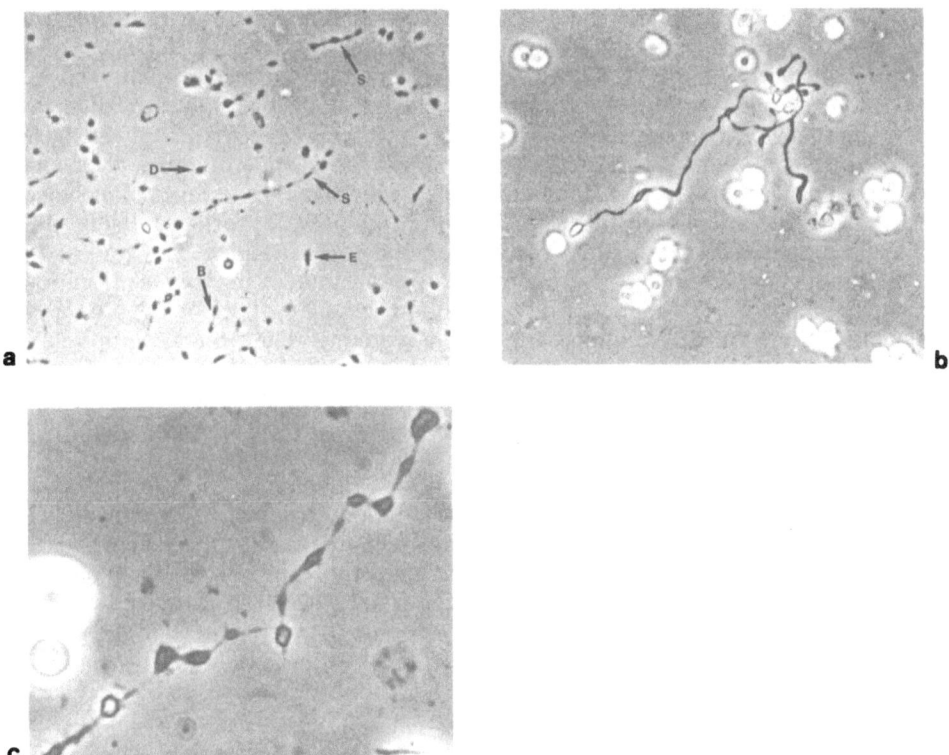

Fig. 5.2. Phase microscope images of proplatelets in rat PRP prepared 24 hours after injection of APS. **a** Low-power view of rat PRP showing numerous non-discoid platelets (*S*, strings; *B*, beaded forms; *E*, elongated platelets; *D*, discoid platelets). **b** Medium-power view of one long convoluted proplatelet showing several branch points. **c** High-power view of a linear proplatelet showing incipient platelet regions separated by cytoplasmic constrictions.

Proplatelets in Peripheral Blood

Although the evidence for the formation of proplatelets by megakaryocytes is now overwhelming, there was little published evidence until recently that such forms existed in the peripheral blood. Thiery and Bessis (1956) included a photograph of citrated rat platelets which showed some fusiform specimens resembling the incipient platelets seen in proplatelet chains. Kraytman (1973) studied the morphology of dog platelets prepared in citrate–formaldehyde and noted that approximately 2.4% of platelets from normal dogs were large elongated forms of variable shape. The recovery period after acute thrombocytopenia induced by extracorporeal circulation of blood through a glass bead column was marked by the appearance of "stress platelets", which were generally larger than normal but included forms with two or even three lobes joined by thin threads of cytoplasm. The author suggested that these forms were megakaryocyte fragments but did not discuss the way in which they were formed. Bessis (1977) reported finding "platelet rosaries" in the blood of patients suffering from thrombopathies, thrombocytopenic purpuras or thrombocythaemias, but not in normal blood.

In out own studies rat platelet-rich plasma (PRP) was prepared using acid–citrate–dextrose containing 20 μg/ml prostaglandin E_1, pH 6.7 ($ACDE_1$), 1 ml per 5 ml of blood (Tong et al. 1987). Atypical platelet forms (proplatelets) were defined as follows: elongated forms were those with length greater than three times the width; beaded forms showed two or three well-demarcated cytoplasmic masses separated by constrictions or slender cytoplasmic threads; strings were longer processes with more than three beads which were sometimes branched and often folded on themselves. Fig. 5.2(a) shows the prevalence of proplatelets in rat PRP prepared 24 hours after acute thrombocytopenia induced by anti-platelet serum (APS). Examples of string forms are shown under higher magnification in Fig. 5.2(b) and (c). Fig. 5.3 shows the more detailed views of rat proplatelets obtainable with electron microscopy. The scanning electron micrograph in Fig. 5.3(a) shows that after APS treatment strings, beaded and elongated forms are commonly found in rat PRP preparations. Fig. 5.3(b) is a transmission electron micrograph of a similar preparation showing a string form cut longitudinally together with discoid platelets and some red cell fragments.

Table 5.1 shows that the total percentage of all atypical forms increased from about 6% in normal rat blood to 17–18% in blood withdrawn 24 hours after APS treatment. In general the proplatelets after APS treatment appeared to be longer and to have a greater number of beads than those in normal rat blood. The frequencies of each form did not differ significantly between aortic and vena cava blood, suggesting that proplatelets were capable of passing through the pulmonary vasculature, although some proplatelet production by pulmonary megakaryocytes could not be ruled out.

Table 5.1. Classification of platelet morphology in PRP from normal and APS-treated rats ($ACDE_1$ anticoagulant)

Platelet forms (% of total)	Normal, IVC (N=6)	Normal, aortic (N=6)	24 hours post-APS IVC (N=6)	24 hours post-APS aortic (N=6)
Discoid	93.9±2.0	94.5±2.9	81.8±6.7	83.4±3.4
Elongated	5.0±1.5	3.6±2.4	14.3±4.5***	10.6±1.7***
Beaded	0.6±0.3	1.2±0.6	2.1±1.0**	4.6±2.6*
String	0.7±0.2	0.9±0.8	1.9±2.3	1.6±0.4
All non-discoid (proplatelets)	6.3±1.7	5.6±3.0	18.3±6.8**	16.6±3.5***

PRP, platelet rich plasma; APS, anti platelet serum; $ACDE_1$, acid–citrate–dextrose + prostagandin E_1; IVC, inferior vena cava.
Differential counts were performed under phase microscopy at ×250 magnification. The total counted in each sample ranged from 1700 to 2400 in normal rats and 200 to 990 in APS rats. Results shown are percentages of platelets in PRP (mean±SD). At 24 hours after APS, the whole blood platelet counts were 9.5±4.3% (IVC) and 8.0±2.4% (aortic) of the pretreatment platelet counts. Statistical comparisons were made using independent t tests: *$p<0.02$, **$p<0.01$, ***$p<0.001$. Based on data presented in Tong et al. (1987).

Mean platelet volume (MPV) increased about 45% one day after APS treatment and declined thereafter. Calculation shows that this rise in volume could be fully accounted for if the new proplatelet forms had on average a volume equal to five times the normal MPV. While most of the string forms had volumes greater than this, the average proplatelet volume was probably less. Neverthe-

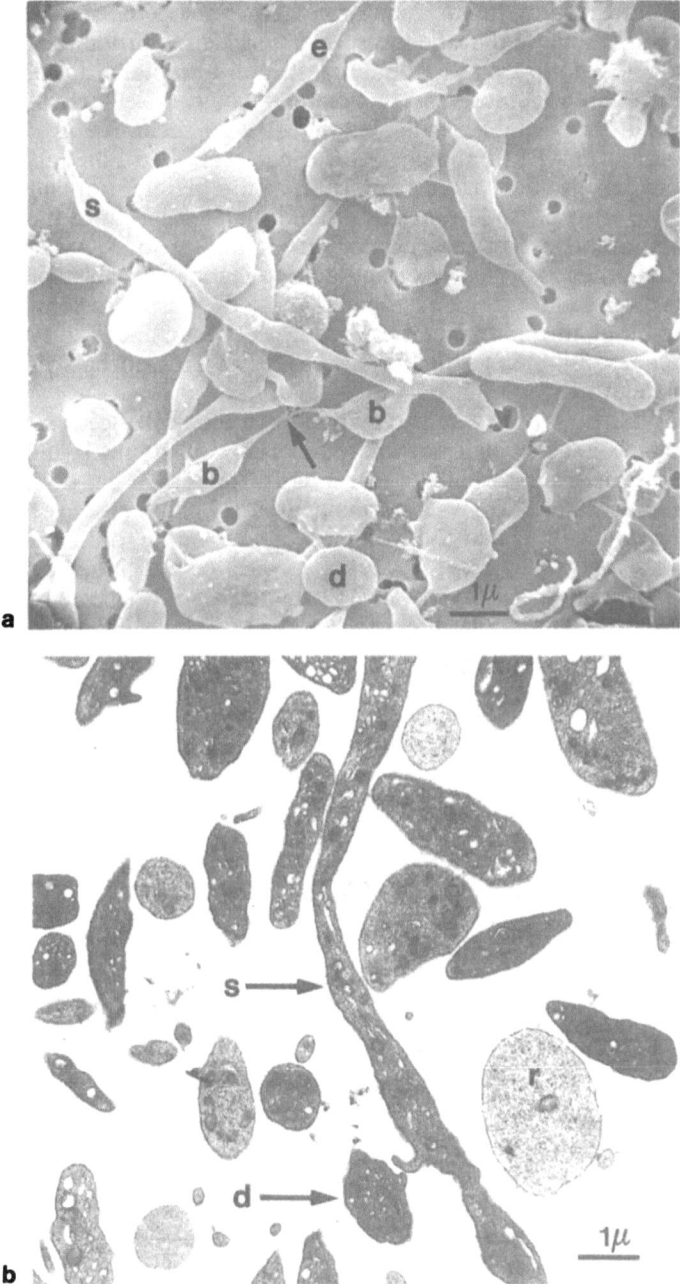

Fig. 5.3. Electron micrographs of rat platelets prepared 24 hours after APS treatment. **a** Scanning electron micrograph after filtration of the platelets onto a nucleopore polycarbonate filter (pore size 0.6 μm). Numerous proplatelets are visible (s, strings; b, beaded forms; e, elongated platelets; d, discoid platelets). The *arrow* shows a thin cytoplasmic strand joining two parts of a beaded proplatelet. Some debris is also present. **b** Transmission electron micrograph showing one long string proplatelet (s) together with discoid platelets (d) and some red cell fragments (r).

less, proplatelets would certainly make a major contribution to the increased MPV seen at this time. Assuming that the life-span of circulating proplatelets is relatively short (minutes–hours) they would constitute a rapidly declining proportion of the platelet population as the platelet count rose after APS treatment. Thus it is not surprising that the peak in MPV has been reported to occur as early as 6 hours after APS treatment (Trowbridge et al. 1986) since at this time proplatelets may constitute a larger proportion of the platelet population than subsequently. It is also possible that the discoid platelets produced after proplatelet fragmentation are larger than normal during this period. Kraytman (1973) reported the emergence of large normal-looking platelets in addition to putative proplatelets after acute thrombocytopenia in the dog. The acceleration of proplatelet formation by thrombopoietin preparations (Leven and Yee 1987) may also be accompanied by changes in the properties of these proplatelets, resulting in larger platelet progeny.

Trowbridge (1987) has pointed out that certain aperture impedence systems used for platelet volume analysis will not allow recording of atypical voltage pulses such as those arising from proplatelet forms. Our Coulter ZF has no such editing circuits. The multichannel analyser normally uses 512 channels to record volumes in the range 1–34 fl. Thus the volumes of very large proplatelets (volumes greater than ten normal platelets) would be truncated by this apparatus and so our estimate of MPV may be slightly low (Penington and Tong 1987). It is very interesting that Savage et al. (1988) reported no increase in MPV after the induction of acute thrombocytopenia in baboons by extracorporeal circulation of blood through a glass bead column. This may indicate that their apparatus had editing circuits which excluded the atypical signals from proplatelets.

Handagama et al. (1987a) also studied proplatelets from normal and acutely bled rats. These authors defined proplatelets as elongated cytoplasmic strands greater than ten platelets in length (20 μm) and measured a threefold increase in these forms in mixed venous blood 24 hours after acute blood loss, but no increase above controls at 12 or 48 hours. Interestingly, these authors reported much lower frequencies of these long string forms in left ventricular blood at all times and suggest that they may be efficiently fragmented in the lung.

Previous reports of proplatelets in the peripheral blood are rare and may relate to the fragility or aggregability of these forms. Handagama et al. (1987a) reported that the recovery of proplatelets was minimal without the use of the platelet inhibitors adenosine and theophylline in their citrated buffer. We have routinely used PGE_1 in our preparations for the same reason. A further reason may relate to the routine use of EDTA as an anticoagulant. We found that rat platelets prepared in EDTA were sphered and the characteristic proplatelet forms were no longer detectable. Radley and Hartshorn (1987) showed that beaded proplatelets rapidly retracted into a ball when stimulated by ADP, and Radley and Haller (1982) showed proplatelet processes still attached to megakaryocytes retracted when exposed to cold or vinicristine – both agents known to disrupt microtubules. It is likely that EDTA also causes the extended proplatelets to retract into spherical macrothrombocytes. Alternatively, EDTA may accelerate proplatelet fragmentation, although this seems less likely. In any case, the routine use of EDTA as anticoagulant may explain the few reports of proplatelet forms in blood smears. The "megathrombocytes" which have been observed (Garg et al. 1971) may be sphered proplatelets or individual platelets from the tail of the usual log-normal volume distribution.

Fragmentation of Proplatelets

The final step of fragmentation of proplatelets into individual platelets does not appear to occur readily in the in vitro systems which have been described, although detachment of segments occurred to some extent in the systems of Handagama et al. (1987b) and Leven and Yee (1987). Detachment of proplatelet segments from the endothelium of the marrow sinusoids may involve a contractile process at the transcellular pore, perhaps assisted by the blood flow through these vessels. It seems reasonable to assume that the very high shearing stresses subsequently experienced by the highly asymmetrical proplatelets in small arterial vessels could lead to final detachment at the attenuated constriction sites. It is possible that changes in the biochemical environment may facilitate this process. Shaw (1988) has pointed out that cytokinesis is often strongly dependent on oxidative phosphorylation and it may be that a more oxygen-rich environment such as the lungs may accelerate proplatelet fragmentation.

Alternative Mechanisms for Platelet Release

Several alternative mechanisms for platelet formation have been suggested by other authors. Trowbridge, Martin and Slater have suggested that the pulmonary blood vessels may play a unique role in platelet production (Trowbridge et al. 1982; Slater et al. 1983; Martin et al. 1983b). Trowbridge (1988) has presented the image of whole megakaryocytes or smaller fragments of megakaryocyte cytoplasm becoming repeatedly trapped astride capillary Y-junctions in the lung and thereby suffering successive binary divisions. This author has then shown that such a process could lead to the observed log-normal distribution of platelet volume if it is assumed that the proportions into which the cytoplasm is divided vary randomly around a mean of 50% and if the probability of division varies from 1.0 for fragment volumes $\geqslant$20 fl down to zero for fragment volumes $\leqslant$3.0 fl.

Radley (1988) has criticized several aspects of this account. Although megakaryocytes are sometimes released from the bone marrow substantially intact and low numbers of megakaryocytes can be found in the peripheral circulation, the formation of proplatelet processes in the bone marrow and the presence of residual bare megakaryocyte nuclei in the marrow have been well verified (Bunting 1909; Behnke 1969; Becker and De Bruhn 1976; Radley and Haller 1983). Radley (1988) has also criticized the image of megakaryocytes repeatedly caught astride vessel bifurcations. Given the motility of these cells, deformation along the long axis of thin blood vessels seems a more likely option. In fact the process of proplatelet formation observed in the bone marrow and in culture is also likely to occur in other parts of the circulation and this was observed to occur in the small number of megakaryocytes which migrated out of lung explants (Radley 1988).

Although Trowbridge (1988) has largely ignored proplatelet formation in his model, the mathematical analysis he develops may be equally applicable to the process of proplatelet fragmentation, even though the image of the long beaded proplatelet differs from the globular megakaryocyte fragments he describes. The fragmentation of proplatelets up to 500 μm in length (Handagama et al. 1986) would involve numerous independent binary divisions which could occur at a range of possible sites along each segment. These constriction sites seem to be distributed in a very irregular fashion (see Fig. 5.2(c)) although this cannot be assumed to be a perfectly random distribution.

Some earlier workers proposed that the invaginated membrane in mature megakaryocytes demarcated incipient platelets which were then released by a disintegration of the megakaryocyte cytoplasm along cleavage planes determined by this demarcation membrane system (Yamada 1957). Apparent fragmentation of spherical megakaryocytes into platelets has been reported after long-term culture in semi-solid media (McLeod et al. 1976; Williams et al. 1978) or after cyto-centrifugation (Zucker-Franklin and Petursson 1984; Straneva et al. 1986). These treatments may cause deterioration or artefactual fragmentation of megakaryocytes. Observations on perfusion-fixed bone marrow or short-term liquid cultures of megakaryocytes are much more likely to show physiological mechanisms of platelet release.

Other workers have suggested that platelets are shed by budding from the surface of megakaryocytes (Djaldetti et al. 1979). Although megakaryocytes frequently show a variety of surface blebs, these probably indicate cell motility, injury sustained during isolation from marrow (White 1989), or fixation artefact (Behnke 1969). Transmission electron micrographs are frequently presented in which megakaryocytes appear to be shedding platelets from their surfaces (Behnke and Tinggaard Pedersen, 1974; Williams et al. 1978). In many cases these represent thin sections through convoluted proplatelets which are still attached to adjacent megakaryocytes. Tavassoli and Aoki (1989) used serial sections to show that this was the case for numerous "platelets" they observed in marrow sinusoids.

When Do Individual Platelets Begin to Exist?

The idea that individual platelets are pre-formed in the megakaryocyte has been very persistent since Yamada (1957) first described the "demarcation membrane system". The origin of this notion is quite understandable. Pulvertaft (1958) reported that under the phase microscope mature megakaryocytes have a mottled appearance very similar to that of a platelet aggregate, while Behnke (1969) pointed out that the dilation of the demarcation membrane system in these cells often gives the impression that the cytoplasm has been divided into platelet-sized territories. The latter worker, however, never witnessed the release of platelets from a spherical megakaryocyte and reported that the apparent division of the cytoplasm into platelet areas subsided as soon as pseudopod formation began.

Other workers have suggested that the cytoplasm of the mature megakaryocyte is demarcated into cylindrical processes which are the nascent proplatelets (Becker and De Bruyn 1976). In this view the proplatelets are thought to unwind from the megakaryocyte in the way that a ball of string unwinds (Weiss 1965).

Radley and Haller (1982) rejected both these notions and suggested that the demarcation membrane system simply acts as a fluid store of membrane which is progressively evaginated and reorganized to cover the extending proplatelets. Rapid re-invagination of membrane was shown to occur when proplatelets retracted under the influence of cold or vincristine (Radley and Haller 1982). These investigators have suggested that individual platelets may simply be defined by the positions of the cytoplasmic constrictions in the proplatelets.

Although nascent platelets are probably not defined by the demarcation membrane system, something of the notion of preformed platelets may need to be retained. If platelets were purely random fragments of megakaryocyte cytoplasm, one might expect a certain percentage of bizarre and dysfunctional forms in addition to some very small forms, but in fact such forms generally only appear in pathological states. The presence of the expanded, beaded regions in the proplatelet processes suggests the presence of an underlying framework defining the platelet regions. Transmission electron micrographs have revealed that these expanded regions contain most of the platelet organelles. Fig. 5.4 shows a convoluted proplatelet from an APS-treated rat which has been incubated with mepacrine, a fluorescent marker of platelet dense granules. The fluorescent granules are not randomly located but are clustered in the incipient platelet regions and found only rarely in the connecting cytoplasmic strands. Loftus et al. (1984) studied unsectioned platelet whole mounts using high-voltage transmission electron microscopy and showed an intricate three-dimensional network of fine actin filaments which appeared to connect and encompass all the cytoplasmic organelles. Fox and Phillips (1983) concluded that 40%–50% of the actin in unstimulated platelets existed in the form of microfilaments and this proportion increased to 60%–80% after stimulation by thrombin. This actin-based cytoskeleton may hold organelles together like bunches of grapes and help to define the nascent platelets. Although such platelet cores would ensure that each platelet contained at least a minimum complement of organelles, varying amounts of membrane and cytoplasm might be associated with these substructures. Radley et al. (1987) expressed doubts about the existence of such substructures after they treated proplatelet processes with thrombin and observed bands of microfilaments forming a cylinder along the axis of certain processes without any evidence of segmentation into individual platelet territories. However, transmission electron microscopy of thin sections is a relatively poor tool for visualizing microfilaments (Mattson and Zuiches 1981; Pryzwansky

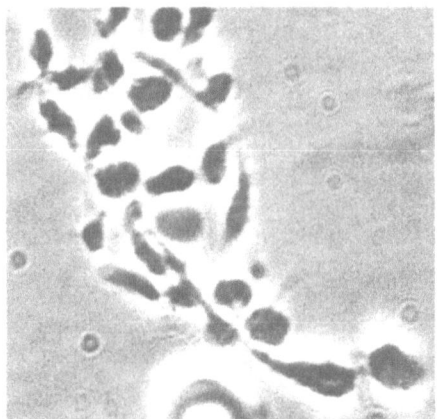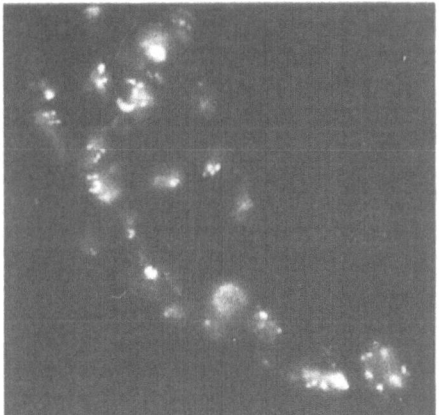

a   b

Fig. 5.4.   High-power view under phase of a single tangled proplatelet from rat PRP 24 hours after APS treatment. **a** Normal illumination showing many incipient platelet regions separated by thin cytoplasmic threads. **b** Same field epi-illuminated with blue light. Prior treatment with the fluorescent marker mepacrine has revealed the clusters of dense granules in the expanded platelet regions.

1987) and analysis of proplatelets by whole mount methods may reveal further underlying structure.

Proplatelets and Platelet Volume Heterogeneity

The recent developments in our understanding of platelet formation give us a new perspective from which to analyse various aspects of platelet heterogeneity. The existence of the broad log-normal distribution of platelet volume points to a degree of randomness in platelet formation which may reflect the manner in which megakaryocyte processes are fragmented. Paulus et al. (1986) analysed the normal platelet volume distribution in great detail and showed that the small deviation from log-normality in the tail of the distribution may be explained by the presence of a small number of unfragmented proplatelet segments.

While it is possible that the wide dispersion in platelet volume may simply be an unavoidable consequence of the mechanism of platelet formation, it may also have some relationship to platelet function. Platelets normally fufil their destiny by rapidly forming a continuous carpet over denuded subendothelium or packing together tightly to form a haemostatic plug. In both these situations, it is likely that closer packing may be attained if the flowing blood contains a wide distribution of platelet sizes. While larger platelets might adhere initially, smaller platelets might then fit into spaces too small for the larger platelets. Even though platelet shape change, fibrin formation and retraction eventually consolidate a haemostatic plug, the stability of the initial aggregate may be enhanced by the tighter packing available within a heterogeneous platelet population.

In addition to analysing the dispersion in platelet volume, we must also attempt to explain the systematic patterns in MPV such as the inverse relationship between MPV and platelet count (Levin and Bessman 1983). Several studies have shown that MPV is an important determinant of platelet function. Larger platelets normally survive longer in the circulation (Thompson et al 1983b; Chamberlain and Penington 1988b), but they aggregate more readily in vitro (Karpatkin 1978; Haver and Gear, 1981; Thompson et al. 1983a) and are selectively consumed during extensive haemostasis in vivo (Yamazaki et al. 1980; Thompson 1985). Since the body has to achieve efficient haemostasis while avoiding thrombosis, the platelet count is adjusted in inverse relationship to MPV in order to achieve a similar total platelet mass and a similar haemostatic efficiency in different individuals (Thompson and Jabubowski 1988).

The way in which MPV is controlled is unclear at present. Consideration of the process of proplatelet formation suggests that MPV may be governed by the average thickness of the proplatelets as well as the average distance between the constriction sites. It is interesting that Handagama et al. (1986) observed that proplatelet processes from canine megakaryocytes appeared thicker than those of rats, given that the MPV of dog platelets is about 40% greater than that of rat platelets (Eason et al. 1986). While the factors governing the average distance between proplatelet constrictions are unknown at present, it is possible that the average thickness of the proplatelet is governed by the supply of invaginated membrane in the megakaryocyte.

In order to examine this concept let us consider a mature spherical megakaryocyte with a diameter of 30 μm and a nucleus occupying 14% of the cell volume (Penington et al. 1976). If the cytoplasm of this megakaryocyte is converted into a single cylindrical proplatelet with a diameter of 3 μm, a simple geometrical calculation reveals that the amount of surface membrane required will be approximately 6× the amount of membrane covering the megakaryocyte. On the other hand, if the final proplatelet diameter is 1.5 μm, the proplatelet will be 4× longer and the amount of membrane required will be 12× the amount of membrane covering the spherical megakaryocyte. Thus it is possible that the final thickness of the proplatelet may be limited by the amount of invaginated membrane available in the megakaryocyte. There is evidence that the large platelets found in ITP have reduced amounts of invaginated membrane (Boneu et al. 1982b) which presumably also derives from the demarcation membrane of the megakaryocyte. Paulus et al. (1979) have already suggested that the large platelets found in Mediterranean macrothrombocytosis and the May–Hegglin anomaly may arise from a limitation on the amount of demarcation membrane in the megakaryocytes. Jackson (1989) pointed out that although large membrane complexes are frequently found in the megakaryocytes and platelets of giant platelet syndromes, such as that of the Wistar–Furth rat, this membrane may not be available for evagination onto the platelet surface. In support of this idea, Stenberg and Levin (1989) have published a photograph showing that some areas of the demarcation membrane system in megakaryocytes of the Wistar–Furth rat do not communicate with the extracellular space.

Penington et al. (1976) reported that the amount of demarcation membrane increased with megakaryocyte ploidy in the steady state and suggested that the 32N megakaryocytes gave rise to smaller, less-dense platelets than the 8N megakaryocytes. In the present context we would predict that the 32N megakaryocytes would give rise to thinner proplatelets than the 8N megakaryocytes, although this relationship might be altered during accelerated thrombopoiesis. A recent review by Corash (1989) has revealed the present lack of consensus concerning the relationship between MPV and megakaryocyte size and ploidy in both normal and pathological states. Although it has been suggested that membrane availability may be the immediate determinant of MPV, other mechanisms may operate. The proplatelet theory of platelet formation provides a conceptual framework within which future experiments may be devised. In vitro studies of platelet formation by cultured megakaryocytes of defined size and ploidy may throw further light on the determination of platelet heterogeneity.

Platelet Density Heterogeneity and Platelet Ageing

The relationship between platelet age and platelet density has been a controversial topic for well over a decade. The possibility of a relationship between platelet density and age was probably suggested by the prior discovery that erythrocyte density increased steadily with cell age (Leif and Vinograd 1964). This relationship is now well accepted, although there is still active discussion of possible mechanisms for this rise in erythrocyte density (see Clark, 1988, for a comprehensive review). The lack of agreement in platelet density studies mainly reflects the difficulties of isolating platelets in an unactivated state, the variety of density gradient procedures which have been employed, and the use of platelets from different species. We have focused our efforts on the characterization of human platelet density subpopulations and the relationship between platelet density and platelet age in normal human subjects.

Preparation of Platelet Density Subpopulations

Some of the early workers in this field used density-gradient materials which were immiscible with water (Karpatkin 1969a; Minter and Ingram 1970) or hyperosmotic (Booyse et al. 1968) and the duration and force of centrifugation were sometimes insufficient to achieve density equilibrium. Many recent workers have used discontinuous gradients, which take longer to reach equilibrium and suffer from crowding effects at the interfaces. Martin and co-workers pointed out the artefacts which may arise from the use of these methods and concluded that continuous gradients of Percoll were the best available alternative (Martin and Trowbridge 1982; Martin et al. 1983a).

In our studies we have used continuous Percoll gradients made up in a modified Tyrode's (MT) buffer based on that employed by Rand et al. (1981). This buffer contains citrate, glucose and bovine serum albumin and we adjust the pH to 6.7 to help dampen platelet reactivity. Our centrifugation conditions (3500 g × 60 min) appear to be theoretically adequate for the majority of platelets to reach density equilibrium (Martin and Trowbridge 1982) and empirically we found no significant change in the density distribution when we doubled the force or duration of centrifugation (Chamberlain and Penington 1988a). We routinely harvested over 90% of the platelets from 21 ml of blood by diluting and centrifuging the red cell column three times before pooling the diluted PRP. We minimized platelet activation by adding PGE_1 and theophylline to the ACD anticoagulant and added additional PGE_1 before each of two pelleting steps in the procedure.

After centrifugation in the linear Percoll gradient the platelets formed a wide band which appeared as a unimodal bell-shaped distribution after photometric scanning (Fig. 5.5). The detailed shape of this continuous density distribution contains considerably more information than is available from the few steps of a discontinuous gradient. The continuous density distribution was arbitrarily divided into five fractions, each containing approximately 20% of the platelets. These density subpopulations together with a sample of the unfractionated total population were then subjected to biochemical and morphometric analysis.

Morphometric Analysis of Platelet Density Subpopulations

Fig. 5.6 shows scanning electron micrographs for the low-density (LD) platelets (fraction 1) and the high-density (HD) platelets (fraction 5) prepared by Dr Priti Seth in our department. The heterogeneity of platelet volume is very apparent in both these fractions. The elongated platelets may be young platelets which have recently separated from proplatelet chains. The frequency of elongated platelets in the LD fraction was 2%–3% while the frequency of these forms in the HD fraction was <1.0%.

In agreement with most other investigators we found that MPV was correlated with platelet density, even though platelets in each density fraction showed a wide distribution of volume. Although this result could have arisen artefactually if

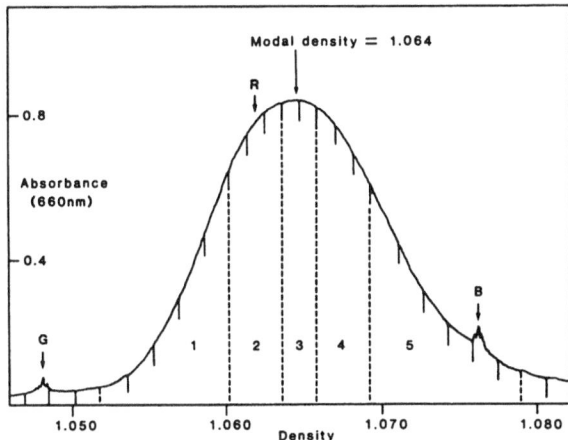

Fig. 5.5. Photometric record of a normal human platelet density distribution prepared on a linear Percoll gradient. The letters indicate the position of the green, red and blue density marker beads (Pharmacia) while the short downward strokes indicate the subsequent division of the gradient into 0.4-ml fractions. Fractions were pooled as indicated to give five regions containing approximately equal numbers of platelets. Reprinted from Chamberlain and Penington (1988).

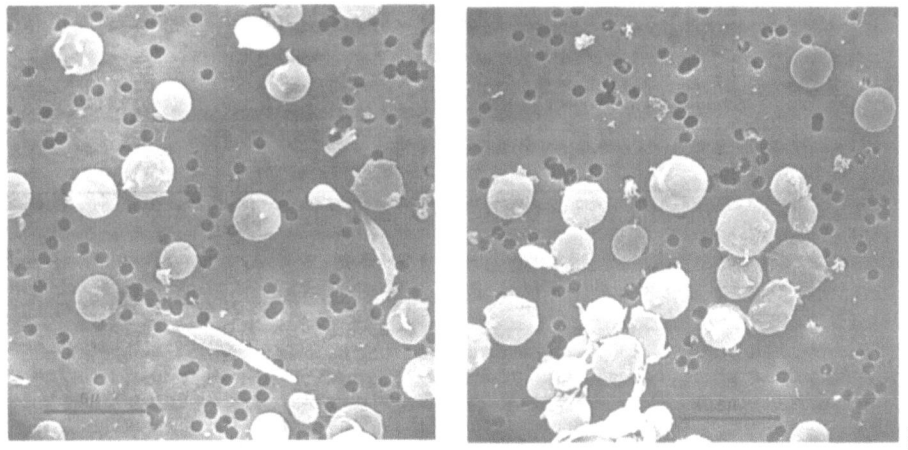

Fig. 5.6. Scanning electron micrographs of platelet density subpopulations after fixation and filtration onto nucleopore polycarbonate filters (pore size 0.6 μm). Some debris is present in both fields. **a** LD subpopulation showing variation in platelet size and the presence of two atypical spindle-shaped platelets. **b** HD subpopulation also showing great variation in platelet size.

density equilibrium had not been reached, we found that the ratio of MPV in the extreme fractions (HD/LD = 1.4) was unaffected when twice the normal centrifugal force was employed (Chamberlain and Penington 1988a). The correlation between MPV and platelet density is likely to reflect some aspect of thrombopoiesis and may relate to the observed differences in cytoplasmic composition in megakaryocytes of different ploidy (Penington et al. 1976).

Transmission electron micrographs of the different density subpopulations were subjected to morphometric analysis using a computerized image analyser [Chamberlain et al. 1988a). The morphology of platelets prepared for electron microscopy was improved by allowing them to recover in a nutrient buffer at 37 °C for 30 minutes before fixation. One hundred randomly selected platelet sections were measured in each subpopulation from seven normal subjects. Some of the platelets showed small pseudopodia but most of the platelets were discoid with circumferential microtubule bands and random organelle distribution. The HD platelet sections had a significantly greater mean cross-sectional area than the LD platelet sections, reflecting the difference in MPV. The LD platelets were significantly more elongated in cross-section than the HD platelets, which seemed more rounded, probably reflecting their greater organelle content. Table 5.2 shows the concentrations of various subcellular structures in the different density subpopulations. The open canalicular system (OCS) occupied a slightly greater percentage of the cross-sectional area in the LD platelets compared to the HD platelets. The HD platelets were found to contain significantly greater concentrations per unit area of α-granules, dense granules, mitochondria and glycogen aggregations compared to the LD platelets. Our results also showed that there was a significant increase in the size of both dense granules and α-granules as platelet density increased (Table 5.3). We were surprised to find the opposite trend for the size of mitochondria and suggested that this may have indicated a degree of mitochondrial swelling in the LD platelets. These platelets have smaller reserves of glycogen and may be more susceptible to the stresses of in vitro processing. Fig. 5.7 shows platelets from the extreme density fractions which

Table 5.2. Organelle concentration/unit area in platelet cross-sections

Organelle	Total pop.	F1	F3	F5
OCS (% area)	12.1 ±4.0	13.6 ±3.6	11.9 ±3.3	11.1 ±3.9**
Glycogen (% area)	1.65±0.89	0.30±0.19	1.02±0.32	3.92±2.12**
α-Granules (n)	2.79±0.46	2.50±0.39	2.87±0.31	3.10±0.41**
Dense granules (n)	0.11±0.04	0.10±0.03	0.13±0.05	0.13±0.04**
Mitochondria (n)	0.62±0.19	0.57±0.13	0.66±0.15	0.70±0.20*

The results are mean±SD ($N=7$) for the total platelet population and density fractions 1, 3 and 5. (% area), percentage of cross-sectional area occupied by aggregations of glycogen particles or the empty structures of the open canalicular system (OCS). (n), number of organelles per square micrometre of cross-sectional area. Statistical comparisons of F1 (LD) and F5 (HD) were made using paired t tests: *$p<0.05$, **$p<0.01$. Based on data published in Chamberlain et al. (1988a).

Table 5.3. Cross-sectional area of platelet organelles ($\times 10^{-2}$ μm)

Organelle	Total pop.	F1	F3	F5
α-Granules	2.93±0.35	2.66±0.36	2.83±0.27	3.18±0.30**
Dense granules	2.38±0.36	1.95±0.36	2.41±0.33	2.65±0.47*
Mitochondria	3.59±0.60	3.84±0.65	3.42±0.66	3.26±0.70***

The results are mean±SD ($N=7$). Statistical comparisons of F1 (low-density platelets) and F5 (high-density platelets) were made using paired t tests: *$p<0.05$, **$p<0.01$, ***$p<0.001$. Based on data published in Chamberlain et al. (1988a).

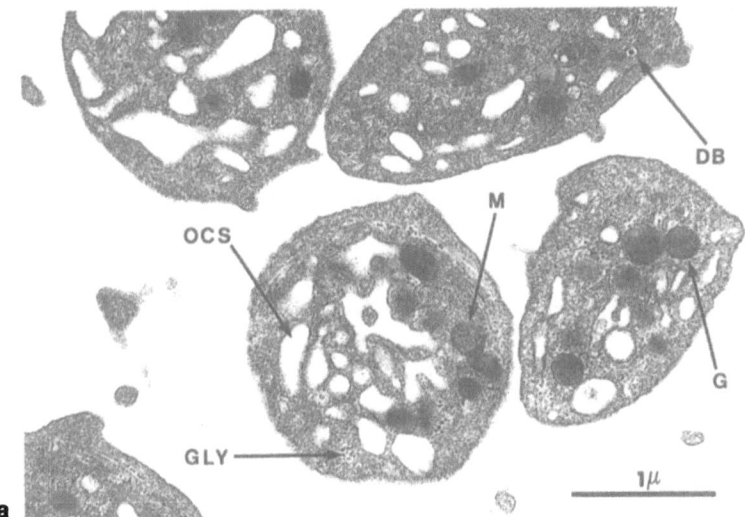

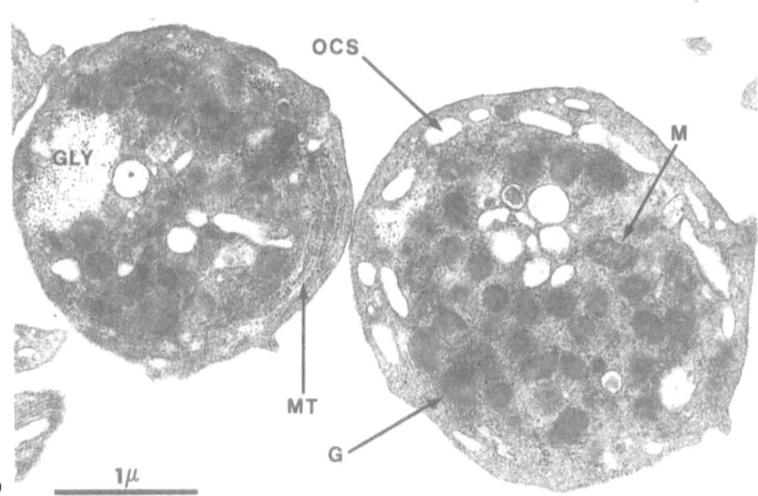

Fig. 5.7. Transmission electron micrographs of platelets from the extreme density subpopulations which illustrate some of the major features of each. Ultrastructural features include: open canalicular system (*OCS*), marginal microtubules (*MT*), mitochondria (*M*), α-granules (*G*), dense bodies (*DB*) and glycogen (*GLY*). **a** LD platelets showing a more prominent OCS but a relative deficiency of granules and glycogen. **b** HD platelets showing abundant granules and glycogen particles.

illustrate some of these trends: the LD platelets contain relatively more OCS while the HD platelets contain greater concentrations of granules, mitochondria and glycogen.

Our morphometric results differed from those reported by Corash et al. (1977) in several ways. These workers reported that the OCS occupied at least 50% of the cross-sectional area in many of their LD platelets, while it only occupied about 10% of the area in their HD platelets. We found that the OCS occupied

13.6±3.6% of the cross-sectional area in the LD platelets and 11.1±3.9% of the area in the HD platelets, and platelets containing more than 50% OCS were rare. The total granule content reported by Corash et al. (1977) for the HD subpopulation (6.5±1.4/section) agreed with our result (7.1±1.2) but the result for the LD subpopulation (2.0±0.5) was only half the value we obtained (5.0±1.0). Even though Corash et al. (1977) selected slightly narrower cuts for their extreme subpopulations (15% rather than 20%), the combination of dilated OCS and low granule content suggests that their LD subpopulation may have contained significant numbers of degranulated platelets. This is relevant to their finding that there was no significant difference in the number of mitochondria in cross-sections from the extreme density subpopulations. Contamination of the LD subpopulation with HD platelets which had undergone the release reaction would have artefactually increased the mitochondrial content of this fraction.

Duyvené de Witt et al. (1987) carried out a morphometric analysis of platelet density subpopulations using a different approach. Instead of analysing single thin sections from numerous different platelets, these workers analysed complete sets of serial sections from six platelets in each of four density fractions. They reported that both MPV and total granule concentration increased with platelet density, but the concentration of mitochondria and the percentage of volume occupied by the OCS were similar in each density fraction. The advantage of using full sets of serial sections is that a three-dimensional reconstruction of the platelets is possible and the total number of organelles per platelet can be counted. However, the small number of platelets studied and the lack of information concerning how these platelets were selected cause one to question whether the samples were truly representative of each density subpopulation.

Biochemical Properties of Platelet Density Subpopulations

Our own morphometric observations were reinforced by measurements of appropriate biochemical markers. Fig. 5.8 shows selected biochemical results expressed as concentrations to allow for the differences in MPV between the density fractions (shown in Fig. 5.8(a)). The HD platelets contained significantly higher concentrations of α-granule proteins (β-thromboglobulin, von Willebrand factor), dense granule markers (5-HT, calcium), mitochondrial marker enzymes (monoamine oxidase, cytochrome oxidase, glutamate dehydrogenase and NADP-dependent isocitrate dehydrogenase) and glycogen (Chamberlain and Penington 1988a; Chamberlain et al. 1989b).

We made a special study of the mitochondria because Corash et al. (1984) had reported a similar rise in monoamine oxidase (MAO) activity with platelet density but interpreted this in the light of their morphometric data suggesting that the number of mitochondria did not vary with density (Corash et al. 1977). In order to explain these data they suggested that both platelet density and platelet MAO activity declined with platelet age. We found that the activity of MAO and three other mitochondrial marker enzymes were extremely well correlated in the different density fractions, suggesting the presence of different numbers of mitochondria rather than stages in enzyme deterioration, since it is unlikely that four very different enzymes would decay at exactly the same rates (Fig. 5.9). These biochemical results were supported by the morphometric findings already described.

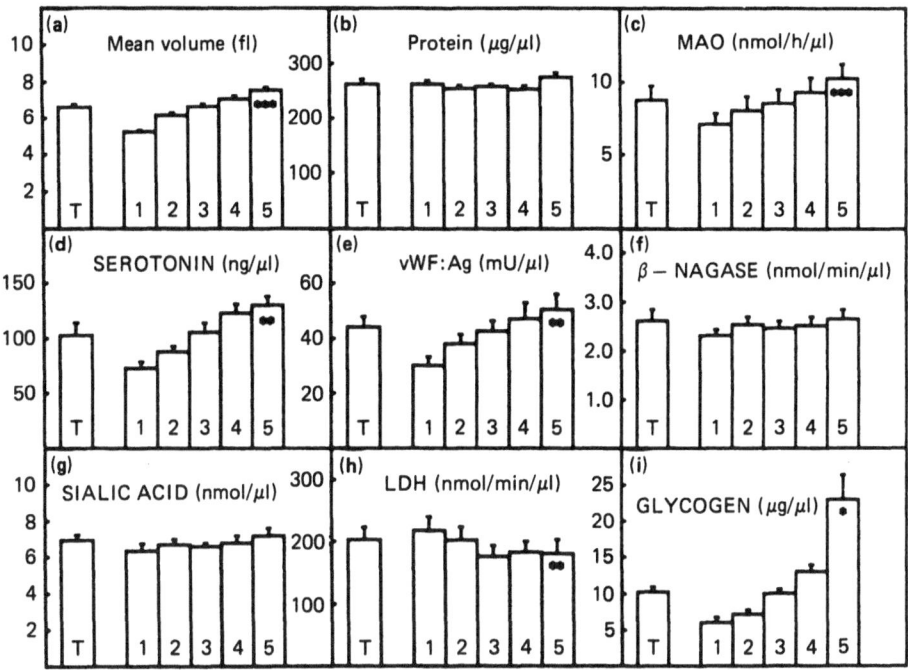

Fig. 5.8. Mean platelet volumes and concentrations of subcellular constituents in the total platelet population (T) and the five density subpopulations (mean±SEM, $N=7$–28). Platelet density increases from fraction 1 (LD) to fraction 5 (HD). Statistical comparisons were made using the paired sign test: $^{*}p<0.05$, $^{**}p<0.01$, $^{***}p<0.001$. Combination of histograms presented in Chamberlain and Penington (1988a) and Chamberlain et al. (1989b).

Fig. 5.8 shows the results of some of our other biochemical measurements on the platelet density subpopulations. We were a little surprised that total protein concentration did not differ significantly in the different subpopulations. Presumably the lower concentration of α-granule proteins in the LD platelets is compensated by relatively greater amounts of membrane and cytoplasmic proteins. The results of Rand et al. (1981) and Corash et al. (1984) also seem to show similar protein concentrations in all density subpopulations. The concentrations of lysosomal enzymes (β-glucuronidase and β-N-acetylglucosaminidase) were not significantly different in the density subpopulations and this was also reported by Corash et al. (1984). Lysosomes are smaller and less dense than α-granules and probably make an insignificant contribution to platelet density. We found that the concentration of total sialic acid did not differ between the subpopulations, in agreement with the results of Rand et al. (1981) but contrasting with those reported by Soslau and Giles (1982), who speculated that platelets may lose sialic acid while undergoing a decrease in density with age.

We found that the concentrations of the cytosolic enzymes lactate dehydrogenase (LDH) and glucose-6-phosphate dehydrogenase (G6PD) were slightly higher in the LD platelets compared to the HD platelets (significant at $p<0.01$ for LDH only). These results contrast markedly with those reported by Karpatkin and Strick (1972), who found the concentration of LDH in the LD platelets to be half that in the HD platelets while G6PD had similar concentrations in both

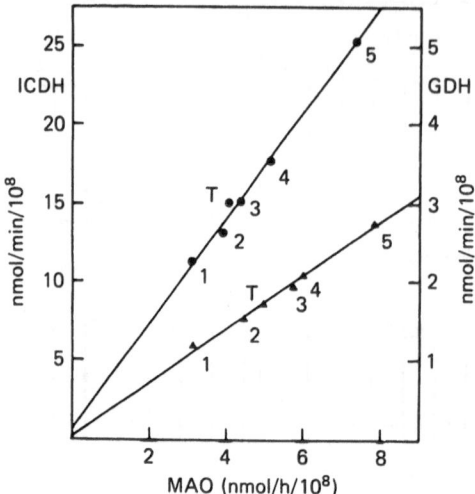

Fig. 5.9. Correlation between isocitrate dehydrogenase (ICDH) and monoamine oxidase (MAO) activities (●) and between glutamate dehydrogenase (GDH) and MAO activities (▲) when both enzymes of each pair were assayed in the same samples of total platelet population (T) and corresponding density fractions (1–5). ($R=0.99$, $p<0.001$, for both regressions). Reprinted from Chamberlain and Penington (1988a).

subpopulations. The authors considered that LDH activity declined with time and so their results supported the thesis that LD platelets were senescent. Our results appear to be more supportive of the antithesis, although they may simply reflect the greater amount of organelle-free cytoplasm in the LD platelet population.

The results of our structural studies seem to support the view that the importance of different subcellular structures as determinants of platelet density depends on their density, size and relative abundance. Several investigators have suggested that α-granule content is a major structural determinant of platelet density (Vicic and Weiss 1983; Van Oost et al. 1984). Our own results support this view but the steep gradient between glycogen content and platelet density (Table 5.2, Fig. 5.8 (i)) suggests that glycogen content also has a very significant influence. The other structural correlations suggest that significant but probably smaller contributions are made by the content of OCS, mitochondria and dense granules.

Functional Properties of Density-Separated Platelets

Only a limited amount of work has been done on the functional properties of platelet density subpopulations. Karpatkin (1969b) reported that HD platelets aggregated more quickly and released greater quantities of ATP, ADP and platelet factor 4 than LD platelets in response to stimulation by ADP, thrombin and adrenaline. More recent studies using gentler preparation methods have not reported such large differences in function between the density subpopulations.

Martin et al. (1981) briefly reported some aggregometer experiments in which stimulation with 0.5 mM arachidonate produced 22 ng/10^8 of thromboxane B_2 in the HD platelets compared to 10 ng/10^8 in the LD platelets, while the response to thrombin stimulation was similar in all subpopulations. Nubile et al. (1987) reported a greater extent of aggregation in response to ADP in the LD platelets compared to the HD platelets, while the responses to collagen and adrenaline were slightly greater in the HD platelets. Caranobe et al. (1982) reported no significant difference in 5-HT uptake between their density subpopulations, while Corash et al. (1984) reported a lower rate of 5-HT transport in the LD platelets but found that LD and HD platelets lost similar percentages of their dense bodies in response to thrombin. More recently, we found that uptake of labelled 5-HT and release in response to thrombin (0.1 and 1.0 units/ml) did not differ significantly between the density subpopulations (Chamberlain et al. 1989a). These more recent studies clearly show that platelets of all densities are functionally active and they give little support to the contention of Karpatkin (1969b) and Corash et al. (1984) that the LD platelets are a relatively senescent subpopulation.

Age-Dependent Properties of Platelets

There are few studies comparing the properties of young and old platelets during steady-state thrombopoiesis. Hirsh et al. (1968) used [^{35}S]sulphate as a cohort label in rabbits and reported that young platelets showed greater adherence to collagen fibres both in vitro and in vivo but did not appear to be selectively aggregated by ADP. Haver and Gear (1981), however, did report greater aggregation by young, [^{75}Se]selenomethionine-labelled rat platelets after ADP stimulation, while Thompson et al. (1984) reported that young baboon platelets were more susceptible to thrombin-induced aggregation than relatively old platelets.

Studies in humans are rare, but Johnson et al. (1971) investigated a patient whose thrombopoiesis could be switched on by plasma infusions. Relatively young platelets were obtained 4 days after infusion and older platelets were obtained 18–21 days after infusion. The older platelets were associated with longer bleeding times, decreased platelet adhesiveness and deficient platelet factor 3 availability. No structural differences between young and old platelets were observed by electron microscopy. Other studies on platelet ageing have been flawed by the assumptions that stress platelets obtained after acute thrombocytopenia are equivalent to normal young platelets or that the platelets surviving irradiation or cytotoxic drug treatment are equivalent to normal old platelets (Ginsberg and Aster 1972; Bolton et al. 1980; Blajchman et al. 1981; Steiner and Vancura 1985). The steady-state studies suggest that platelets become functionally less responsive as they age, but this may be due to subtle changes and there is no evidence for large structural changes during normal platelet ageing.

Despite this, Karpatkin (1972) and Corash et al. (1977, 1984) have expressed the view that human platelets normally decrease in density and progressively lose granule contents as they age in the circulation. This hypothesis may be tested by examining the loss of β-thromboglobulin (βTG) from platelet α-granules during normal ageing. βTG is thought to be completely platelet-specific and if it is released into the plasma by leakage, platelet activation or lysis, it suffers first-order elimination with a half-life of about 100 minutes (Dawes et al. 1978). Estimates of platelet βTG content in normal subjects have ranged from 2.5 μg/10^8 (Han et al. 1980) to 7.0 μg/10^8 (Fabris et al. 1984) and estimates of free plasma βTG have ranged from 6.0 ng/ml (Files et al. 1981) to 33 ng/ml (Fabris et al. 1984). Here we will select average values of 5.0 μg/10^8 and 20 ng/ml.

Under steady-state conditions, the rate of βTG secretion (R_s) is equal to the rate of elimination (R_e) and the latter is given by the expression $R_e = k[\beta TG]$, where $k = \log_e 2/t_{\frac{1}{2}}$ and $t_{\frac{1}{2}} = 100$ minutes. It follows that $R_s = 0.693 \times 20/100 = 0.14$ ng/ml per minute or 200 ng/ml per day. Thus the secretion of βTG over the average platelet life-span of 9 days is about 1.8 μg/ml of PRP. Assuming a normal whole blood platelet count of 250×10^9/l or 4.2×10^8/ml of plasma, the platelet βTG content will be 21 μg/ml. Thus the βTG secretion over 9 days will be approximately 1.8/21 or 9% of the total βTG content of the platelets. However, it has been estimated that up to 18% of human platelets are destroyed randomly without reaching their potential life-span (Hanson and Slichter 1985). It is reasonable to expect that a substantial proportion of these would release their βTG content intravascularly during haemostatic interactions. In addition, the original estimate of free plasma βTG concentration is probably too high because it will include some contribution from release in vitro. Thus the figure of 9% should be taken as an upper limit for general βTG loss from surviving platelets and the actual figure may be closer to zero. Since LD platelets contain less than 50% of the βTG content of LD platelets (Chamberlain et al. 1989a), it is clear that loss of granule contents during platelet ageing cannot account for most of the heterogeneity in platelet α-granule contents.

Our structural studies gave no support to the suggestion that the LD platelets were a relatively senescent platelet population; in fact, two results seemed to suggest that the LD platelets were a slightly younger subpopulation. We counted the number of dense granules in platelets using the fluorescent marker mepacrine and found that the concentration of dense granules was positively correlated with platelet density (Chamberlain et al. 1989b). We then found that the 5-HT content per granule in the LD platelets was only two-thirds that of the content in the HD platelets. Since 5-HT is known to be accumulated from the plasma during the platelet life-span (Mezzano et al. 1984a), this may indicate that the LD platelets are a slightly younger population. On the other hand, the electron micrographs showed that the dense granules in the LD platelets appeared to be about 25% smaller than the dense granules in the HD platelets, so this may account for the difference in 5-HT content. The second piece of evidence was the increased LDH concentration in the LD platelets but, as indicated above, this may simply reflect the reduced organelle content of these platelets. In order to analyse properly the relationship between platelet density and platelet age, platelets of defined ages need to be labelled in some way.

Platelet Population Labelling by MAO Inhibition

Most of the investigators who have concluded that platelet density decreases with platelet age have performed platelet labelling experiments in rabbits (Karpatkin 1969a; Corash and Shafer 1982; Packham et al. 1985). We wished to avoid the problem of species differences and performed our labelling experiments in human subjects using a method which avoids both ex vivo handling of platelets and the injection of radioactive materials (Chamberlain et al. 1988b). The method is very similar to the use of aspirin for the irreversible inhibition of platelet cyclo-oxygenase, but in this case the mitochondrial enzyme MAO is inhibited by one of the irreversible MAO inhibitors which are currently prescribed for depression. We decided to avoid the aspirin method because the cyclo-oxygenase assay is complex and aspirin is known to interfere with platelet function. On the other hand, MAO assays are straightforward and reliable and the platelet samples can be frozen before assay. There is no evidence that a single dose of an MAO inhibitor affects platelet function.

The use of MAO inhibitors to label platelet populations rests on a number of assumptions. MAO is located in the outer membrane of mitochondria but is coded by nuclear genes (Bach et al. 1988). Synthesis of this enzyme during the circulating life of the platelet is assumed to be insignificant (Kieffer et al. 1987). Tranylcypromine blood levels fall to less than 2% of maximum after 12 hours (Simpson et al. 1985) and are assumed to be negligible after 24 hours. MAO inhibition persisting beyond this time is assumed to be irreversible (Silverman 1983). It follows that recovery of platelet MAO activity is a measure of the replacement of circulating platelets by newly formed platelets containing uninhibited enzyme.

The main disadvantage of using irreversible MAO inhibitors at present is that they can cause potentially serious hypertensive reactions and so clinical supervision is required during their administration. Hypertensive reactions follow the ingestion of amine-containing foods or medicines so these must be avoided for 24 hours preceding and 7 days following the ingestion of the drug. We gave 10 normal subjects a single 20-mg dose of tranylcypromine (Parnate), which is the most potent of the traditional MAO inhibitors. There was a significant rise in supine systolic blood pressure in the group from 119 ± 10 to 128 ± 14 mmHg one day after drug ingestion, but this fell back to normal on subsequent days. In future the possibility of hypertensive reactions may be completely avoided by the availability of the MAO-B specific inhibitor deprenyl (Selegiline), which is now being incorporated into treatment regimes for Parkinson's disease (Jarrott and Vajda 1987). This drug is a potent, irreversible inhibitor of platelet MAO (which is the B form of the enzyme) but spares the A form of the enzyme, which therefore remains available to metabolize dietary amines.

The Recovery of MAO Activity in Platlet Density Subpopulations After Irreversible MAO Inhibition

Platelet MAO activity was measured in the total platelet population and in the five density subpopulations before drug ingestion (day 0) and 1,2,3,5,8 and 15 days afterwards. The MAO activities on day 15 did not differ significantly from the activities measured on day 0 and so the means of these two days were used as the baseline values. Mean MAO activity in the total platelet population was reduced to 21% of normal one day after drug ingestion and showed only a slight rise on day 2. This lag phase is thought to be due to inhibition of MAO activity in the megakaryocyte compartment. From day 2 to day 8 the MAO activity

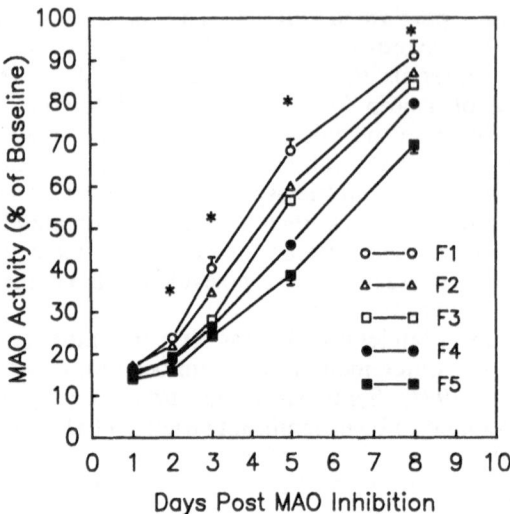

Fig. 5.10. Recovery of MAO activity in the platelet density subpopulations after inhibition by 20 mg of tranylcypromine on day 0 (mean±SEM, $N = 10$). Each MAO activity has been expressed as a percentage of the corresponding baseline activity. Error bars have only been shown for fraction 1 (LD) and fraction 5 (HD). Statistical comparisons of the percentage activities in fractions 1 and 5 were performed using paired sign tests: *$p < 0.01$. Based on data presented in Chamberlain et al. 1989a.

increased in a near-linear fashion and curve-fitting of the data points in this segment gave estimates of the megakaryocyte–platelet regeneration time (MPRT) (Chamberlain et al. 1988b). Further analysis of these data revealed a correlation between this measure of mean platelet life-span and mean platelet volume (Chamberlain and Penington 1988b).

The return of MAO activity in the density subpopulations showed different patterns to that found in the total platelet population (Chamberlain et al. 1989a). Fig. 5.10 shows the MAO activities in the density subpopulations expressed as percentages of their baseline values. While there were no significant differences in percentage MAO activity on day 1, between days 1 and 5 the rates of recovery in MAO activity were inversely proportional to platelet density. A lag phase was evident between days 1 and 2 in all density fractions but its extent appeared greater in the denser fractions. The extent of MAO recovery in the LD subpopulation (fraction 1) was significantly greater than the recovery in the HD subpopulation (fraction 5) on days 2, 3, 5 and 8 ($p < 0.01$, sign test). By day 8, MAO activity in the LD platelets had reached baseline in 4 out of the 10 subjects, while this had not occurred in any of the HD samples.

Interpretation of Labelling Studies of Density-Separated Platelets

The patterns of recovery of MAO activity in the different density subpopulations were very similar to the recovery patterns for human platelet cyclo-oxygenase activity after aspirin inhibition (Boneu et al. 1980; Mezzano et al. 1981;

McDonald and Ali 1983). The latter authors suggested two main interpretations of their results, which we have also tested against our own data. The simplest interpretation is that platelet life-span is correlated with platelet density. Thus the more rapid return of enzyme activity in the LD subpopulation would result from higher platelet turnover in this subpopulation. Mezzano et al. (1981) reported as counter-evidence to this view that labelled platelet subpopulations enriched in LD platelets survived in vivo for longer periods than subpopulations enriched in HD platelets. Boneu et al. (1982a) also eschewed this view since they found none of the expected narrowing of density distributions of radiolabelled platelets with time. If platelet turnover was correlated with platelet density, the regeneration curves for MAO activity in the density subpopulations would differ in slope but have essentially the same shape (linear or slightly concave downwards). Examination of Fig. 5.10 shows a slight increase in slope between days 5 and 8 for the two most dense fractions and this pattern is best explained by the second interpretation, which states that platelets increase slightly in density as they age. In this case the turnover of platelets in the LD subpopulation appears to be more rapid because platelets are being lost from this fraction by increasing their density as well as by removal from the circulation.

Supportive evidence for the latter hypothesis was obtained by Mezzano et al. (1981, 1984a) and Boneu et al. (1982a) using ^{51}Cr-labelled platelets. These authors reported that after reinfusion of a labelled total platelet population, the LD platelets lost radioactivity rapidly while the radioactivity of the HD platelets did not begin to decline for several days. Boneu et al. (1982a) also showed that the whole density distribution of the labelled platelets appeared to shift to higher densities during the first three days after reinfusion, and a similar result was reported by Martin and Penington (1983) in Japanese monkeys and Savage et al. (1986) in baboons.

We have found only one labelling study providing evidence that human platelets decline in density with age. Amorosi et al. (1971) labelled platelets in vivo using [^{75}Se]selenomethionine and found that the label was preferentially incorporated into dense platelets during the first few days after infusion. The use of discontinuous gradients of water-immiscible oils to separate the platelets and the small number of subjects studied reduce the value of this study in comparison with the opposing results obtained in all the other studies.

With this one exception, the labelling studies performed in humans support the concept of a slight increase in platelet density with age. In direct contrast to this, studies in rabbits using cohort labels (Charmatz and Karpatkin 1974; Rand et al. 1981; Corash and Shafer 1982) or total population labels (Rand et al. 1983; Packham et al. 1985) have consistently supported the hypothesis that young rabbit platelets are relatively dense and become less dense as they age in the circulation. There is evidence that rabbit platelets differ significantly from human platelets in several other ways. Rabbit platelets contain more dense granules than human platelets despite their smaller size; they circulate for less than one-third the human platelet life-span (Rand et al. 1983) and a much higher percentage of them appear to be destroyed randomly (Trowbridge and Martin 1983). Extrapolation from rabbit platelets to human platelets should be undertaken with caution. Results of labelling studies in other species have varied: baboons (Savage et al. 1986) and Japanese monkeys (Martin and Penington 1983) appear to follow the human pattern, while rhesus monkeys (Corash et al. 1978) and dogs (Mezzano et al. 1984b) appear to follow the rabbit pattern.

Possible Mechanisms for the Increase in Human Platelet Density with Platelet Age

The results of our labelling study may be explained by a shift in the whole density distribution to higher density during the circulating life of the platelets, although we cannot rule out the possibility that there is also a positive correlation between platelet life-span and platelet density. The radiolabelling experiments of Boneu et al. (1982a) and Watson and Ludlam (1986) in humans, Martin and Penington (1983) in monkeys and Savage et al. (1986) in baboons have shown density rises of 0.001–0.003 g/cm^3 when comparing a relatively aged population with a normal mixed platelet population. The total shift in density over the life-span of the platelet might be about twice this value – i.e. an average of about 0.004 g/cm^3. This represents a shift of about 10%–15% of the total width of the normal human density distribution (Martin et al. 1983a). We have suggested two possible mechanisms for such an increase in density (Chamberlain et al. 1989a).

The first possible mechanism would involve a slight shrinkage of the platelets due to a redistribution of water and electrolytes. Using the formula derived by Holme and Murphy (1983) for such transitions, a density change of 0.004 g/cm^3 would involve a decrease in volume of about 7%. Such a shrinkage could be caused by a change in the activity of ion pumps or leakage pathways in the plasma membrane. It is possible that the structural rearrangement of newly released platelets from elongated or teardrop shapes to the discoid form may involve some shrinkage and re-invagination of surface membrane.

The second mechanism would involve an increase in the glycogen content of platelets as they age in the circulation. Glycogen is moderately abundant in platelets and its density has been estimated by isopycnic centrifugation in aqueous media to be very high (1.6 g/cm^3) (Scott and Still 1970). The process of proplatelet formation has an absolute dependence on glycolysis (Handagama et al. 1987c) and is quite likely to lead to some depletion of glycogen stores and a consequent reduction in the density of the newly formed platelets. As the glycogen stores are repleted over subsequent days, the platelets may show a slight shift to higher densities. There is some evidence that the young platelets produced in response to acute thrombocytopenia have an increased content of glycogen (Ginsberg and Aster 1972). However, these platelets should not be taken as typical of normal young platelets since increased glycogen content has also been observed in the megakaryocytes after acute thrombocytopenia (Penington and Streatfield 1975). Increased platelet glycogen content has been observed after corticosteroid treatment (Payne 1981) and the rise after acute thrombocytopenia may also be a response to stress hormones. Morphometric analysis of the glycogen content of normal proplatelets should help to test this hypothesis.

Although platelet glycogen content may increase during the platelet life-span, most of the other structural determinants of platelet density are only formed during thrombopoiesis and are not likely to change significantly during the normal platelet life-span. The variation in properties such as the α-granule content may simply reflect a degree of randomness during platelet formation. The observations of Penington et al. (1976) that the organelle concentration in megakaryocyte cytoplasm seemed to be inversely related to megakaryocyte ploidy may also explain some of the variation in platelet composition. However, the relationship between the cytoplasm composition of megakaryocytes and platelets has been made less clear by the large rearrangements of megakaryocyte cytoplasm which are now thought to occur during proplatelet formation (Radley and Haller 1982). In vitro studies of platelet-forming megakaryocytes of defined ploidy should ultimately help to answer these questions.

Platelet Density Heterogeneity in Pathological States

Knowledge of the normal platelet density distribution and its determinants provides a firm basis for understanding the changes in platelet density which may arise in pathological states. Reduced platelet density has been reported after platelet storage in vitro (Holme and Murphy 1983), after cardiopulmonary bypass (Van Oost et al. 1983), in patients suffering from inherited platelet disorders (Vicic and Weiss 1983), acquired myeloproliferative disorders (Caranobe et al. 1980), cancer (Boneu et al. 1984) and diabetes (Collier et al. 1986). Increased platelet density has been reported within the first 12 hours after myocardial infarction (Martin et al. 1983c). Since platelet density is a complex property with many possible determinants, these findings cannot be interpreted without further measurements. In our own study on platelet changes after cardiopulmonary bypass, we found a significant decrease in modal platelet density without any alteration in mean platelet volume or platelet glycogen content. Platelet degranulation during bypass was confirmed by an eight-fold rise in plasma βTG concentration and a significant decrease of 22% in platelet βTG content. Direct counts of dense granules using mepacrine fluorescence also showed a significant decrease from a mean count of 6.0 to 5.0 granules/platelet (Chamberlain, Tong and Penington, unpublished observations). While degranulation was the likely cause of the density change in this situation, Collier et al. (1986) reported that the decreased platelet density in diabetic subjects was accompanied by normal levels of α-granule and dense granule markers. Platelets from these patients may have decreased glycogen levels, while the increase in platelet density after myocardial infarction may reflect increased glycogen levels induced by elevated levels of corticosteroid hormones (Payne 1981). The decrease in platelet density during in vitro storage probably reflects a combination of decreased glycogen content (Murphy and Gardner 1971), swelling (Holme and Murphy 1983), degranulation and lysis (Kalmin et al. 1983). Changes in the platelet density distribution may indicate clinically significant platelet activation, altered platelet metabolism or altered thrombopoiesis. It is clear, however, that interpretation of density changes requires further measurements to identify the key factors involved in each case.

Conclusions

While consensus in the field of platelet heterogeneity has not yet been achieved, the studies outlined above give strong support to certain views about the origin of platelet heterogeneity while leaving a range of other questions open for future investigation. The ability of megakaryocytes to extend long beaded processes in vitro, the detailed observations on proplatelet formation in bone marrow by scanning electron microscopy and the observation of detached proplatelet segments in the peripheral circulation all give strong support to the proplatelet theory of platelet formation. We need to develop a better understanding of the factors determining the position of the constriction sites in the proplatelet chains and of the actual process of fragmentation. These and other questions concerning the ultrastructure of proplatelets may best be answered by studying megakaryocytes in liquid culture stimulated by thrombopoietin preparations (Levin and Yee 1987). We also need further information on the life-span of proplatelets in vivo and whether or not they are sequestered in the lungs or other sites in the body. We also need more consistent data regarding the concentration of megakaryocytes in the lungs and peripheral circulation.

We believe that our studies show that human platelets do not decrease in density with age, in contrast to the reported behaviour of rabbit platelets. In humans the LD platelets are probably a slightly younger population than the HD platelets, but most platelet properties are determined during thrombopoiesis and any changes during the platelet life-span are probably minor under normal conditions. Platelet density analysis may still be a useful method of detecting certain platelet abnormalities such as significant in vivo degranulation. Further measurements will be needed in such cases to eliminate the ambiguity of platelet density changes.

This research was supported in part by grants from the National Heart Foundation of Australia and from the National Health and Medical Research Council of Australia.

References

Amorosi E, Garg SK, Karpatkin S (1971) Heterogeneity of human platelets. IV. Identification of a young population with [^{75}Se]selenomethionine. Br J Haematol 21:227–232

Bach AWJ, Lan NC, Johnson DL et al. (1988) cDNA cloning of human liver monoamine oxidase A and B: molecular basis of differences in enzymatic properties. Proc Natl Acad Sci 85:4934–4938

Ballem PJ, Segal GM, Stratton JR, Gernsheimer T, Adamson JW, Slichter S (1987) Mechanisms of thrombocytopenia in chronic autoimmune thrombocytopenic purpura. J Clin Invest 80:33–40

Becker RP, De Bruyn PPH (1976) The transmural passage of blood cells into myeloid sinusoids and the entry of platelets into the sinusoids: a scanning electron microscopic investigation. Am J Anat 145:183–206

Behnke O (1969) An electron microscope study of the rat megakaryocyte. II. Some aspects of platelet release and microtubules. J Ultrastruct Res 26:111–129

Behnke O (1970) Microtubules in disk-shaped blood cells. Int Rev Exp Pathol 9:1–92

Behnke O, Tinggaard Pedersen N (1974) Ultrastructural aspects of megakaryocyte maturation and platelet release. In: Baldini MG, Ebbe S (eds) Platelets: production, function, transfusion and storage. Grune & Stratton, New York, pp 21–31

Bessis M (1977) Blood smears reinterpreted. Springer, Berlin Heidelberg New York

Blajchman MA, Senyl AF, Hirsh J, Genton E, George JN (1981) Hemostatic function, survival and membrane glycoprotein changes in young versus old rabbit platelets. J Clin Invest 68:1289–1294

Bolton AE, Amess JAL, Lekhwani CP, Elliot P (1980) β-Thromboglobulin content of human blood platelets. Scand J Haematol 25:25–29

Boneu B, Sie P, Caranobe C, Nouvel C, Bierme R (1980) Malondialdehyde (MDA) reappearance in human platelet density populations after a single intake of aspirin. Thromb Res 19:609–620

Boneu B, Vigoni F, Boneu A, Caranobe C, Sie P (1982a) Further studies on the relationship between platelet buoyant density and age. Am J Haematol 13:239–246

Boneu B, Robert A, Sie P et al. (1982b) Coulter counter studies of hypotonic-induced macrothrombocytosis in normal subjects and in idiopathic thrombocytopenic purpura patients. Br J Haematol 51:305–311

Boneu B, Bugat R, Boneu A, Eche N, Sie P, Combes P-F (1984) Exhausted platelets in patients with malignant solid tumours without evidence of active consumption coagulopathy. Eur J Cancer Clin Oncol 20:899–903

Booyse FM, Hoveke TP, Rafelson ME (1968) Studies on human platelets. II. Protein synthetic activity of various platelet populations. Biochim Biophys Acta 57:660–663

Bunting (1909) Blood-platelet and megalokaryocyte reactions in the rabbit. J Exp Med 11:541–522

Caranobe C, Sie P, Nouvel C, Laurent G, Pris J, Boneu B. (1980) Platelets in myeloproliferative disorders. II. Serotonin uptake and storage: Correlations with mepacrine labelled dense bodies and with platelet density. Scand J Haematol 25:289–295

Caranobe C, Sie P, Boneu B (1982) Serotonin uptake and storage in human platelet density subpopulations. Br J Haematol 52:253–258

Chamberlain KG, Penington DG (1988a) Monoamine oxidase and other mitochondrial enzymes in density subpopulations of human platelets. Thromb Haemostas 59:29–33

Chamberlain KG, Penington DG (1988b) Correlation between megakaryocyte–platelet regeneration time and mean platelet volume. Thromb Res 50:739–744

Chamberlain KG, Froebel M, Macpherson J, Penington DG (1988a) Morphometric analysis of density subpopulations of normal human platelets. Thromb Haemostas 60:44–49

Chamberlain KG, Tong M, Chiu E, Penington DG (1988b) The use of monoamine oxidase inhibition to estimate megakaryocyte–platelet regeneration time (MPRT). Thromb Res 49:425–435

Chamberlain KG, Tong M, Chiu E, Penington DG (1989a) The relationship of human platelet density to platelet age: platelet population labelling by monoamine oxidase inhibition. Blood 73:1218–1225

Chamberlain KG, Seth P, Jones MK, Penington DG (1989b) Subcellular composition of platelet density subpopulations prepared using continuous Percoll gradients. Br J Haematol 72: 199–207

Charmatz A, Karpatkin S (1974) Heterogeneity of rabbit platelets. I. Employment of an albumin density gradient for the separation of a young platelet population identified with ^{75}Se-seleno-methionine. Thromb Diath Haemorrh 31:485–492

Clark MR (1988) Senescence of red blood cells: progress and problems. Physiol Rev 68:503–554

Collier A, Watson HHK, Matthews DM, Strain L, Ludlam CA, Clarke BF (1986) Platelet-density analysis and intraplatelet granule content in young insulin-dependent diabetics. Diabetes 35:1081–1084

Corash L (1989) The relationship between megakaryocyte ploidy and platelet volume. Blood Cells 15:81–107

Corash L, Shafer B (1982) Use of asplenic rabbits to demonstrate that platelet age and density are related. Blood 60:166–171

Corash L, Tan H, Gralnick HR (1977) Heterogeneity of human whole blood platelet subpopulations. I. Relationship between buoyant density, cell volume, and ultrastructure. Blood 49:71–87

Corash L, Shafer B, Perlow M (1978) Heterogeneity of human whole blood platelet subpopulations. II. Use of a subhuman primate model to analyse the relationship between density and platelet age. Blood 52:726–734

Corash L, Costa JL, Shafer B, Donlon JA, Murphy D (1984) Heterogeneity of human blood subpopulations. III. Density-dependent differences in subcellular constituents. Blood 64:185–193

Dawes J, Smith RC, Pepper DS (1978) The release, distribution, and clearance of human β-thromboglobulin and platelet factor 4. Thromb Res 12:851–861

De Bruyn PPH (1981) Structural substrates of bone marrow function. Seminars Haematol 18:179–193

Djaldetti M, Fishman P, Bessler H, Notti I (1979) SEM observations on the mechanism of platelet release from megakaryocytes. Thromb Haemostas 42:611–620

Duyvené de Wit LJ, Badenhorst PN, Heyns A du P (1987) Ultrastructural morphometric observations on serial sectioned human blood platelet subpopulations. Eur J Cell Biol 43:408–411

Eason CT, Pattison A, Howells DD, Mitcheson J, Bonner FW (1986) Platelet population profiles: significance of species variation and drug-induced changes. J Appl Toxicol 6:437–441

Eldor A, Levine RF, Caine YG, Hyam E, Vlodavsky I (1986) Megakaryocyte interaction with the subendothelial extracellular matrix. Prog Clin Biol Res 215:399–404

Fabris F, Randi ML, Casonato A, Zanon RDB, Bonvicini P, Girolami A (1984) Clinical significance of beta-thromboglobulin in patients with high platelet count. Acta Haemat 71:32–38

Files JC, Malpass TW, Yee EK, Ritchie JL, Harker LA (1981) Studies of human platelet α-granule release in vivo. Blood 58:607–618

Fox JEB, Phillips DR (1983) Polymerization and organization of actin filaments within platelets. Seminars Haematol 20:243–260

Garg SK, Amorosi EL, Karpatkin S (1971) Use of the megathrombocyte as an index of megakaryocyte number. New Engl J Med 284:11–17

Ginsberg AD, Aster RH (1972) Changes associated with platelet aging. Thromb Diath Haemorrh 27:407–415

Ginsberg MH (1981) Role of platelets in inflammation and rheumatic disease. Adv Inflammation Res 2:53–71

Haller CJ, Radley JM (1983) Time-lapse cinemicrography and scanning electron microscopy of platelet formation by megakaryocytes. Blood cells 9: 407–418

Han P, Butt RW, Turpie AGG, Walker WHC, Genton E (1980) Beta-thromboglobulin radioimmunoassay: a laboratory characterization and evaluation. J Immunoassay 1:211–227

Handagama PJ, Jain NC, Kono CS, Feldman BF (1986) Scanning electron microscopic studies of megakaryocytes and platelet formation in the dog and rat. Am J Vet Res 47:2454–2460

Handagama PJ, Feldman BF, Jain NC, Farver TB, Kono CS (1987a) Circulating proplatelets: isolation and quantitation in healthy rats and in rats with induced acute blood loss. Am J Vet Res 48:962–965

Handagama PJ, Jain NC, Feldman BF, Kono CS (1987b) Scanning electron microscope study of platelet release by canine megakaryocytes in vitro. Am J Vet Res 48:1003–1006

Handagama PJ, Feldman BF, Jain NC, Farver TB, Kono CS (1987c) In vitro platelet release by rat megakaryocytes: effect of metabolic inhibitors and cytoskeletal disrupting agents. Am J Vet Res 48:1142–1146

Handagama PJ, Jain NC, Feldman BF, Farver TB, Kono CS (1987d) In vitro platelet release by rat megakaryocytes: effect of heterologous antiplatelet serum. Am J Vet Res 48:1147–1149

Hanson SR, Slichter SJ (1985) Platelet kinetics in patients with bone marrow hypoplasia: evidence for a fixed platelet requirement. Blood 66:1105–1109

Haver VM, Gear ARL (1981) Functional fractionation of platelets. J Lab Clin Med 97:187–204

Hirsh J, Glynn MF, Mustard JF (1968) The effect of platelet age on platelet adherence to collagen. J Clin Invest 47:466–473

Holme S, Murphy S (1983) Platelet storage at 22 °C for transfusion: interrelationship of platelet density and size, medium pH, and viability after in vivo infusion. J Lab Clin Med 101:161–174

Jackson CW (1989) Animal models with inherited hematopoietic abnormalities as tools to study thrombopoiesis. Blood Cells 15:237–253

Jarrott B, Vajda FJE (1987) The current status of monoamine oxidase and its inhibitors. Med J Aust 146:634–638

Johnson CA, Abildgaard CF, Schulman I (1971) Functional studies of young versus old platelets in a patient with chronic thrombocytopenia. Blood 37:163–171

Joseph M, Auriault C, Capron A, Vorng H, Viens P (1983) A new function for platelets: IgE-dependent killing of schistosomes. Nature 303:810–812

Kalmin ND, Wilson MJ, Liles BA (1983) In vitro assessment of platelet damage during rotator storage. Am J Clin Pathol 79:719–721

Karpatkin S (1969a) Heterogeneity of human platelets. I. Metabolic and kinetic evidence suggestive of young and old platelets. J Clin Invest 48:1073–1082

Karpatkin S (1969b) Heterogeneity of human platelets II. Functional evidence suggestive of young and old platelets. J Clin Invest 48:1083–1087

Karpatkin S (1972) Human platelet senescence. Ann Rev Med 23:101–128

Karpatkin S (1978) Heterogeneity of human platelets. VI. Correlation of platelet function with platelet volume. Blood 51:307–316

Karpatkin S, Strick N (1972) Heterogeneity of human platelets. V. Differences in glycolytic and related enzymes with possible reference to platelet age. 51:1235–1242

Kieffer N, Guichard J, Farcet J-P, Vainchenker W, Breton-Gorius J (1987) Biosynthesis of major platelet proteins in human blood platelets. Eur J Biochem 164:189–195

Kraytman M (1973) Platelet size in thrombocytopenias and thrombocytosis of various origin. Blood 41:587–598

Larrimer NR, Balcerzak SP, Metz EN, Lee RE (1970) Surface structure of normal human platelets. Am J Med Sci 259:242–256

Leif RC, Vinograd J (1964) The distribution of buoyant density of human erythrocytes in bovine albumin solutions. Proc Natl Acad Sci 51:520–528

Leven RM, Nachmias VT (1988) Microtubule coils occur in intact megakaryocytes. Blood Cells 13:509–511

Leven RM, Yee MK (1987) Megakaryocyte morphogenesis stimulated in vitro by whole and partially fractionated thrombocytopenic plasma: a model system for the study of platelet formation. Blood 69:1046–1052

Levin J, Bessman JD (1983) The inverse relation between platelet volume and platelet number: abnormalities in hematologic disease and evidence that platelet size does not correlate with platelet age. J Lab Clin Med 101:295–307

Levine RF, Fedorko ME (1976) Isolation of intact megakaryocytes from guinea pig femoral marrow. Successful harvest made possible with inhibitors of platelet aggregation: enrichment achieved with a two-step separation technique. J Cell Biol 69:159–172

Lichman MA, Chamberlain JK, Simon W, Santillo PA (1978) Parasinusoidal location of megakaryocytes in marrow: A determinant of platelet release. Am J Haematol 4:303–312

Loftus JC, Choate J, Albrecht RM (1984) Platelet activation and cytoskeletal reorganization: high voltage electron microscopic examination of intact and triton-extracted whole mounts. J Cell Biol 98:2019–2025

Martin JF, Penington DG (1983) The relationship between the age and density of circulating ^{51}Cr labelled platelets in the sub-human primate. Thromb Res 30:157–164

Martin JF, Trowbridge EA (1982) Theoretical requirements for the density separation of platelets with comparison of continuous and discontinuous gradients. Thromb Res 27:513–522

Martin JF, Shaw T, Jakubowski J, Penington DG, Martin TJ (1981) Production of thromboxane B2 by platelets is related to their density. Thromb Haemost 46:198

Martin JF, Shaw T, Heggie J, Penington DG (1983a) Measurement of the density of human platelets and its relationship to volume. Br J Haematol 54:337–352

Martin JF, Slater DN, Trowbridge EA (1983b) Abnormal intrapulmonary platelet production: a possible cause of vascular and lung disease. Lancet i:793–796

Martin JF, Plumb J, Kilby RS, Kishk YT (1983c) Changes in platelet volume and density in myocardial infarction. Br Med J 287:456–459

Mattson JC, Zuiches CA (1981) Elucidation of the platelet cytoskeletal. Ann NY Acad Sci 370:11–21

McDonald JWD, Ali M (1983) Recovery of cyclo-oxygenase activity after aspirin in populations of platelets separated on Stractan density gradients. Prostaglandins Leukotrienes Med 12:245–252

McLeod DL, Shreeve MM, Axelrad AA (1976) Induction of megakaryocyte colonies with platelet formation in vitro. Nature 261:492–494

Mezzano D, Hwang K-L, Catalano P, Aster RH (1981) Evidence that platelet buoyant density, but not size, correlates with platelet age in man. Am J Hematol 11:61–76

Mezzano D, Aranda E, Rodriguez S, Foradori A, Lira P (1984a) Increase in density and accumulation of serotonin by human ageing platelets. Am J Hematol 17:11–21

Mezzano D, Aranda E, Foradori A, Rodriguez S, Lira P (1984b) Kinetics of platelet density subpopulations in splenectomised mongrel dogs. Am J Hematol 17:373–382

Minter FM, Ingram M (1970) Platelet volume: density relations in acutely bled dogs. Br J Haematol 20:55–68

Murphy S, Gardner FH (1971) Platelet storage at 22 °C: Metabolic, morphologic and functional studies. J Clin Invest 50:370–377

Muto M (1976) A scanning and transmission electron microscopic study on rat bone marrow sinuses and transmural migration of blood cells. Arch Histol Jap 39:51–66

Nubile G, Gregoria MD, Ridolfi D, D'Alonzo L, Izzi L (1987) Aggregazione piastrinca indotta da adenosin difosfata, collagene ed adrenalina nelle sottopopolazioni piastriniche umane. Quad Sclavo Diagn 23:331–340

Packham MA, Guccione MA, O'Brien KM (1985) Duration of the effect of aspirin on the synthesis of thromboxane by density subpopulations of rabbit platelets stimulated with thrombin. Blood 66:287–290

Paulus JM, Bury J, Grosdent JC (1979) Control of platelet territory development in megakaryocytes. Blood Cells 5:59–88

Paulus JM, Esch L, Grosdent JC, Goddet A (1986) Deviation from lognormality in platelet volume distributions: inferences about the mechanism of thrombopoiesis. Prog Clin Biol Res 215:417–426

Payne CM (1981) Platelet satellitism. Am J Pathol 103:116–128

Penington DG (1987) Thrombopoiesis. In: Bloom AL, Thomas DP (eds) Haemostasis and thrombosis (2nd edn). Churchill Livingstone, Edinburgh London Melbourne New York, pp 1–8

Penington DG, Streatfield K (1975) Heterogeneity of megakaryocytes and platelets. Ser Haemat 8:22–48

Penington DG, Tong M (1987) Correspondence. Blood 70:600–601

Penington DG, Streatfield K, Roxburgh AE (1976) Megakaryocytes and the heterogeneity of circulating platelets. Br J Haematol 34:639–653

Pryzwansky KB (1987) Human leukocytes as viewed by stereo high-voltage electronmicroscopy. Blood Cells 12:505–530

Pulvertaft RJV (1958) The effect of reduced oxygen tension on platelet formation in vitro. J Clin Pathol 11:535–542

Pulvertaft RJV, Humble JG (1956) Culture de moelle osseuse sur lames tournantes. Rev Hemat 11:349–377

Radley JM (1986) Ultrastructural aspects of platelet production. Prog Clin Biol Res 215:387–398

Radley JM (1988) Commentary. Blood Cells 13:459–461

Radley JM, Haller CJ (1982) The demarcation membrane system of the megakaryocyte: a misnomer. Blood 60:213–219

Radley JM, Haller CJ (1983) Fate of senescent megakaryocytes in the bone marrow. Br J Haematol 53:277–287

Radley JM, Hartshorn MA (1987) Megakaryocyte fragments and the microtubule coil. Blood Cells 12:603–610

Radley JM, Scurfield G (1980) The mechanism of platelet release. Blood 56:996–999

Radley JM, Hartshorn MA, Green SL (1987) The response of megakaryocytes with processes to thrombin. Thromb Haemostas 58:732–736

Rand ML, Greenberg JP, Packham MA, Mustard JF (1981) Density subpopulations of rabbit platelets: size, protein, and sialic acid content, and specific radioactivity changes following labelling with ^{35}S-sulphate in vivo. Blood 57:741–745

Rand ML, Packham MA, Mustard JF (1983) Survival of density subpopulations of rabbit platelets: use of ^{51}Cr- or ^{111}In-labelled platelets to measure survival of least dense and most dense platelets concurrently. Blood 61:362–367

Savage B, Mcfadden PR, Hanson SR, Harker LA (1986) The relation of platelet density to platelet age: survival of low- and high-density ^{111}Indium-labelled platelets in baboons. Blood 68:386–393

Savage B, Hanson SR, Harker LA (1988) Selective decrease in platelet dense granule adenine nucleotides during recovery from acute experimental thrombocytopenia and ensuing thrombocytosis in baboons. Br J Haematol 68:75–82

Scott RB, Still WJS (1970) Glycogen in human blood platelets. Isolation by ultracentrifugation and characteristics of the isolated particles. Blood 35:517–532

Scurfield G, Radley JM (1981) Aspects of platelet formation and release. Am J Hematol 10:285–296

Sharp GA, Weber K, Osburn M (1982) Centriole number and process formation in established neuroblastoma cells and primary dorsal root ganglion neurones. Eur J Cell Biol 29:97–103

Shaw T (1988) The role of blood platelets in nucleoside metabolism: regulation of megakaryocyte development and platelet production. Mutation Res 200:67–97

Silverman RB (1983) Mechanism of inactivation of monamine oxidase by *trans*-2-phenylcyclopropylamine and the structure of the enzyme–inactivator adduct. J Biol Chem 258:14766–14769

Simpson GM, Frederickson E, Palmer R, Pi E, Sloane RB, White K (1985) Platelet monoamine oxidase inhibition by deprenyl and tranylcypromine: implications for clinical use. Biol Psychiatr 20:680–684

Slater DN, Trowbridge EA, Martin JF (1983) The megakaryocyte in thrombocytopenia: a microscopic study which supports the theory that platelets are produced in the pulmonary circulation. Thromb Res 31:163–176

Soslau G, Giles J (1982) The loss of sialic acid and its prevention in stored human platelets. Thromb Res 26:443–455

Steiner M, Vancura S (1985) Asymmetrical loss of sialic acid from membrane glycoproteins during platelet aging. Thromb Res 40:465–471

Stenberg PE, Levin J (1989) Mechanisms of platelet production. Blood Cells 15:23–47

Stranova JE, Goheen MP, Hiu SL, Bruno E, Hoffman R (1986) Terminal cytoplasmic maturation of human megakaryocytes in vitro. Exp Hematol 14:919–929

Tavassoli M, Aoki M (1989) Localization of megakaryocytes in the bone marrow. Blood Cells 15:3–14

Thiery J-P, Bessis M (1956) Mecanisme de la plaquettogenese. Etude 'in vitro' par la microcinematographie. Rev Hematol 2:162–174

Thompson CB (1985) Selective consumption of large platelets during massive bleeding. Br Med J 291:95–96

Thompson CB, Jakubowski JA (1988) The pathophysiology and clinical relevance of platelet heterogeneity. Blood 72:1–8

Thompson CB, Jakubowski JA, Quinn PG, Deykin D, Valeri CR (1983a) Platelet size as a determinant of platelet function. J Lab Clin Med 101:205–213

Thompson CB, Love DG, Quinn PG, Valeri CR (1983b) Platelet size does not correlate with platelet age. Blood 62:487–494

Thompson CB, Jakubowski JA, Quinn PG, Deykin D, Valeri CR (1984) Platelet size and age determine platelet function independently. Blood 63:1372–1375

Tong M, Seth P, Penington DG (1987) Proplatelets and stress platelets. Blood 69:522–528

Trowbridge EA (1987) Correspondence. Blood 70:600

Trowbridge EA (1988) Pulmonary platelet production: A physical analogue of mitosis. Blood Cells 13:451–458

Trowbridge EA, Martin JF (1983) A biological approach to the platelet survival curve with criticism of previous interpretations. Phys Med Biol 28:1349–1368

Trowbridge EA, Martin JF, Slater DN (1982) Evidence for a theory of physical fragmentation of megakaryocytes, implying that all platelets are produced in the pulmonary circulation. Thromb Res 28:461–475

Trowbridge EA, Warren CW, Martin JF (1986) Platelet volume heterogeneity in acute thrombocytopenia. Clin Phys Physiol Meas 7:203–210

Van Oost BA, Van Hien-Hogg IH, Timmermans APM, Sixma JJ (1983) The effect of thrombin on the density distribution of blood platelets: detection of activated platelets in the circulation. Blood 62:433–438

Van Oost BA, Timmermans APM, Sixma JJ (1984) Evidence that platelet density depends on the α-granule content in platelets. Blood 63:482–485

Vicic WJ, Weiss HJ (1983) Evidence that α-granules are a major determinant of platelet density: studies in storage pool deficiency. Thromb Haemostas 50:878–880

Watson HHK, Ludlam CA (1986) Survival of 111-indium platelet subpopulations of varying density in normal and post splenectomised subjects. Br J Haematol 62:117–124

Weiss L (1965) The structure of bone marrow, functional interrelationships of vascular and hematopoietic compartments in experimental hemolytic anemia. J Morphol 117:467–538

White JG (1989) Commentary. Blood Cells 15:48–58

Williams N, Jackson H, Sheridan APC, Murphy MJ, Elste A, Moore MAS (1978) Regulation of megakaryocytosis in long-term murine bone marrow cultures. Blood 51:245–255

Wright JH (1906) The origin and nature of the blood plates. Boston Med Surg J 154:643–645

Wright JH (1910) The histogenesis of blood platelets. J Morphol 21:263–278

Yamada E (1957) The fine structure of the megakaryocyte in the mouse spleen. Acta Anat 29:267–290

Yamazaki H, Motomiya T, Watanabe C, Miyagawa N, Yahara Y, Okawa Y, Onozawa Y (1980) Consumption of larger platelets with decrease in adenine nucleotide content in thrombosis, disseminated intravascular coagulation, and postoperative state. Thromb Res 18:77–88

Zucker MB, Borrelli J (1954) Reversible alterations in platelet morphology produced by anticoagulants and by cold. Blood 9:602–608

Zucker-Franklin D, Petursson S (1984) Thrombocytopoiesis: Analysis by membrane tracer and freeze–fracture studies on fresh human and cultured mouse megakaryocytes. J Cell Biol 99:390–402

6 Characterization of Platelets and Megakaryocytes of the Wistar Furth Rat: An Animal Model with Inherently Large Mean Platelet Volume

C. W. Jackson, S. A. Steward and N. K. Hutson

Introduction

Mean platelet volume (MPV) varies from species to species, but is relatively constant among normal individuals of a given species (von Behrens 1972); however, the mechanisms whereby megakaryocyte cytoplasm is subdivided into platelets and platelet size is determined are not understood. Two hypotheses have been presented concerning this process. First, from ultrastructural studies, Penington et al. (1976) suggested that megakaryocytes of larger DNA content produced smaller platelets. Second, Trowbridge et al. (1984) and Martin et al. (1986) have hypothesized that platelet size is largely determined by fragmentation of megakaryocyte cytoplasm at bifurcations in the pulmonary vasculature and hence platelet size of normal individuals of a given species would be determined by the size of the smallest pulmonary vessels. Neither of these hypotheses has been directly tested.

Information about normal mechanisms has often been gained by study of abnormal individuals. The literature indicates that abnormal MPV is found in several clinical situations. Large MPV is associated with Bernard–Soulier syndrome (Bernard and Soulier 1948) and May–Hegglin anomaly (Godwin and Ginsburg 1974) as well as with other less well-defined thrombocytopathies (Epstein et al. 1972; Murphy et al. 1972; Eckstein et al. 1975; Hansen et al. 1978; Greaves et al. 1987) and in certain ethnic groups (von Behrens 1975a; Paulus 1975; von Behrens 1975b; Paulus and Casals 1978). In contrast, small MPV is present in patients with Wiskott–Aldrich syndrome (Murphy et al. 1972; Baldini 1971). Of these, structural abnormalities have been detected only in the Bernard–Soulier syndrome (deficiency of surface glycoprotein Ib–IX complex) (Nurden and Caen 1975) and in May–Hegglin anomaly (apparent qualitative defect in surface glycoprotein V) (Ricci et al. 1985). These are very rare patients on whom only limited studies can be performed. Recently, we serendipitously found that a small laboratory animal, the Wistar Furth rat, has an abnormally large MPV (Jackson et al. 1988). This chapter reviews and updates our studies of platelets and megakaryocytes in this animal model.

Materials and Methods

All rat strains including Wistar Furth, Wistar Kyoto, Wistar Munich, Wistar, Long–Evans and Sprague–Dawley, were purchased from Harlan Industries Inc., Indianapolis, Indiana. Rats of the Long–Evans strain were usually employed as reference controls because of our considerable data concerning platelets and megakaryocytopoiesis in this strain and because the black-and-white coat colour of Long–Evans rats allows them to be readily distinguished from the white Wistar Furth rats. Platelets were enumerated by phase-contrast microscopy. Other blood cells were quantified with an automated blood cell counter.

MPVs were measured using an electronic particle counter with a 48-μm diameter orifice and a 128-channel analyser. Blood for platelet size analysis was anticoagulated with Na$_2$EDTA at a final concentration of 12.5 mM. Platelets were separated from whole blood in self-generated Percoll (Pharmacia Inc., Piscataway, New Jersey) density gradients to facilitate recovery of the large platelets present in blood of Wistar Furth rats (Jackson et al. 1988). Analysis of platelet size was performed 2–6 hours after blood collection, a time period during which size of human platelets in EDTA-anticoagulated blood has been shown to be stable (Levin and Bessman 1983).

Platelet survival was evaluated after in vitro labelling of Percoll density gradient-isolated platelets with [^{111}In]indium oxine (Amersham Corp., Arlington Heights, Illinois).

The DNA distributions of megakaryocytes in unfractionated marrow were determined by two-colour flow cytometry as described earlier (Jackson et al. 1984). Megakaryocyte concentration and diameter were determined in longitudinal sternal marrow sections. Marrow megakaryocyte turnover time was estimated from [^{3}H]thymidine labelling index curves determined from autoradiograms of bone marrow smears after intravenous injection of 1 μCi/g body weight of [^{3}H]thymidine (specific activity 2.0 Ci/mmol, New England Nuclear, Boston, Massachusetts).

The aggregating ability of platelets in plasma was assessed with a dual-channel platelet aggregometer (Chrono-Log Corp., Havertown, Pennsylvania) using ADP and suspended equine collagen fibrils (Hormon-Chemie München GmbH, Munich, West Germany) as agonists.

For ultrastructural studies, platelets anticoagulated with 0.1 M acid citrate (pH 6.0) and 8 μM prostaglandin E$_1$ were separated from whole blood in Percoll density gradients and fixed in glutaraldehyde and post-fixed in osmium tetroxide. Small pieces of femoral marrow were similarly fixed in glutaraldehyde. In some cases, ruthenium red was added during glutaraldehyde fixation of platelets to examine whether internal membrane complexes were surface connected.

Platelet protein profiles were studied by one-dimensional SDS–polyacrylamide gel electrophoresis. Blood was collected from the dorsal aorta or via cardiac puncture of metofane-anaesthetized rats into syringes containing Na_2EDTA. Platelets were separated either by density gradient centrifugation in Percoll gradients or by differential centrifugation. Platelets were pelleted and washed three times in buffer (0.001 M Na_2EDTA, 0.01 M Hepes buffer and 0.15 M NaCl, pH 7.6). Platelets suspended in EHS buffer were solubilized by boiling for 5 min in one-third volume of gel sample buffer containing 0.125 M Tris–HCl, pH 6.8, 40% glycerol, 8% SDS, 160 mM dithiothreitol and 0.01% bromphenol blue. One-dimensional SDS–polyacrylamide gel electrophoresis was performed in 7.5%–15% linear gradients of acrylamide using the discontinuous buffer system of Laemmli (1970). Gels were stained with Coomassie blue.

Platelet surface glycoprotein profiles of Wistar Furth platelets were compared to those of Wistar, Long–Evans and Sprague–Dawley rats by examination of fluorograms of SDS-solubilized platelets separated by SDS–polyacrylamide electrophoresis after labelling with the periodate/NaB^3H_4 procedure (Liao et al. 1973) which primarily labels sialic acid residues.

Reciprocal bone marrow transplantation was performed between Wistar Furth and Long–Evans rats to determine whether the large MPV of Wistar Furth rats was related to an intrinsic megakaryocyte abnormality or some general metabolic trait. Rats were given a lethal exposure of whole-body irradiation using a ^{137}Cs source and one day later infused with marrow cells of the reciprocal or the same strain (Jackson et al. 1988). MPV was measured after platelet counts had recovered and stabilized.

Acute, severe thrombocytopenia was produced by intraperitoneal injection of heterologous platelet antiserum as previously described (Jackson et al. 1984).

Results

MPV of adult Wistar Furth rats were about twice those of Wistar, Long–Evans and Sprague–Dawley rats and two other Wistar substrains, while platelet count in the adult Wistar Furth rats was only one-third that of the other three strains and the Wistar Munich substrain and one-half that of the Wistar Kyoto substrain (Table 6.1). In contrast to the relatively constant MPV with age in Long–Evans rats (~4 fl), the mean platelet volume of Wistar Furth rats increased with age, from 6 fl at 3 weeks to 7 fl at 10 weeks, 8 fl at 18–22 weeks, and >9 fl at 52 weeks (Jackson et al. 1988). This increase in MPV with age was associated with a proportional decrease in platelet count, so that circulating platelet mass remained relatively constant.

Megakaryocyte concentration in marrow sections was about 30% lower in Wistar Furth compared to Wistar and Long–Evans rats, while average megakaryocyte diameter did not significantly differ among the three strains (Table 6.2).

DNA distributions of Wistar Furth megakaryocytes determined by two-colour flow cytometry were not significantly different from those of Long–Evans rats; 16N was the major DNA peak in both strains (Jackson et al. 1988).

Megakaryocyte turnover rate in Wistar Furth and Long–Evans rats, as estimated from labelling index curves generated from examination of megakaryo-

Table 6.1. Platelet counts and mean platelet volumes of Wistar Furth rats versus those of other rat strains

Rat strain	No. of rats	Platelet count $\times 10^3/mm^3$	MPV
Wistar Furth	17	308± 51[a]	8.5±1.4 (37)[b]
Wistar	11	1081± 68	4.0±0.3
Wistar Kyoto	4	640± 54	3.9±0.1
Wistar Munich	4	1064± 50	4.1±0.3
Long–Evans hooded	17	896±128	4.2±0.3 (30)
Sprague–Dawley	7	926± 82	4.1±0.2

Numbers in parentheses indicate number of rats studied when the number was different from that indicated in column 2.
[a] Mean±1 SD.
[b] MPV in this table were from adult animals ≥10 weeks of age.

Table 6.2. Marrow megakaryocyte concentration and size

Rat strain	No. of rats	Megakaryocyte concentration/ high-power field[b]	Average megakaryocyte diameter $(\mu m)^c$
Wistar Furth	7	4.5±0.6[a,d]	18.4±0.5
Wistar	5	6.7±0.5	18.4±0.5
Long–Evans	7	6.6±0.8	19.0±0.8

[a] Mean±1 SD.
[b] Megakaryocytes were counted in 17–88 (median 38) high-power fields for each rat.
[c] Diameters of 50 megakaryocytes were measured for each rat. Megakaryocyte diameter in fixed marrow sections is reduced due to shrinkage so that the average diameters reported here should only be considered relative.
[d] Average megakaryocyte concentration of Wistar Furth rats was significantly different from that of Wistar and Long–Evans rats ($p < 0.001$).

cytes in autoradiograms of marrow collected at increasing intervals after in vivo injection of [³H]thymidine, was not different (Jackson et al. 1988).

Platelet survival time, as measured by the in vivo disappearance of radioactivity after transfusion of platelets labelled in vitro with [¹¹¹In]indium oxine, was similar in Wistar Furth and Long–Evans rats (Jackson et al. 1988).

Reciprocal crosses of Wistar Furth × Long–Evans rats yielded offspring which all had mean platelet volumes like those of Long–Evans rats, indicating that the large platelet phenotype of Wistar Furth rats was inherited as an autosomal recessive characteristic. Backcrosses of these F_1 offspring with Wistar Furth rats yielded offspring among which the ratio of those with large MPV to those with normal MPV was approximately 1 : 1, suggesting that a difference at a single allele was responsible for the large platelet phenotype (Jackson et al. 1988).

Platelets of Wistar Furth rats showed similar aggregation responses to ADP and collagen as did those of Long–Evans rats (Jackson et al. 1988).

Ultrastructural analysis revealed that platelets of Wistar Furth rats frequently contained large abnormal membrane complexes, often larger than 1 μm in diameter (Jackson et al. 1988). No granules or other organelles were observed in these membranous regions. These membrane complexes stained with ruthenium red, indicating that they were surface connected. Such membrane mazes were not observed in Long–Evans platelets. Microtubules appeared to be normally distributed in Wistar Furth platelets.

The cytoplasm of Wistar Furth megakaryocytes often contained similar membrane complexes and disordered demarcation membrane arrangements (Jackson et al. 1988).

Wistar Furth platelets also differ from Wistar platelets in their protein profiles, as studied by one-dimensional SDS–polyacrylamide gel electrophoresis. Wistar Furth platelets consistently show decreased quantities of proteins with apparent molecular weights of 60 000, 16 000 and 8500 (Fig. 6.1). The membrane glycoprotein pattern of Wistar Furth platelets, studied by mild periodate treatment followed by labelling with [^{3}H]sodium borohydride and fluorography, revealed no abnormalities in the major glycoprotein bands (Jackson et al. 1988).

Reciprocal bone marrow transplantations were performed between Wistar Furth and Long–Evans rats to establish whether the large MPV phenotype of Wistar Furth rats results from an intrinsic characteristic of the megakaryocytic series or is related to a more general metabolic trait of these rats. MPV of recipient rats after marrow reconstitution were like those of the marrow donor strain, indicating that the large platelet phenotype is an intrinsic characteristic of Wistar Furth megakaryocytes (Jackson et al. 1988).

MPV of Wistar Furth rats increased in response to platelet antiserum-induced, acute, severe thrombocytopenia (platelet counts to <5% of baseline at 24 hours) in a similar fashion to that of Long–Evans rats; however, recovery of Wistar Furth platelet counts to pretreatment levels required 5 days, compared to 4 days for platelets of Long–Evans rats (Jackson et al. 1988). This slower platelet recovery of Wistar Furth rats may be attributed to the smaller shift to the right in megakaryocyte DNA distribution seen in response to thrombocytopenia in this strain compared to that in Long–Evans rats (Jackson et al. 1988). Megakaryocyte concentration increased to a similar degree in both rat strains after induction of this degree of thrombocytopenia.

Discussion

The primary determination of platelet size must take place during megakaryocyte maturation. Abnormally large platelets most likely result from incomplete or disordered subdivision of megakaryocytes into platelets. The Wistar Furth rat has macrothrombocytopenia (large MPV with reduced platelet count) with increased platelet size heterogeneity. Paulus et al. (1979) have reported that platelet size heterogeneity is inversely related to platelet count even in healthy subjects. He suggested that large MPV results from diminished or incomplete demarcation membrane formation and that the increased platelet size heterogeneity associated with larger MPV occurs because platelet demarcation is erratic when it is incomplete. The autosomal recessive inheritance pattern of the large MPV in Wistar Furth rats would be consistent with a qualitative or quantitative abnormality in some component necessary for subdivision of megakaryocyte cytoplasm into platelets. Consistent deficiencies in three proteins with apparent molecular

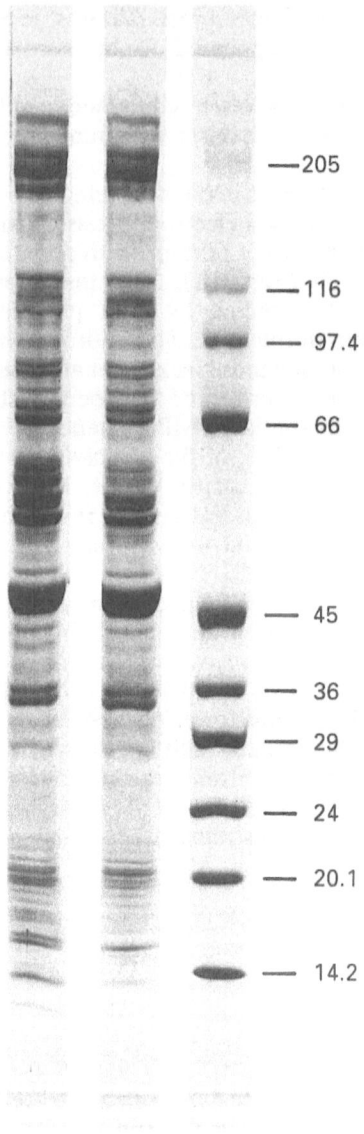

W   WF

Fig. 6.1. Comparison of protein profiles of SDS-solubilized platelets from Wistar Furth and Wistar rats separated in 7.5%–15% linear gradients of acrylamide by SDS–polyacrylamide electrophoresis and stained with Coomassie blue. *W*, Wistar platelets; *WF*, Wistar Furth platelets. The numbers on the right are molecular weights (in thousands) of molecular weight markers (*right-hand lane*) electrophoresed in parallel with the platelets.

weights of 60 000, 16 000 and 8500 were detected in platelets of Wistar Furth rats by SDS–polyacrylamide gel electrophoresis. Whether the large MPV of Wistar Furth rats is related to a deficiency of one or more of these proteins cannot be determined at this point. The large platelets seen in classical Bernard–Soulier syndrome are deficient in the glycoprotein Ib–IX complex (Nurden and Caen 1975). Whether the large platelets in this syndrome are a direct result of a deficiency of the glycoprotein Ib–IX complex cannot be discerned at this point. Glycoprotein Ib does not appear to be decreased in Wistar Furth rat platelets as studied by periodate-[^{3}H]borohydride labelling (Jackson et al. 1988). Nevertheless, the report by Fox (1985) that some membrane glycoproteins such as glycoprotein Ib are linked to the platelet membrane skeleton raises the possibility that these large membrane–skeletal protein complexes may play a role in platelet size determination.

Our observation that the MPV of recipients after reciprocal marrow transplants between the Wistar Furth and Long–Evans strains is like that of the marrow donor suggests that the macrothrombocytopenia of Wistar Furth rats results from an intrinsic megakaryocyte abnormality; however, the age-related increase in MPV in Wistar Furth rats suggests that the extent of expression of the megakaryocyte abnormality is influenced by some age-related metabolic trait such that less subdivision of megakaryocyte cytoplasm occurs with increasing age, resulting in larger platelets.

In addition to the abnormally large MPV, Wistar Furth rats also showed about a 30% lower marrow megakaryocyte concentration than Wistar and Long–Evans rats. The larger MPV would not seem to be the consequence of lower megakaryocyte concentration in the Wistar Furth strain since the mouse mutants W/W^v (Ebbe et al. 1973a) and S1/S1^d (Ebbe et al. 1973b), with low megakaryocyte concentrations, produce platelets with normal mean platelet volumes. It should also be pointed out that in contrast to those of W/W^v (Ebbe et al. 1973a) and S1/S1^d (Ebbe et al. 1973b; Ebbe et al. 1986) mice, megakaryocytes of Wistar Furth rats do not show increased size and DNA content (Jackson et al. 1988).

Megakaryocytes of Wistar Furth rats also have a muted response to acute, severe thrombocytopenia in that although the proportion of 32N and 64N megakaryocytes increases, the megakaryocyte DNA distribution never shows a shift from 16N to 32N as the major DNA peak after 2–3 days as do rats of the Long–Evans (Jackson et al. 1988) and Sprague–Dawley (Penington and Olsen 1970) strains. This muted megakaryocyte response probably explains the slower post-thrombocytopenia platelet recovery rate in Wistar Furth rats (Jackson et al. 1988). The reason for this reduced megakaryocyte response is not clear, but of the possibilities, reduced responsiveness of Wistar Furth megakaryocytes to thrombopoietic-stimulating factor seems the most likely.

A number of patients have been reported with hereditary macrothrombocytopenia, some with associated platelet functional defects (Bernard and Soulier 1948; Epstein et al. 1972; Murphy et al. 1972; Eckstein et al. 1975; Greaves et al. 1987), some without (Godwin and Ginsberg 1974; von Behrens 1975a, b; Paulus 1975; Hansen et al. 1978). The largest group of such patients would appear to be those with Mediterranean macrothrombocytopenia who have a large MPV with reduced platelet count and normal platelet function (von Behrens 1972) and survival (Paulus and Casals 1978). By electron microscopy, the equatorial arrangement of microtubules in platelets of these patients is more haphazard than normal (von Behrens 1975b), but the maze-like membrane complexes observed in Wistar Furth platelets (Jackson et al. 1988) and in other thrombocytopenias (Epstein et al. 1972; Breton-Gorius 1975) have not been observed (Paulus et al. 1974). The age-related increase in MPV we observed in Wistar Furth rats was not seen in patients with Mediterranean macrothrombocytopenia (von Behrens 1975b). Dohle bodies were not detected in Wistar Furth granulocytes, suggesting that this rat model is not analogous to the May–Hegglin anomaly in man. Renal disease and deafness associated with macrothrombocytopenia in a group of patients reported by Epstein et al. (1972) and others (Eckstein et al. 1975; Hansen et al. 1978) has not been detected in Wistar Furth rats. Thus, the characteristics of the macrothrombocytopenia in Wistar Furth rats do not entirely mimic those reported in any of the clinical hereditary macrothrombocytopenias but, of these, they probably most closely resemble Mediterranean macrothrombocytopenia.

What this rat model has revealed about determination of platelet size can be summarized as follows:

1. Platelet size is primarily determined during megakaryocyte maturation and is an intrinsic characteristic of megakaryocytes of a given strain. This is based on our observation that MPV after reciprocal bone marrow transplantation between Wistar Furth and Long–Evans rats were like those of the marrow donors.

2. The autosomal recessive inheritance pattern of the large MPV phenotype in Wistar Furth rats suggests that large platelets can result from quantitative or qualitative abnormalities of some structural component(s). The decreases in some protein bands in Wistar Furth platelets may represent such abnormalities.

Further characterization of the protein deficiencies of Wistar Furth platelets and study of their possible association with the large MPV phenotype in these rats may yield further insights into the process of platelet formation.

Supported in part by US Public Health Service grants HL 31598, CA 21765 and CA 20180 awarded by The National Institutes of Health, Department of Health and Human Services and by the American Lebanese Syrian Associated Charities.

References

Baldini MG (1971) Increased platelet destruction: hereditary intrinsic defects. In: Paulus JM (ed) Platelet kinetics. North-Holland, Amsterdam, pp 287–295

Bernard J, Soulier J (1948) Sur une nouvelle variste de dystrophie thrombocytaire hemorragipare congenitale. Sem Hop Paris 24:3217

Breton-Gorius J (1975) Development of two membrane systems associated in giant complexes in pathological megakaryocytes. Ser Haematol 8:49–67

Ebbe S, Phalen E, Stohlman F, Jr (1973a) Abnormalities of megakaryocytes in W/W^v mice. Blood 42:857–864

Ebbe S, Phalen E, Stohlman F, Jr (1973b) Abnormalities of megakaryocytes in Sl/Sl^d mice. Blood 42:865–871

Ebbe S, Bentfeld-Barker M, Adrados C et al. (1986) Functionally abnormal stromal cells and megakaryocyte size, ploidy, and ultrastructure in Sl/Sl^d mice. Blood Cells 12:217–232

Eckstein JD, Filip DJ, Watts JC (1975) Hereditary thrombocytopenia, deafness, and renal disease. Ann Intern Med 82:639–644

Epstein CJ, Sahud MA, Piel CF et al. (1972) Hereditary macrothrombocytopathia, nephritis and deafness. Am J Med 52:299–310

Fox JEB (1985) Linkage of a membrane skeleton to integral membrane glycoproteins in human platelets: Identification of one of the glycoproteins as glycoprotein Ib. J Clin Invest 76:1673–1683

Godwin HA, Ginsburg AD (1974) May–Hegglin anomaly: a defect in megakaryocyte fragmentation? Br J Haematol 26:117–128

Greaves M, Pickering C, Martin J, Cartwright I, Preston FE (1987) A new familial giant platelet syndrome with structural, metabolic and functional abnormalities of platelets due to a primary megakaryocyte defect. Br J Haematol 65:429–435

Hansen MS, Behnke O, Pedersen NT, Videbak A (1978) Megathrombocytopenia associated with glomerulonephritis, deafness and aortic cystic medianecrosis. Scand J Haematol 21:197–205

Jackson CW, Brown LK, Somerville BC, Lyles SA, Look AT (1984) Two-color flow cytometric measurement of DNA distributions of rat megakaryocytes in unfixed, unfractionated marrow cell suspensions. Blood 63:768–778

Jackson CW, Hutson NK, Steward SA et al. (1988) The Wistar Furth rat: an animal model of hereditary macrothrombocytopenia. Blood 71:1676–1686

Laemmli UK (1970) Cleavage of structural proteins during the assembly of the head of bacteriophage T4. Nature (London) 227:680

Levin J, Bessman JD (1983) The inverse relation between platelet volume and platelet number. J Lab Clin Med 101:295–307

Liao T-H, Gallop PM, Blumenfeld OO (1973) Modification of sialyl residues of sialoglycoprotein(s) of the human erythrocyte surface. J Biol Chem 248:8247–8253

Martin JF, Slater DN, Trowbridge EA (1986) Evidence that platelets are produced in the pulmonary circulation by a physical process. In: Levine RF, Williams N, Levin J, Evatt BL (eds) Megakaryocyte development and function. Liss, New York, pp 405–416

Murphy S, Oski FA, Naiman JL, Lusch CJ, Goldberg S, Gardner FH (1972) Platelet size and kinetics in hereditary and acquired thrombocytopenia. N Engl J Med 286:499–504

Nurden AT, Caen JP (1975) Specific roles for platelet surface glycoproteins in platelet function. Nature 255:720–722

Paulus JM (1975) Platelet size in man. Blood 46:321–336

Paulus JM, Casals FJ (1978) Platelet formation in Mediterranean macrothrombocytosis. Nouv Rev Franc Hemat 20:151–154

Paulus JM, Breton-Gorius J, Kinet-Denoel C, Boniver J (1974) Megakaryocyte ultrastructure and ploidy in human macrothrombocytosis. In: Baldini MG, Ebbe S (eds) Platelets: production, function, transfusion and storage. Grune & Stratton, New York, p 131–141

Paulus JM, Bury J, Grosdent JC (1979) Control of platelet territory development in megakaryocytes. Blood Cells 5:59–88

Penington DG, Olsen TE (1970) Megakaryocytes in states of altered platelet production: Cell numbers, size and DNA content. Br J Haematol 18:447–463

Penington DG, Streatfield K, Roxburgh AE (1976) Megakaryocytes and the heterogeneity of circulating platelets. Br J Haematol 34: 639–653

Ricci G, Manservigi R, Albonici L, Zavagli G, Cassai E (1985) Evidence for glycoprotein abnormality in platelets from patients with May–Hegglin anomaly. Thromb Haemostas 54:862–865

Trowbridge EA, Martin JF, Slater DH et al. (1984) The origin of platelet count and volume. Clin Phys Physiol Meas 5:145–170

von Behrens WE (1972) Evidence of phylogenetic canalization of the circulating platelet mass in man. Thromb Diath Haemorrh 27:159–172

von Behrens WE (1975a) Splenomegaly, macrothrombocytopenia and stomatocytosis in healthy Mediterranean subjects (splenomegaly in Mediterranean macrothrombocytopenia). Scand J Haematol 14:258–267

von Behrens WE (1975b) Mediterranean macrothrombocytopenia. Blood 46:199–208

Technical Questions

Martin: Did you measure platelet mass?
Jackson: In the normal Wistar Furth rat?

Martin: Yes.

Jackson: The platelet mass is about 30% lower, in agreement with the 30% lower megakaryocyte number in that rat strain.

Martin: Did you study bleeding times?

Jackson: No, we have not done that. However, I would not expect to see a bleeding abnormality in these animals because surgery has been performed many times, not by us but by others, and no abnormality has been reported.

7 The Circulating Megakaryocyte, Platelet Volume Heterogeneity and Thrombopoiesis

E. A. Trowbridge

The Concept of Bone Marrow Thrombopoiesis: How Did It Start?

In 1906 Wright used a Romanowsky polychrome stain to establish that blood platelets were detached fragments of megakaryocyte (MK) cytoplasm. Subjective assessment of fixed thin sections viewed through a light microscope led him to conclude: "Loss of cytoplasm occurs chiefly by the detachment of buds or plate-like fragments, from pseudopods, or of whole pseudopods." The presence of MKs with pseudopodia, in the marrow, has been confirmed using electron microscopy (Behnke 1969; Becker and De Bruyn 1976; Muto 1976; Lichtman et al. 1978; Slater et al. 1983a). Filamentous extensions of MK cytoplasm have been observed in culture (Thiery and Bessis 1956; Radley and Scurfield 1980; Haller and Radley 1983; Radley and Hartshorn 1987). It has been assumed that they correspond to the cytoplasmic protrusions seen by Wright (1906, 1910) in his sections. Unfortunately, MKs have never been observed producing platelets in the marrow, or in culture for that matter, from pseudopodia. The in vivo studies have been constrained by the necessity to interpret dynamic events by static representations. The culture studies allow megakaryocytes to be observed dynamically by microcinematography, but introduce conditions that may not apply in vivo. Radley and Hartshorn (1987) state: "This system has so far not revealed details of the sequence in which release occurs, since the spontaneous rupture of the processes or liberation of individual platelets has not been observed regardless of monitoring for long periods by time-lapse cinematography." Indeed, it has been suggested that failure to produce platelets from the cytoplasmic processes, containing putative platelets, observed in culture, may be an artefact produced by a reaction to the culture medium (White 1987). Nevertheless the subjective interpretation imposed by Wright in 1906 still dominates present-day thinking and teaching about platelet production and its influence on platelet heterogeneity. This is most surprising, when all the facts that are available are considered and a logical interpretation is applied to the data.

The Megakaryocyte Demarcation Membrane System and Platelet Territories

Megakaryocytes are large polyploid cells, with a wide range of volumes. Some MKs are as small as 1000 fl while others are over 50 000 fl in size. This means they are 10–500 times as large as the average size of the human red blood cell. Approximately four-fifths of this volume is cytoplasm, which contains various organelles and an extensive invaginated demarcation membrane system (DMS). The expression DMS was used after Yamada (1957) suggested that this membrane delineated future platelets in the MK cytoplasm. Three-dimensional freeze–fracture studies by Shaklai and Tavassoli (1978) confirmed earlier two-dimensional electron microscopic observations by Behnke (1968) that the DMS nearly always appears as a tubular arrangement. The membrane does not surround a volume of cytoplasm and so does not delineate platelets in a three-dimensional sense. Recognizing this deficiency in the argument for predelineation of "platelet territories" Shaklai and Tavassoli (1978) proposed a mechanism of tubular fusion followed by membrane fission to explain how a tubular system can be transformed into the flat membranes that are necessary for enclosure of the cytoplasm of the platelet. The biological control mechanism for this process was not discussed.

Radley and Haller (1982) have suggested that DMS may be a misnomer. In their in vitro studies they observed longitudinally arranged microtubules and a limited amount of invaginated membrane in thin sections of MK cytoplasmic processes. However, when cells with similar filamentous processes were treated with vincristine or exposed to low temperature the microtubules disassembled, the attenuated processes retracted, and an extensive tubular system was reformed. Radley and Haller (1982) argued that the tubular invaginations act as a membrane reserve for the attenuated processes, rather than delineating platelets. They proposed that the membrane reserve undergoes evagination during formation of the filamentous processes. This seems an attractive hypothesis for channels that are long, single tubes, even when tortuous and branched. However, the freeze–fracture studies of Shaklai and Tavassoli (1978) show this not to be the case. The invaginated system exists as a complex of interacting channels involving fusion and branching so that there is communication between many of the invaginations. White (1983) has suggested that this complex of intracytoplasmic tunnels would be torn apart in simple evagination. In addition the process of evagination, loss of DMS and cytoplasmic attentuation does not explain the presence of the interconnecting system of canaliculi in the platelet. This complex of interacting channels, just as in the MK, can stretch from one side of the cell to the other (White, 1983). Despite these apparent inconsistencies the process of growth and demarcation of "platelet territories" has been proposed as a mechanism for platelet volume heterogeneity (Paulus et al. 1979). This model does not address the problem of platelet release from the MK nor does it identify the mechanism of biological control over the growth and demarcation which is supposed to determine platelet size.

The surface area of the MK alone is not sufficient to provide the total surface area of the platelets it produces. Based on the simplest geometrical shape of a sphere, the volume of the MK, V_M, is related to its surface area, A_M, by the equation

$$A_M = (4 \pi)^{1/3} (3 V_M)^{2/3}$$

For the sake of argument, if this MK produces 1000 platelets then the mean volume of these platelets will be $V_M/1000$. Thus the mean surface area of the platelets, A_P, will be given by

$$A_P = (4 \pi)^{1/3} (3 V_M/1000)^{2/3}$$

The total surface area, A_T, of the 1000 platelets that make up the cytoplasm is

$$A_T = 1000 A_P = 1000 (4 \pi)^{1/3} (3 V_M/1000)^{2/3}$$

Hence $A_T/A_M = 1000^{1/3} = 10$. Thus, there must be 10 times the surface area of the plasma membrane of the MK available for each platelet to have a surface membrane. If the MK produces fewer than a 1000 platelets, these will be larger platelets and the demand for surface membrane will be less than a factor of 10. Conversely, if more than 1000 platelets are produced from the MK then the platelets will be smaller, but the total surface membrane of the platelets will be greater than 10 times that of the surface membrane of the MK. It seems that the DMS is the only source of membrane reserve available but, as later sections of this chapter will show, the membrane evagination suggested by Radley and Haller (1982) is not a prerequisite for platelet production. The DMS is continuous with the boundary plasma membrane (Behnke 1968; MacPherson 1972) and shares histochemical and ultrastructural characteristics with both the outer coat and the surface-connected canalicular system of the platelet (Behnke 1968, 1969; Zucker-Franklin and Petursson 1986). Hence, in normal circumstances, the amount of DMS synthesized by the MK is much more than that needed for the simple requirement of providing the surface coat of the platelet. This observation also suggests that development of the DMS may not be related directly to platelet production by territory delineation, but may be simply a consequence of the unique position of the MK in cell biology.

The MK undergoes endoreduplication in the later stages of maturation. Binary chromosomal reduplication occurs without concomitant nuclear and cytoplasmic division. Hence the nuclear DNA content of the cell follows a binary geometrical progression with each endoreduplication to produce a polyploid cell. The normal mitotic cell is diploid, but before cytokinesis sufficient new plasma membrane is synthesized to provide a surface covering for the two daughter cells created from the original mother cell. If A_M is the surface area of membrane just before cytokinesis and V is the volume of the cell at that instant, then $A_M = (4\pi)^{1/3} (3V)^{2/3}$, based on the simplest geometry of a sphere. However, the size of the mother cell, V, must be twice the size, $V/2$, of each the two daughter cells it is about to produce, assuming minimal protein synthesis to produce cytoplasm after cytokinesis. If A_C is the surface area of the daughter cell then $A_C = (4\pi)^{1/3} (3V/2)^{2/3}$. The total area of cell membrane after cytokinesis will be $2A_C = 2^{1/3} A_M$. Hence the cell has to generate 26% more membrane just before cytokinesis to provide the necessary surface covering (Penington 1981). In the MK the cytoplasm does not divide but, if the cell is still programmed to produce the appropriate amount of membrane, a 4N megakaryocyte will possess 26% more membrane than the 2N cell. However, it will not need this excess 26% to surround the cytoplasm because the cell has not divided into two. The only way this extra membrane can be accommodated is by invagination within the cytoplasm. As far as membrane synthesis is concerned the 4N MK is equivalent to two 2N cells, each of which is programmed to produce 26% more membrane at the next endoreduplication. Hence the 8N cell has 52% more membrane than it needs to cover its outer surface. Continuing this argument, 16N cells have 104% excess membrane and the membrane in 32N cells is in excess by 208%. This analysis may explain why Penington et al. (1976) observed a greater amount of DMS in 32N MKs than in 8N cells. These workers also separated platelets by density and observed that the most dense platelets were larger than the least dense platelets. The former cells had less canalicular system than the latter cells. On this basis they argued that the large most dense cells arise from 8N MKs and the small least dense cells come from 32N MKs. How this happens, in other words what is the mechanism of thrombopoiesis, was not discussed. If platelets are produced in the marrow from cytoplasmic protrusions and the invaginated DMS is not an integral part of the MK cytoplasmic processes in the marrow (Radley and Haller 1982) then it is difficult to see how the different amounts of DMS seen in the different MK ploidy classes influence platelet size. The concepts of platelet production from MK cytoplasmic processes and DMS predetermination are incompatible. Nevertheless, the histochemical and ultrastructural similarities between the DMS and the platelet surface coat, mentioned earlier, do suggest that the DMS has some part to play in thrombopoiesis. It follows that an alternative explanation must be found for the MK pseudopodia observed in marrow sections and in culture. Behnke (1969), in his electron microscopic study of rat MKs, identified this problem and also hinted at an alternative reason for the cytoplasmic processes. He reported:

Despite an extensive search we were never able to obtain pictures that might be interpreted as the liberation of "platelet areas" from a spherical megakaryocyte. With the formation of cytoplasmic extensions the apparent subdivision of the cytoplasm into "platelet areas" subsides. Naturally electron micrographs only give instantaneous records of the dynamic process taking place during platelet liberation; an alternative interpretation of the cytoplasm of a megakaryocyte protruding into the sinusoid is that the megakaryocyte shown was fixed in the initial stage of diapedesis through the sinusoidal wall and that the whole cell was entering the circulation.

Diapedesis and Sinusoidal Megakaryocytes

Tavassoli and Aoki (1981) have provided direct electron microscopic evidence that MKs in their entirety migrate through the vessel wall. MKs, like other haemopoietic cells, develop and mature in the extravascular compartment of the marrow. Hence to enter the circulation they must pass through the sinus endothelial barrier separating the marrow from the blood. The migratory pathway of the selective transmural diapedesis of other haemopoetic cells is usually transcellular. For example, De Bruyn et al. (1971) have described the selective entry of mature myeloid cells into bone marrow sinusoids. Farr and De Bruyn (1975) have documented the selective return of lymphocytes from the circulation into the lymphatic tissue via the postcapillary venular endothelium. Diapedesis occurs through relatively rigid endothelial apertures, with a diameter of 3–4 μm, and not between the junction of two endothelial cells. Therefore, migrating cells must be deformable before they can pass this barrier and enter the circulation.

This presents a problem if the nucleus of the haemopoietic cell is relatively rigid. For example, the nuclear material in the red cell can be extruded during its passage across the endothelial barrier (Tavassoli and Crosby 1973). The size of the bone marrow MK with a mean diameter of 25 μm, and the presence of a multilobed nucleus, suggests that migration of the entire cell into the circulation through an opening of 3–4 μm demands a marked degree of deformability of both the cytoplasm and nucleus. Nevertheless, the pictures presented by Tavassoli and Aoki (1981) show an entire MK, complete with nucleus, squeezing through an endothelial cell. Serial sections through the area of migration indicate continuity of membrane below the endothelial aperture, whose maximum width was 6 μm. This event was not unique; transendothelial passage of other MKs was also observed. In addition MKs frequently extended cytoplasmic projections into the lumen, but these projections could be classified into two separate groups. The most frequent type were small, short, multiple projections of length 1–2 μm. These processes were free from organelles. Similar processes have been reported in a more recent study by Slater et al. (1983a). The second type of projection contained the normal spectrum and concentration of cytoplasmic organelles. These processes were larger, usually single, and less frequent than the organelle-free projections. Tavassoli and Aoki (1981) concluded, like Behnke (1969) before them, that the latter projections may represent an early stage of diapedesis. In contrast, they argued that the organelle-free processes were not linked to cell delivery, but were more likely to serve as an "anchorage" or a "monitoring" system for the extravascular cell. They drew an analogy with a similar "anchorage" and "screening" system demonstrated by cordal macrophages in the spleen (Tavassoli and Weiss 1973). Without organelles, it is unlikely that these processes could give rise to individual platelets by "budding".

Becker and De Bruyn (1976) coined the phrase "proplatelet" cytoplasm to describe the long (120 μm) cylindrical cytoplasmic projections with a diameter of 2.5 μm that they observed emanating from some bone marrow MK in the rat. Based on a mean MK diameter of 20.9 μm obtained from Harker (1968) and a nuclear diameter half that of the MK diameter, they calculated that the volume of cytoplasm associated with an average-sized MK was about 4000 fl. (It should be pointed out at this stage that Harker's fixation technique resulted in cell shrinkage of around 25%.) The cylindrical cytoplasmic process had a volume of 600 fl, so they concluded that about six proplatelets may arise from one MK on average. Becker and De Bruyn (1976) argued that the concept of platelet territories was based on extravascular liberation of platelets. This would then entail transmural diapedesis by individual platelets, a mechanism which they could not confirm by serial section techniques. Hence they postulated that the platelet zones seen in profile in transmission electron microscopy represented sections through maturing proplatelet processes that were intertwined and compacted about the nucleus of the MK. The unravelling of these processes, accompanied by penetration of the sinusoidal lining, then constituted the later stages of MK maturation and platelet production. Unfortunately, the unravelling process has never been observed by Radley and his colleagues in any of their cinematography studies.

More recent evidence (Slater et al. 1983a) has demonstrated that MK cytoplasm is capable of amoeboid movement, leaving the naked nucleus behind in the marrow. Hence, large cytoplasmic fragments as well as entire MKs can leave the extravascular space by transendothelial migration to enter the marrow sinusoids. The cytoplasmic protrusions are compatible with the contractile basis of amoeboid movement, thus providing a chemical control of motility (Taylor et al. 1973). Free calcium ions control contractility, causing the cytoplasm to circulate in a fountain pattern in the form of a "sol–gel" tube. The parallel alignment of microtubules in the direction of the long axis of the cytoplasmic processes observed by Radley and Scurfield (1980) may be a reflection of this contractility. Indeed, even Wright (1906) commented: "The majority of the giant cells are of spherical form, but a minority are of varied and irregular shape by reason of the distortion of their cytoplasm into processes and pseudopod-like prolongation of varying length, form and width, so that they present all the varieties of form and outline shown by a motile ameba."

In a dynamic study of thrombopoiesis of rabbit bone marrow, Kinosita and Ohno (1961) produced evidence that conflicts with that of Wright and subsequent workers. Windows were made in the femur or tibia near the distal end. Organized marrow tissue regenerated into the window area from portions of relatively undisturbed marrow. A thin layer of marrow which appeared on the window glass was transilluminated, examined by phase-contrast microscopy and documented using microcinematography. Kinosita and Ohno (1961) summarized their results in the following way:

The thrombocytic series of cells at varied stages of maturation are found scattered in the marrow tissue. They are seldom in the interior parts of the sinusoidal network meshes, but are usually directly on or near the sinusoidal walls. They show cytoplasmic movement, but are not locomotive, usually remaining about where they have developed. Cytoplasmic processes have never been observed projecting through the walls into the sinusoid lumen. Although a few megakaryocytes sometimes happen to be situated near each other, they are not necessarily at the same stage of maturation. Occasionally, a moderately large megakaryocyte is observed drifting in a wide sinusoid. These, if they do not complete further development in the marrow, may be carried in the systemic and then the pulmonary circulation, finally becoming trapped in an alveolor capillary where they complete development.

The same authors reported that platelets are produced by cytoplasmic disintegration both in the extrasinusoidal and sinusoidal spaces. They reported that the cytoplasmic fragments produced in the extravascular compartment then passed through the sinusoidal walls and were released into the circulation.

The observation of sinusoidal MKs has been confirmed in the rabbit by electron microscopy (Slater et al. 1983a) and in the rat by light microscopy (Warren 1987), but no other studies have reported cytoplasmic disintegration. A plausible explanation for this phenomenon could be MK activation on the glass of the observation window, since platelet and presumably megakaryocyte activation by glass had not been documented at the time of the dynamic study of Kinosita and Ohno (1961). It is clear that Wright (1910) also accepted that entire megakaryocytes as well as cytoplasmic fragments had ready access to the blood stream (see also Behnke 1969), but this aspect seems to be conveniently overlooked by those supporters of bone marrow platelet production when they quote Wright's work.

Circulating Megakaryocytes

The passage of entire MKs across the blood–bone marrow barrier is compatible with the observation of circulating MKs in various vessels in man and other mammals. For example, the vessel most frequently harvested for blood in man is the antecubital vein. Megakaryocytes are rarely seen in smears made from antecubital blood in haematologically normal adults. However, a small number of MKs are present. Hansen and Tinggaard Pedersen (1978) used a saponin haemolysis centrifugation technique and millipore filters to study the circulating MKs in blood from the antecubital vein in healthy adult humans. Twenty-one men and 30 women aged between 21 and 73 years were investigated. Seven MKs/ ml blood (range 1–13) were found in the men and 5 MKs/ml of blood (range 1–20) were found in the women. Of the 441 MKs studied, 99% were naked nuclei or had a thin rim of cytoplasm, but none possessed the copious cytoplasm associated with bone marrow MKs. Using the same technique, Tinggaard Pedersen and Cohn (1981) studied intact MKs in the venous blood as a marker for thrombopoiesis in children. A total of 110 children, aged 0–15 years, were investigated. The average number of MKs decreased from 18/ml of blood in the first year of life to 5–6 MKs/ml of blood after the 6th year. The percentage of intact MKs possessing copious cytoplasm decreased from about 40% in the first year of life to only a few per cent (<5%) after the 10th year. The higher percentage of intact MKs in young children compared with adults, which decreases with age, reflects a decrease in active haemopoietic tissue in the forearm during childhood. Using a dextran sedimentation technique Dago et al. (1971) came to the conclusion that more than 10 MKs/ml of peripheral venous blood was an unusual occurrence. In 33 patients with chronic myeloproliferative disease, Tinggaard Pedersen and Laursen (1983) found a significantly higher number of MKs per millilitre of blood in cubital venous blood than in normal adult humans. In patients with chronic myeloid leukaemia and myelofibrosis an increased number of intact MKs was found, reflecting active haemopoietic tissue in the peripheral part of the upper extremity in these diseases. Tinggaard Pedersen and Petersen (1980) evaluated the number of MKs in the umbilical artery and vein of 22 newborn infants delivered by Caesarean section. In blood from the umbilical artery there were 66 MKs/ml of blood; 25% of these MKs had copious cytoplasm. In contrast in umbilical vein blood there were 47 MKs/ml of blood, of which only 8% possessed copious cytoplasm. There was a significantly smaller concentration of MKs, 28 MKs/ml of blood, of which 8% had copious cytoplasm in aortic blood obtained from 16 newborn infants. The number of MKs in the cubital venous blood of 18 mothers harvested 30 minutes before delivery was 18 MKs/ml of blood. Only 1.5% had copious cytoplasm. When 14 of these mothers were studied 3 months after delivery, the concentration of MKs in cubital venous blood had reverted back to normal levels of 5 MKs/ml of blood. Again only 1.5% of these MKs possessed copious cytoplasm. Efrati et al. (1961) have also reported megakaryocytes in the umbilical vein. Careful assessment of placental material by Dr D. N. Slater (personal communication) has revealed MKs with a full complement of cytoplasm in placental vessels.

Blood has also been sampled from the inferior vena cava, femoral artery and the cubital vein of 17 patients with hypertension (Tinggaard Pedersen 1978). On average, 12, 4 and 5 MKs/ml of blood respectively were found in these vessels. More importantly perhaps, 30% of the MKs in central venous blood possessed copious cytoplasm, whereas MKs in arterial and cubital venous blood had sparse or no visible cytoplasm. The significantly lower concentration of MKs in arterial blood compared with central venous blood suggests that the pulmonary capillary bed filters some of the circulating MKs out of the blood. The concentration and increased percentage of MKs and copious cytoplasm in the aortic blood of newborn infants suggests this filtering function is not so effective as in adults. This can be attributed to the presence of right to left shunts through small vessels in the pulmonary circulation, especially in cases of lung disease such as respiratory distress syndrome.

Kaufman et al. (1965a) and Kallinikos-Maniatis (1969) catheterized patients with various cardiac defects and found MKs in the right atrium and arterial blood. Increased numbers of circulating MKs have been demonstrated in infectious and malignant conditions and after surgery by Scheinin and Koivuniemi (1963), Hume et al. (1964) and Breslow et al. (1968).

More recent studies, using centrifugal flow elutriation to isolate MKs, have confirmed the earlier reports of circulating MKs (Shoff et al. 1987). Blood was obtained from the pulmonary artery and aorta of 20 cardiac catherization patients. Intact MKs, naked nuclei and enucleate MKs (large cytoplasmic fragments) were found in the pulmonary artery. The finding of an intact MK in arterial blood was a rare event and the concentration of naked nuclei and enucleate MKs was reduced significantly in aortic blood.

Circulating MKs in the peripheral blood of humans was first communicated in the English literature by Minot (1922), although earlier isolated reports had appeared in the Italian literature. The presence of these cells was regarded as indicative of marrow disintegration and was not considered to be a normal event. The accumulation of more recent evidence, some of which is quoted above, suggests that circulating MKs are a normal event but that their concentration in the blood does change in pathological states or after acute disturbance to the platelet/MK axis.

The documentation of circulating MKs is not confined to humans since they have also been observed in the blood of other mammals. For example, Tinggaard Pedersen (1971) evaluated the concentration of MK in the blood from the inferior vena cava in adult rats. In 30 rats (15 male, 15 female) 2 MKs/ml of blood were obtained on average; 43% of these MKs possessed copious cytoplasm, 10% had sparse cytoplasm and the remainder were naked nuclei. No correlation between platelet count and MK concentration in central venous blood could be demonstrated. In a subsequent study Tinggaard Pedersen (1972) observed increased concentrations of MK in the inferior vena cava of rats after treatment with vinblastine and demecolcine. A higher percentage of MK with copious cytoplasm was observed in the vinblastine series. After surgery involving a median abdominal incision to expose the inferior vena, increased concentrations of MKs were found in the inferior vena cava of 58 female rats (Tinggaard Pedersen 1973). There was also an increase in platelet count which reached a maximum, 7–11 days after surgery, of about 150% of the initial value. Tinggaard Pederson (1974) also demonstrated that the pulmonary vessels acted as a filter for circulating MKs in rats, as well as in humans. In the inferior vena cava 2 MKs/ml of blood were found on average in 25 rats. In contrast, only 1 MK was seen in 37.5 ml of blood taken from the abdominal aorta of the same 25 rats. This MK was a naked nucleus. In a more recent study, Warheit and Barnhart (1980) investigated the concentration of circulating MKs in the central venous and arterial blood of 15 mongrel dogs, before and after administration of purified bovine thrombin to produce thrombocytopenia. Circulating venous MK concentration rose from an average of 7 MKs/ml of blood of 23 MKs/ml of blood following thrombin infusion. An increase in mean arterial MK count from 2 to 4 MKs/ml of blood was also observed.

Circulating venous MKs generally contained copious amounts of cytoplasm, while arterial MKs essentially were devoid of cytoplasm. Aabo and Hansen (1979) found 4 MKs/ml of central venous blood in rabbit; 40% of these MKs possessed copious cytoplasm. Hansen et al. (1979) infused thromboplastin into 40 male rabbits as a model for intravascular coagulation. Seven rabbits infused with physiological saline and 6 rabbits sacrificed without infusion were used as controls. An immediate decrease in average platelet count of 58% after infusion of thromboplastin was observed. In 13 rabbits infused with thromboplastin the MK concentration in central venous blood was measured. The MK count increased from an average of 3 MKs/ml of blood in the control animals to 8 MKs/ml of blood 20 hours after the onset of infusion. No alterations in the percentage distribution of cytoplasmic MKs and naked nuclei were observed.

All of this evidence, taken together, indicates that a significant number of MKs possessing copious cytoplasm enter the pulmonary circulation, but very few cells with cytoplasm leave this site in normal function. Hence, logic dictates that the cell cytoplasm must be lost in the pulmonary vessels. In addition, the pulmonary vessels filter out these circulating MKs. In pathological conditions, after surgery and in thrombocytopenic animal models the number of circulating MKs increases. All of these phenomena occur in a number of different mammals.

Pulmonary Megakaryocytes

The presence of MKs in the pulmonary vessels was discussed first by Aschoff (1893), before Wright (1906) linked the platelet to the MK. In most cases they were described as naked and degenerating nuclei without cytoplasmic material. The general opinion was that the MKs were migrants from the bone marrow (or spleen in some circumstances) which had lost their cytoplasm in the process of platelet formation before reaching the lungs, or shortly after being trapped in the pulmonary capillaries. This interpretation was questioned by Howell and Dona-hue (1937). They found some pulmonary MKs with "a quite extraordinary wealth of cytoplasmic processes pushing through the capillaries in many directions". They felt that their histological evidence for the participation of these MKs in platelet formation was more convincing than Wright's evidence for bone marrow platelet production. It seemed to be incompatible with the notion that pulmonary MKs were degenerating cells that had been cast off from the marrow. Hence, they postulated that MKs are formed or developed in the lungs themselves from myeloblastic cells. Brill and Halpern (1948) found pulmonary MKs in every one of the 50 autopsy cases that they studied. In some cases MKs were also found in other organs, such as the spleen, kidney, liver and heart. There appeared to be a correlation between the concentration of MKs in the pulmonary capillaries and their occurrence in other organs. They concluded that the presence of pulmonary MKs is dependent upon their delivery into the blood from the bone marrow and their subsequent filtration by the pulmonary capillary bed. Their data suggested that the greater the number of MKs leaving the marrow the greater the number reaching the lungs and, in turn, the greater the number filtering through the pulmonary bed to reach the other organs.

An elegant experiment performed by Kaufman et al. (1965b) demonstrated that the number of pulmonary MKs depended on the central venous blood supply. They performed an end-to-end shunt in dog by connecting the left pulmonary artery to the left subclavian artery, so that the left lung only received arterial blood. One week after surgery, the concentration of MKs in the right lung, which received only central venous blood, was 73 times higher than the concentration of MKs in the left lung that received the arterial blood. When an end-to-side shunt was used, so that the left lung received a mixture of central venous and arterial blood, the ratio of MK concentration in the two lungs reverted back to 1 : 1. In a sham operation, thoracotomy without shunt, the ratio of MK concentrations in the two lungs was again 1 : 1. This experiment makes the hypothesis of MK formation in lung tissue, proposed by Howell and Donahue (1937), unlikely, but does not refute their conclusion that platelets are produced in the pulmonary bed.

A belief that some relationship existed between the incidence of pulmonary MKs and the formation of platelet thrombi, particularly in some instances of thrombotic thrombocytopenic purpura, led Sharnoff and Kim (1958) to review lung sections of 355 subjects for the presence of MKs. Their material included 317 consecutive unselected human autopsies, of which 53 were neonatal deaths. Excluding the neonates the age range of the other autopsies was 1 month to 98 years. In addition, the lungs of 27 mammals of different species were examined, including 14 young healthy rabbits, 4 apes, 1 hog, 1 leopard, 1 mink, 1 beaver, 1 camel, 1 skunk, 1 duiker, 1 eland and 1 squirrel. Sharnoff and Kim (1958) found MKs in all but three of the lung sections of the 355 subjects studied. They concluded that the presence of MKs in the pulmonary microcirculation is not specific to adult humans, but may be noted in all normal mammals. Sharnoff and Kim (1958) state: "The impression gained from these studies would appear to indicate that pulmonary MKs are not 'effete' cells, as they have been designated, but appear to break up in the pulmonary capillary bed into cell fragments or platelets. From the previously described histologic appearance, the impression is gained that the MKs are broken asunder by their division into the anastomosing capillaries."

In two of the three autopsies that had no pulmonary MKs, adrenaline was given as a stimulant shortly before death. Sharnoff and Kim (1958) tried to reproduce this condition in an experimental rabbit model. Ten young female Belgian hares were given a subcutaneous injection of adrenaline. Platelet counts were obtained before and after injection, with the post-injection count being made just before sacrifice. Lung tissues were removed for sectioning. Fourteen normal untreated animals, with 2–3 MKs/cm^2 of section were used as controls. In addition, 4 animals that were given a 1-ml subcutaneous injection of sterile isotonic saline were used as controls for the injection itself. The adrenaline appeared to cause a striking disappearance of MKs from the lungs. In 7 out of 10 of the experimental animals no pulmonary MKs could be found. In the remaining 3 animals a total of 4 MKs were found in several square centimetres of lung tissue section. In contrast the 4 control animals who received saline revealed an average of 2–3 MKs/cm^2 of section, as did the 14 untreated controls. The platelet count in the ten adrenaline-treated animals increased from 460×10^9 platelets/l of blood to 690×10^9 platelets/l of blood, after injection, whereas the saline controls averaged $590 \times$

10^9 platelets/l of blood before injection and 610×10^9 platelets/l of blood after injection. No significant alteration in red cell count was observed. Sharnoff and Kim (1958) concluded that the adrenaline-induced disappearance of the pulmonary MKs indicated they were transient cells. The concomitant significant rise in platelets in the peripheral blood was taken as support for the hypothesis of Howell and Donahue (1937) that the pulmonary capillary bed may be a site of break-up of the MKs into platelets.

Tinggaard Pedersen (1974) used lung perfusion through the left atrium and retrograde perfusion through the pulmonary artery to demonstrate the filtering capacity of the pulmonary bed for circulating MKs. Three different, but associated, experiments were performed. The first, of simple perfusion and retrograde perfusion, was performed on 3 rats. On a further 3 rats, sodium nitrite was added, in small amounts at a time, to the perfusate for both perfusion directions. Finally, in 3 further rats, sodium nitrite and intermittent brief increases in perfusion pressure were applied in perfusion through the left atrium, while intermittent applications of slight suction, as well as sodium nitrite, were applied to the pulmonary artery. In the first simple perfusion experiment, 3 naked nuclei, showing signs of nuclear degeneration, were found in 100 ml of perfusate from the left atrium. In contrast, 157 MKs were recovered in the same volume of perfusate from the pulmonary artery, an average of 52 MKs/rat. In perfusion with added sodium nitrite, 100 ml of perfusate yielded 4 "naked nuclei" showing signs of degeneration and a total of 488 MKs from the pulmonary artery, an average of 163 MKs/rat. With sodium nitrite and intermittent pressure only 6 MKs, again with signs of nuclear degeneration, were obtained from the left atrium. With periodic slight suction and sodium nitrite, 827 MKs were obtained in 100 ml of perfusate, an average of 276 MKs/rat. The application of sodium nitrite and increased haemodynamic pressure did not result in the passage of more MKs through the pulmonary vessels to the left atrium. Hence MK retention in the pulmonary vessels can be explained in mechanical terms. The size of the pulmonary capillaries prevents the escape of the large MK nuclei. Tinggaard Pedersen (1974) concluded that his data supported the possibility that megakaryocyte nuclei are also fragmented in the precapillaries of the pulmonary bed and thereafter cannot be perceived as MKs in the arterial blood.

Warheit and Barnhart (1980) used scanning and transmission electron microscopy correlations on single cells to identify pulmonary MKs after thrombin infusion in 15 mongrel dogs. Thrombin was infused to augment the number of MKs travelling from the bone marrow to the lung. Cryofractured sections of tissue were viewed in the scanning electron microscope, mapped according to location, and subsequently embedded for transmission electron microscopy. Their data showed that platelet-forming MKs, i.e. MKs possessing an abundance of cytoplasm, become lodged in the pulmonary vasculature.

Ultrastructural studies by Slater et al. (1983b) have confirmed the presence of mature MKs in the pulmonary arteries and naked nuclei in the pulmonary capillaries of a man who died from disseminated intravascular coagulation associated with extensive burns. Hansen and Aabo (1978) investigated 365 consecutive hospital autopsies and 21 forensic autopsies in previously healthy individuals who had died suddenly, for the presence of pulmonary MKs. They also studied the correlation between pulmonary MKs and microthrombosis. They found that those diseases and clinical conditions related to intravascular coagulation had an increased number of pulmonary MKs compared with the controls in the forensic series. This conclusion was supported in an animal model of experimentally induced consumption coagulopathy by thromboplastin infusion in rabbit (Hansen et al. 1979). These observations are supported by a more recent study by Wells et al. (1984), who counted pulmonary MKs in 22 patients dying from extensive burns. In contrast, Hansen and Aabo (1978) found a decreased number of pulmonary MKs in 55 autopsies of both acute (43) and chronic (12) leukaemia, although an increased number of circulating MKs in this disease had been reported by Oelhafen as early as 1914. Abnormal, dwarf MKs have been reported in chronic myeloid leukaemia (Breton-Gorius et al. 1972, 1973; Popescu 1974; Maldonado 1974), so that these cells might not be filtered as effectively by the pulmonary circulation. In addition, if they are retained in the lung their small size and low ploidy, giving a low intensity of stain, may make them difficult to distinguish from other cells. Evidence that MK nuclear size can be a determinant of pulmonary MK concentration was presented by Slater et al. (1983a). They administered six consecutive daily injections of anti-rabbit serum raised in goat to rabbits, to stimulate the platelet/MK axis. The MKs, their nuclei, and the platelets produced, increased in size (Martin et al. 1982). The concentration of pulmonary MKs increased by a factor of 6 compared to control animals injected with goat serum. Megakaryocytes in the pulmonary vessels of rabbit have also been reported by Resl et al. (1987).

Bendix-Hansen and Aabo (1981) investigated the distribution of intrapulmonary MKs in healthy and diseased subjects. They found that in disease the highest MK counts were found in the superior lobe, but there was a uniform distribution of MK counts in the healthy subjects. This difference was attributed to the altered blood supply to the lungs of patients lying in bed. Pulmonary MKs have been linked to the pathogenesis of adult respiratory distress syndrome (Kadas and Szele 1981) and asthma (Slater et al. 1985; Martin et al. 1987). Finally, Sharma and Talbot (1986) found that MKs were invariably present in post-mortem lung tissue and were increased in association with impaired lung function, shock, thrombo-embolism and in cigarette smokers.

If, as the evidence above suggests, circulating MKs and MKs that lose their cytoplasm in the pulmonary circulation are a normal occurrence in mammalian cell biology (Resl et al. 1987), then they may be related intimately to the mechanism of platelet production and the observed heterogeneity of platelet volume.

Platelet Volume Heterogeneity

Both platelets and MKs possess characteristics that are not found in normal mitotic cells. As stated previously, the MK is a large polyploid cell that demonstrates a significant heterogeneity in size and nuclear DNA content. In contrast, the platelet is a small cytoplasmic fragment that circulates anucleate. This cell is not produced by mitosis, since the platelet itself never possesses nuclear material, but it has a metabolically active surface membrane and its cytoplasm contains those organelles that are also found in MK cytoplasm. The cytoplasm is infiltrated by a canalicular system that has its origin in the demarcation membrane system of the MK. Normal, inactivated platelets have the shape of an oblate spheroid. They are maintained in this form by a cytoskeleton based on a circumferential band of microtubules.

Measurement of platelet volume is now a routine procedure in the majority of haematology laboratories. However, different laboratories may use particle-sizing systems that utilize different physical principles. Some systems use aperture-impedance techniques to size platelets, while others use optical techniques.

For aperture-impedence sizing, platelets are suspended in an electrically conducting medium. The cell suspension is forced by a siphoning mechanism to flow through a small aperture with an electrode on either side. As the cell, which behaves as an insulator, passes through the aperture it changes the conductance between the electrodes. This produces a current pulse of short duration which has a magnitude proportional to "cell size". However, the shape of the cell may cause an electrical "shadow" in the electric field of the aperture. It is thought that it is the volume of this "shadow", which may be larger than the geometrical volume of the cell, that is registered as the cell size.

Optical flow cytometers utilize the physical principal that an incident light beam is scattered by diffraction and refraction as it passes through a cellular suspension. The amount and angle of forward scatter depends on the wavelength of the incident light, the shape and size of the cells, and the relative refractive indices of the cells and the suspending medium. If the cell diameter is small compared with the wavelength of the incident beam, then the light is scattered predominantly by diffraction; if the cell diameter is large compared with the wavelength of the incident light then light is scattered predominantly by refraction. Unstained blood cells absorb a negligible amount of light. In early flow cytometers a tungsten halogen lamp was used to produce a $10 \ \mu m \times 100 \ \mu m$ illuminated slit field which was then imaged in the centre of a sheathed flow unit. Later models employ a laser light source. The wavelength of the light source is approximately 5×10^{-7} m, while platelet diameters are $1-4 \times 10^{-6}$ m. Hence, these cells have diameters that are about two to eight times greater than the wavelength of the incident light beam. As a consequence light is scattered in the forward direction by both diffraction and refraction, with refraction probably being the dominant scattering mechanism.

Microscopic planimetry techniques on blood smears (see Fig. 7.1) have also been used to estimate platelet size. These three techniques rely on totally different physical principles yet they all produce platelet volume distributions with a common feature; the distributions are asymmetric with a positive skew. A comparison between platelet volume measurement by aperture impedence, light transmission and planimetry techniques has shown excellent correlation ($r = 0.94$) in normal subjects and also in a variety of pathological conditions (Holme et al. 1981). This suggests that the asymmetry and positive skew in the platelet volume distribution is not an artefact of one particular measurement technique. Nevertheless, significant artefacts can occur during platelet volume measurement. A major source of differences in mean platelet volume and heterogeneity when measured by different techniques stems from the different anticoagulants that are employed. In routine haematology the most commonly used anticoagulant is ethylene diamine tetra-acetic acid (EDTA). The dipotassium salt (K_2EDTA) is normally used for its superior solubility. It has been suggested that EDTA produces a rapid change in platelet shape (Zucker and Borelli 1954),

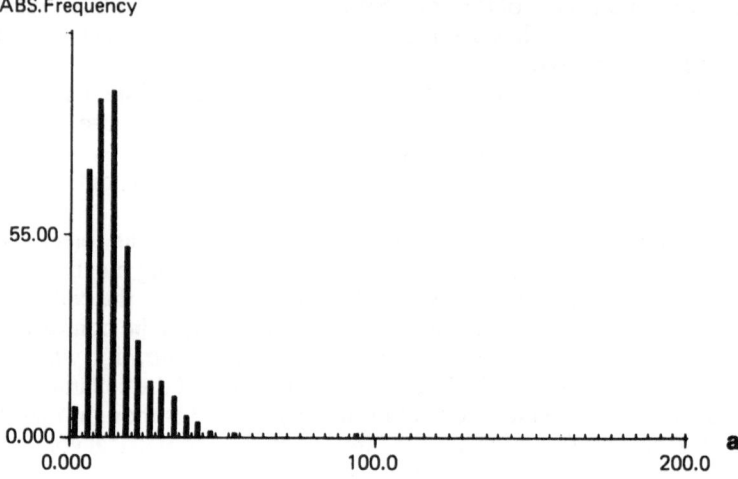

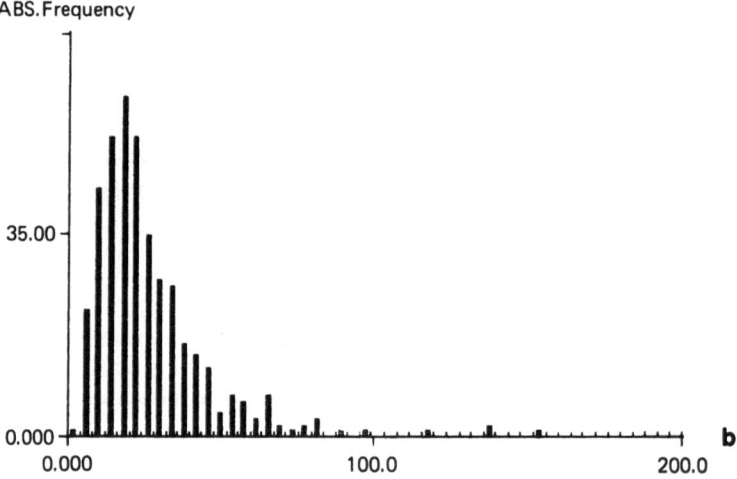

Fig. 7.1. Area distributions of platelets anticoagulated with EDTA for 3 hours ± 15 minutes, on blood smears measured by planimetry using a Kontron Videoplan Image Analysis system. The upper figure shows platelets from a haematologically normal subject; the platelets in the lower figure were harvested from a patient with a myeloproliferative disorder. The measurements were made by Mark Woods.

followed by a gradual increase in platelet size during the first few hours after venepuncture (Zeigler et al. 1978). Evidence which supports this concept has been presented by Holme and Murphy (1980). By measuring the optical density of platelet-rich plasma in an aggregometer and mean platelet volume by aperture impedance methods they demonstrated an immediate shape change and an apparent volume increase in platelets collected in EDTA, followed by a decrease in optical density but an increase in mean platelet volume after 3 hours' storage in EDTA. It has been proposed that EDTA increases the intracellular cyclic AMP concentration (Suvorov and Markosyan 1981). Cyclic AMP alters the permeability of the plasma membrane of platelets. Increase in intracellular fluid, associated with changes in membrane permeability, would cause the cell to swell, but it would also cause a reduction in the relative refractive indices of the cell cytoplasm and suspending medium. As the limiting condition is approached, when the refractive indices of the cell cytoplasm and suspending fluid are equal, no refraction of light and hence negligible light scattering would occur. For this reason, although the geometrical volume of the cell may increase with time, the volume measured by optical methods would decrease with time. This conclusion is reflected in a recent study of the variation of platelet size with storage time in EDTA when measured by aperture impedance (Coulter S Plus) and light-scattering (Technicon H6000) technology (Trowbridge et al. 1985). Over a period of 39 hours platelet volume increased when measured by the S Plus yet decreased on the H6000 (Fig. 7.2). No asymptotic limit for platelet volume was reached in this time. In the same study no change in mean platelet volume with time was observed when sodium citrate and prostaglandin E_1 was used as anticoagulant, although a small decrease in platelet count with time may occur (Trowbridge et al. 1985).

By careful monitoring of the conditions of anticoagulation, pH, gradient osmolarity, time from blood sampling to testing, platelet recovery from whole blood and electrical filtering of the signal from the aperture impedance system, measurement of the platelet volume distribution of a representative sample of the

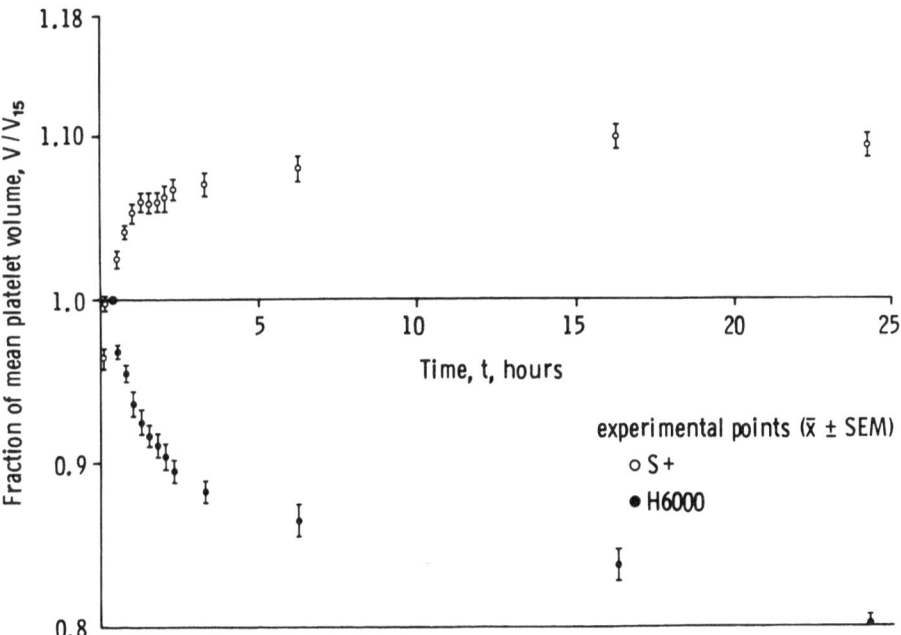

Fig. 7.2. The variation of mean platelet volume, for 29 normal volunteers, with storage time in EDTA when measured on aperture impedance and flow cytometric systems. Platelets increased in size when measured by aperture impedance, but the same platelets decreased in size when measured by light scatter. Reproduced with permission from the Institute of Physics, *Clin. Phys. Physiol. Meas.* 1985, 6:221–238.

cells circulating in the blood can be achieved with the minimum of artefact (Martin et al. 1982, 1983).

Under these conditions, in normal physiology, platelet count and mean volume appear to be derived from a bivariate Gaussian distribution in different mammals (Trowbridge et al. 1984, 1989; Warren 1987). This means that platelet counts are drawn from one Gaussian distribution, while mean platelet volumes are drawn from a second Gaussian distribution, but the two distributions are significantly correlated. For this reason reference regions in the plane of platelet count and mean platelet volume are specified by ellipses (see Fig. 7.3). This method of analysis, or augmentations to it (Warren 1987), is a rigorous statistical evaluation of data presented as nomograms in earlier studies (Bessman et al. 1981; Levin and Bessman 1983).

The regions defined by the ellipses are different for different animals. The associated platelet volume distributions provide a signature of steady-state thrombopoiesis. If subjects with platelet count and mean volume are chosen that lie within the ellipse that defines 2SD (based on the bivariate distribution) from the average platelet count and mean volume for the sample, the average platelet volume distribution for the group, with appropriate 95% confidence limits, can be constructed. Fig. 7.4 shows the average distributions of 9 rats and 13 men, with the shaded areas denoting the 95% confidence limits. The volume distributions,

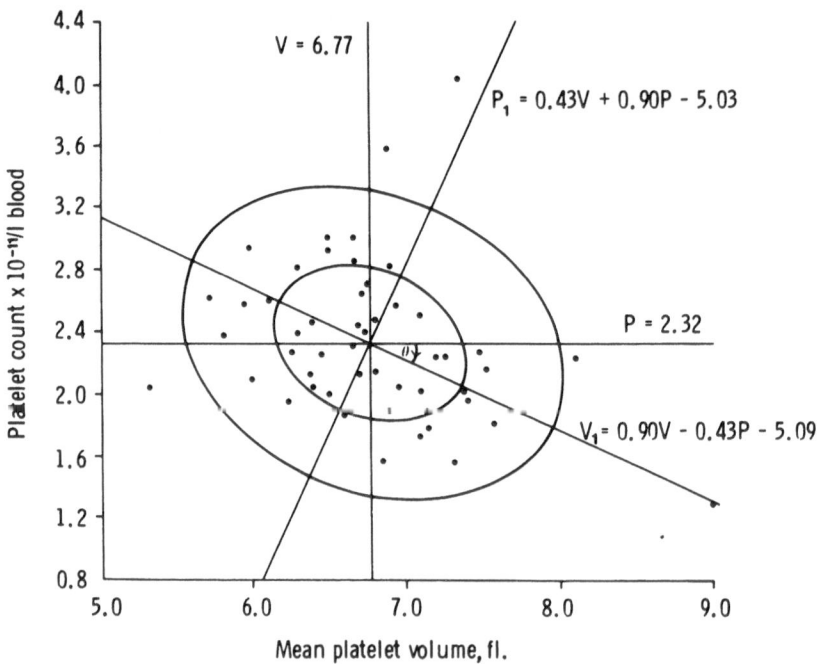

Fig. 7.3. The bivariate Gaussian distribution of platelet count and mean volume for 51 normal volunteers. The volume and count are correlated significantly so the regions of equal dispersion about the bivariate mean ($P = 232 \times 10^9$ platelets/l blood, $V = 6.77$ fl) are represented by ellipses. The inner and outer ellipses represent 1 SD and 2 SD from the mean, respectively. Reproduced with permission from the Institute of Physics, *Clin. Phys. Physiol. Meas.* 1984, 5:145–170.

PLATELET VOLUME DISTRIBUTION SIGNATURE

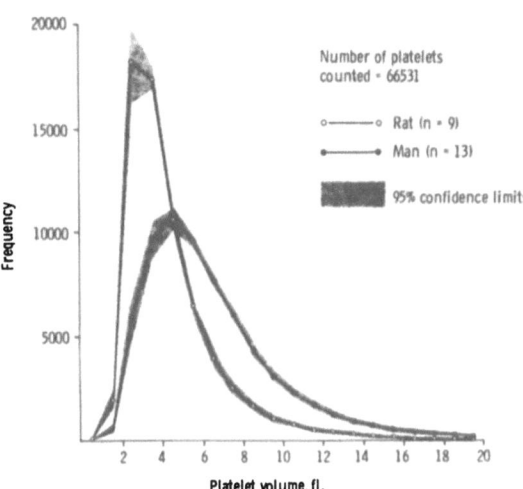

Fig. 7.4. Average platelet volume distribution in man (n=13) and rat (n=9) obtained from subjects drawn from a region inside the inner ellipse in Fig. 7.3 (i.e. 2 SD from the bivariate mean) in man and an identical region of dispersion in rat. Reproduced with permission from the Insitute of Physics, *Clin. Phys. Physiol. Meas.* 1984, 5:145–170.

as expected, are asymmetric with a positive skew. In man, this asymmetry can be removed, to a greater extent, by taking a logarithmic transformation. The distribution of log-volumes is then approximately Gaussian. This procedure is attractive because it allows the entire volume distribution to be described by only two parameters: the mean and the standard deviation of the log-volumes. Indeed, a log-Gaussian platelet volume distribution is fitted to the raw data on commercially available aperture impedence systems. Such asymmetry is not associated with the volume distributions of mitotic cells, which are usually Gaussian and hence symmetric. Paulus et al. (1979) have argued that the log-Gaussian distribution arises from demarcation and growth of platelet territories in the megakaryocyte. However, the freeze–fracture studies identified earlier in this chapter and the disappearance of membrane during pseudopodia formation make this hypothesis unlikely. In addition, the platelet volume distribution deviates significantly from log-Gaussian in other mammals, for example the rat (Fig. 7.4; Trowbridge et al. 1986). The logarithmic transformation will remove a significant proportion of the inherent asymmetry, but the skewness and kurtosis (Table 7.1) of the log-volumes are significantly different from those found in a Gaussian distribution (see Table 7.2). Nevertheless, the heterogeneity in platelet volume appears to be a characteristic of thrombopoiesis, not cell ageing as was first thought. Experimental evidence obtained by McDonald et al. (1964) suggested that young platelets were large platelets that became progressively smaller with time spent in the circulation. More recent evidence has indicated that there is no correlation between platelet size and age (Thompson et al. 1983). The former supposition arose because the investigators did not distinguish between the dynamic response of the platelet/MK control system to a sudden

Table 7.1.   Statistical parameters used in the evaluation of platelet volume distributions

Mean:	measure of central tendency
Coefficient of variation:	$\dfrac{SD}{mean} \times 100$, measure of dispersion
Skewness:	measure of asymmetry
Kurtosis:	measure of convexity
For a Gaussian distribution: skewness = 0, kurtosis = 3	

Table 7.2.   The measures of asymmetry and convexity of experimental platelet volume distributions

	Skewness	Kurtosis
True log-normal	0	3
Man, adult ($n = 52$)	0.0240±0.0047	2.762±0.013
Man, foetus ($n = 50$)	0.0657±0.0133	2.798±0.012
Rabbit ($n = 7$)	0.759 ±0.0446	4.025±0.083
Rat ($n = 41$)	0.727 ±0.0086	3.547±0.023

$\bar{x} \pm$ SEM. All values are highly significant: $p<0.001$, Mann–Whitney U test.

depletion of circulating platelets and the normal steady-state behaviour of the same system.

The heterogeneity of the platelet volume distribution can be manipulated by acute perturbation of the platelet/MK axis (Fig. 7.5; Trowbridge et al. 1986). These changes take place before any significant changes in MK size (Warren 1987) and MK nuclear DNA content (Warren 1987; Corash et al. 1987) are observed in the bone marrow.

Chronic perturbations of the platelet–MK axis also alter the volume heterogeneity (Fig. 7.6). When rabbits are fed on a high-cholesterol diet for 12 weeks, their MKs increase in size, the platelet count increases, and mean platelet volume decreases, with a concomitant alteration in platelet volume heterogeneity (Martin et al. 1985).

Any realistic model of platelet production should be capable of explaining these observations in a quantitative manner.

Pulmonary Thrombopoiesis: A Simple Mechanism

At various times since 1937, when Howell and Donahue first suggested that platelets were produced in the pulmonary circulation, this site has been proposed for thrombopoiesis. For example, Kaufman et al. (1965a, b), Crosby (1976), and Tinggaard Pedersen (1974, 1978) have proposed that all or some of the circulating platelets are produced in the lungs. These proposals have not proved popular in

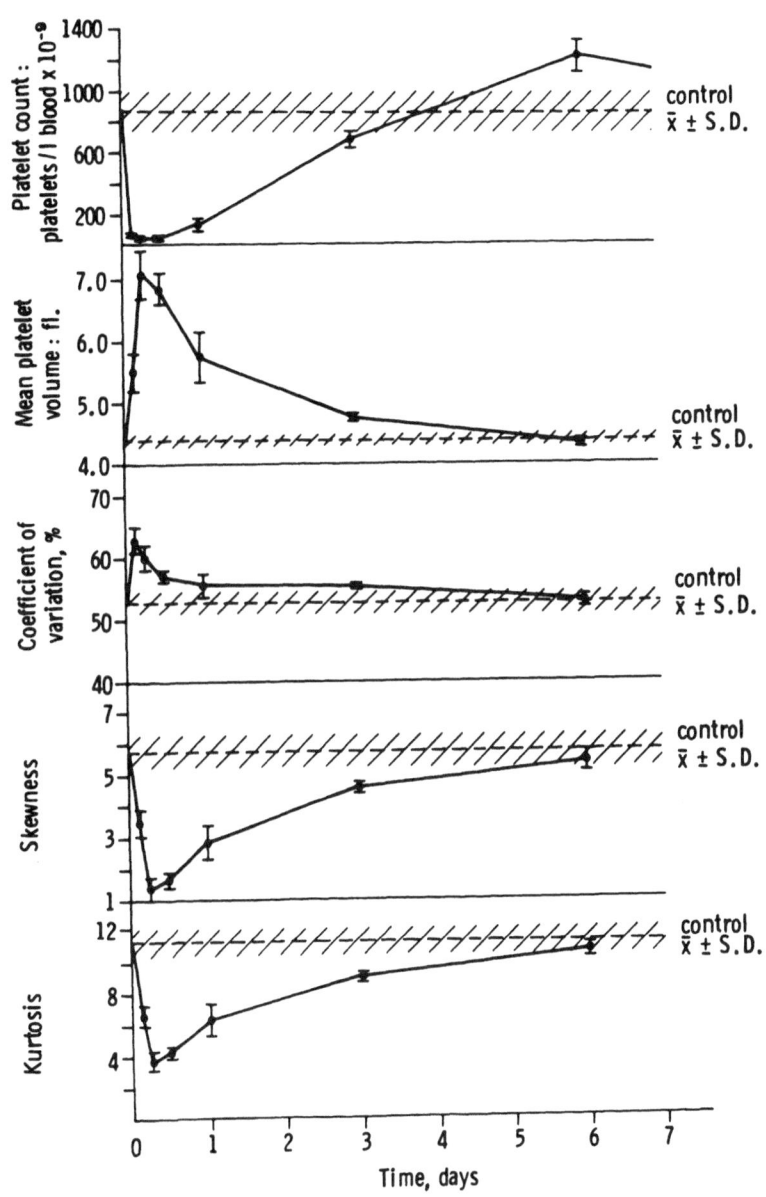

Fig. 7.5. The variation of platelet count, mean volume, volume ceofficient of variation, skewness and kurtosis with time in rat after a single injection of anti-platelet serum ($n = 5$ at each time point, control $n = 42$). Reproduced with permission from the Institute of Physics, *Clin. Phys. Physiol. Meas.* 1986, 7:203–210.

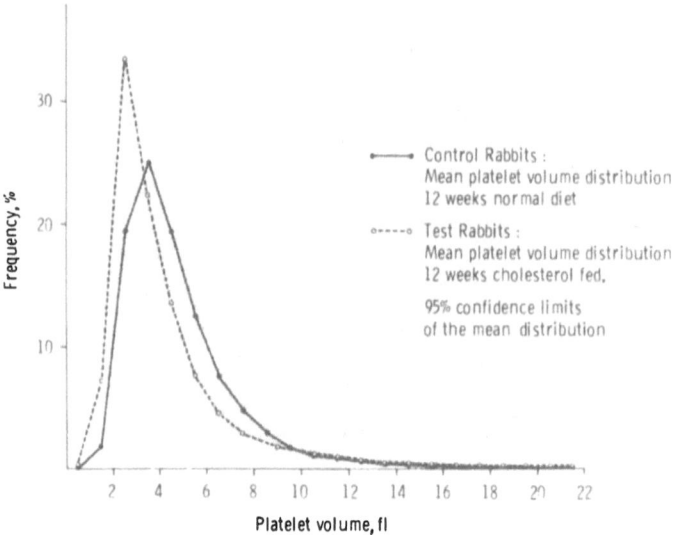

Fig. 7.6. The average platelet volume distribution of rabbits ($n = 5$) fed on a high-cholesterol diet for 12 weeks and controls ($n = 5$) fed on a normal diet for the same time period. Reproduced with permission from *Arteriosclerosis* 1985, 5:604–612.

the absence of a specific production mechanism. However, based on the natural architecture of the pulmonary circulation a simple mechanism does exist, by which the platelet volume distribution can be generated from the MK cytoplasmic volume distribution.

The process of platelet production starts with whole MKs or large cytoplasmic fragments devoid of nuclear material squeezing through the blood–bone marrow. This has been described in detail earlier in this chapter and is depicted schematically in Fig. 7.7. These cells and fragments of cytoplasm are then carried away by the blood into the veins and eventually appear in the central venous blood that drains into the right side of the heart. Throughout this journey, the blood vessels encountered by the MK gradually increase in size. After leaving the right ventricle of the heart, the cells enter the pulmonary circulation. This is a dichotomously branching system. The arborization is extensive, with 300×10^6 branches arising from the single pulmonary artery at the precapillary arteriole level of the pulmonary microcirculation in man (Singhal et al. 1973). The anatomy of the pulmonary capillary system resembles parallel sheets separated and supported by avascular posts rather than the cylindrical capillaries found in the systemic microcirculation (Fung and Sobin 1969). The distance between adjacent supporting posts is thought to be about 4 μm. As the megakaryocyte is carried along in the pulmonary blood, it enters vessels whose diameters progressively decrease in size. Eventually, the cell approaches a pulmonary vessel with similar dimensions to that of itself. For example, a spherical MK with volume 20 000 fl has a diameter of 34 μm, which is much bigger than the diameter of many of the pulmonary vessels. At this stage, based on geometrical size, the MK can do one of three things. It can halt its excursion through the pulmonary bed and occlude the vessel, or it can deform and squeeze through the pulmonary microcirculation in a similar manner to that of its exit through the endothelial cell

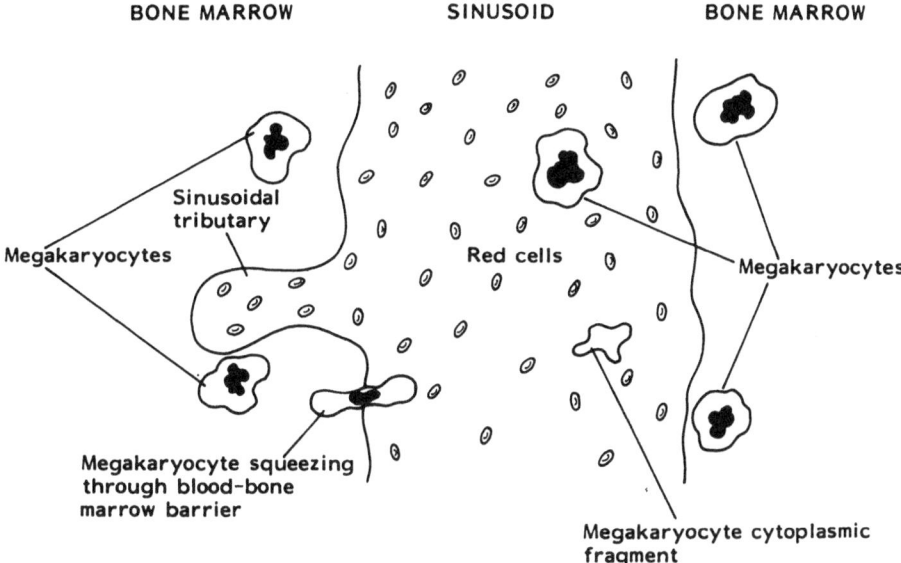

Fig. 7.7. A schematic representation of the bone marrow, showing a megakaryocyte in the act of diapedesis. An entire megakaryocyte and a large cytoplasmic fragment are shown in the marrow sinusoid. The diagram is based on the observation of rat marrow sections prepared by Christopher Warren. Reproduced with permission from *Blood Cells* 1988, 13:451–458.

pores in the bone marrow. Alternatively the cell can divide to produce volumes which are small enough to allow an uninterrupted passage into the next set of smaller vessels. Of the three alternatives the experimental evidence points to the latter. Megakaryocytes with a full complement of cytoplasm are rarely seen occluding the smaller pulmonary vessels with electron microscopy. If vessel occlusion was the natural predominant role of circulating MKs then some interruption of pulmonary blood flow might be expected. Nevertheless a marked degree of filtering of megakaryocyte naked nuclei does occur at this site (Tinggaard Pedersen 1978). If the MK deforms and squeezes through the pulmonary microcirculation without losing its cytoplasm the number of circulating MK with copious cytoplasm should be the same in both central venous and arterial blood. This is not the case (Tinggaard Pedersen 1978; Shoff et al. 1987).

If fragmentation of the MK cytoplasm occurs at a dichotomous branch of a mother vessel into two daughter vessels, the most natural division is binary. One volume of cytoplasm enters one daughter vessel and the other volume enters the other daughter vessel. Whether the nucleus enters into this process is not clear, but experimental evidence presented by Tinggaard Pedersen (1974) suggests some nuclear fragmentation may occur.

If the cytoplasmic volume is unable to make further progress, based on the geometrical size of the cytoplasm and the vessel, the probability of division must be one. However, smaller cytoplasmic volumes may contact the bifurcations of larger vessels as shown in Fig. 7.8. The cytoplasmic volume does not necessarily have to divide to make progress but may do so given the correct conditions. Repetition of this process produces a sequence of random binary divisions. In this

PULMONARY MICROCIRCULATION

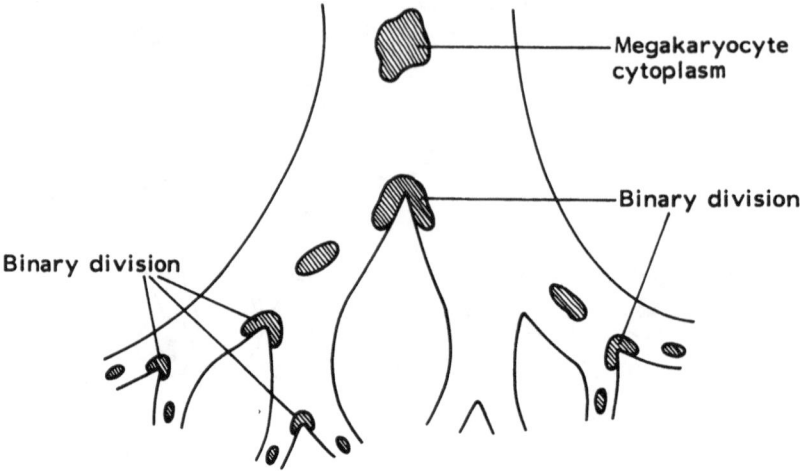

Fig. 7.8. A schematic diagram of the proposed sequence of binary divisions of megakaryocyte cytoplasm in the pulmonary circulation. An electron micrograph of a megakaryocyte astride a bifurcation has been published previously (Trowbridge et al. 1984).

way cellular division into two is retained, and the platelets are produced by a physical analogue of mitosis.

The mechanism of pulmonary platelet production depends on two stochastic processes. The first is the probability of division. Large particles have a probability of division of one that reduces gradually to zero with each subsequent division as the particles decrease in size. However, other parameters such as the pulmonary architecture, pulmonary haemodynamics, the biochemistry ambient and its interaction with the surface membrane, the cytoplasmic morphology and the ability to polymerize the microtubular cytoskeleton may all contribute to the probability of division. In particular the system of interconnected channels enveloped by the demarcation membrane system may act as cleavage sites during the binary division. This would explain the histochemical similarities between the DMS in the MK and the plasma membrane and the surface-connected canalicular system in the platelet (see earlier). In addition fracture along cleavage sites delineated by the DMS would provide a link between the large platelets and abnormal MK DMS morphology seen in the May–Hegglin syndrome (Godwin and Ginsburg 1974) and the animal model of the Wistar Furth rat (Jackson et al. 1988).

After division into two the cytoplasmic particles will be distributed randomly about one half of the original volume in normal platelet production. This is the second stochastic characteristic in the production process. The arrangement of avascular posts, rather like a pin-ball machine, may control the final stages of the sequence of binary divisions, resulting in the circulating cell which has such a small size at the lower end of the volume distribution.

This hypothesis can be tested experimentally by measuring the MK cytoplasmic volume distribution entering the pulmonary circulation in a specific animal. Each volume is then subjected to an appropriate sequence of random binary divisions, and the resulting distribution is compared with the platelet volume distribution circulating in the blood of the same animal.

The probability of division can be expressed by a probability function that depends on a single parameter, λ. As the particles get smaller the probability of division reduces from one to zero at a predetermined lower threshold. The randomness of the division into two particles can be expressed as a Gaussian distribution with mean 0.5 and an appropriate standard deviation, S. Pulmonary platelet production can then be simulated by a computer.

In practice, MKs in central venous blood are difficult to harvest and measure.

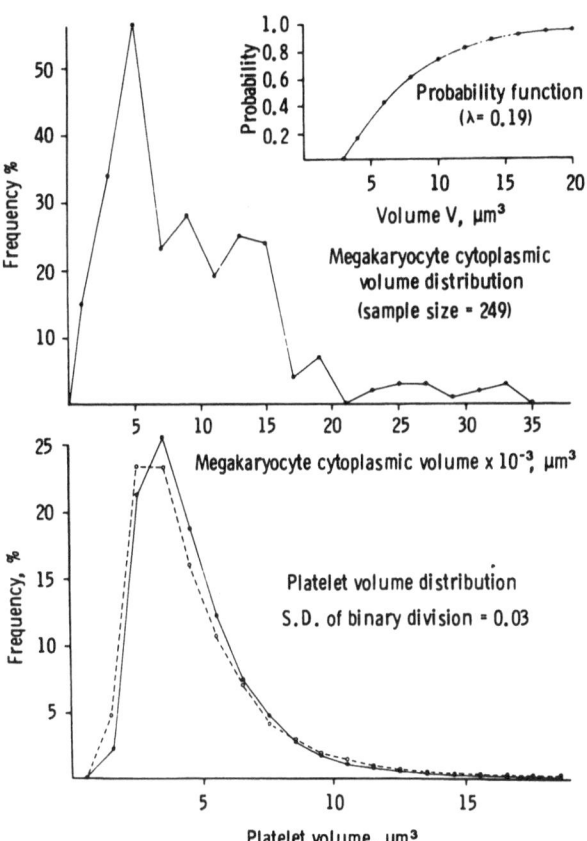

Fig. 7.9. The megakaryocyte cytoplasmic volume distribution of a rabbit (*upper panel*). The experimental (●——●) and theoretical (○----○) platelet volume distributions in the same animal (*lower panel*). The theoretical distribution was obtained from the megakaryocyte cytoplasmic volumes by a sequence of random binary divisions based on the probability function shown in the inset. The probability of a binary division is unity for volumes above 20 fl, decreasing to a value of zero (i.e. no further divisions occur) for cytoplasmic volumes below 3 fl. The standard deviation of the Gaussion distribution of possible volumes produced by the binary division was set at 0.03. The experimental results were obtained by Christopher Warren and the computer program was written by Peter Harley. Reproduced with permission from *IMA J. Math. Appl. Med. Biol.* 1988, 5:45–63.

Hence MK cytoplasmic volume distributions have been constructed from planimetric measurements of MKs in bone marrow sections (Trowbridge et al. 1984). Fig. 7.9 shows the result of the simulation of the production procedure in rabbit. Similar results have been obtained for rat and man (Trowbridge and Harley 1988).

The measurement of MK cytoplasmic volume in the marrow is based on at least two assumptions. The first assumption relies on steady-state thrombopoiesis. Marrow MKs produce future platelets and not those platelets circulating in the blood at the time of measurement. However, in the steady state the MK sample in the marrow should not change with time, and so those MKs which produced the circulating platelets should not be different from those MKs measured at the time of sampling. The second assumption relies on the fact that MKs sampled from one site in the marrow, for example the femur in the rat or the iliac crest in man, is representative of the MK population at other marrow sites.

A recent study (Gladwin et al. 1988) has shown that the second assumption is not valid. Human MK samples from the rib are significantly larger and have a different cytoplasmic volume distribution from MKs in the posterior iliac crest (Fig. 7.10). Nevertheless when the same stochastic characteristics are imposed on the two different-sized cytoplasmic samples, as would be the case in their passage through the pulmonary circulation, identical platelet volume distributions are obtained (Fig. 7.11).

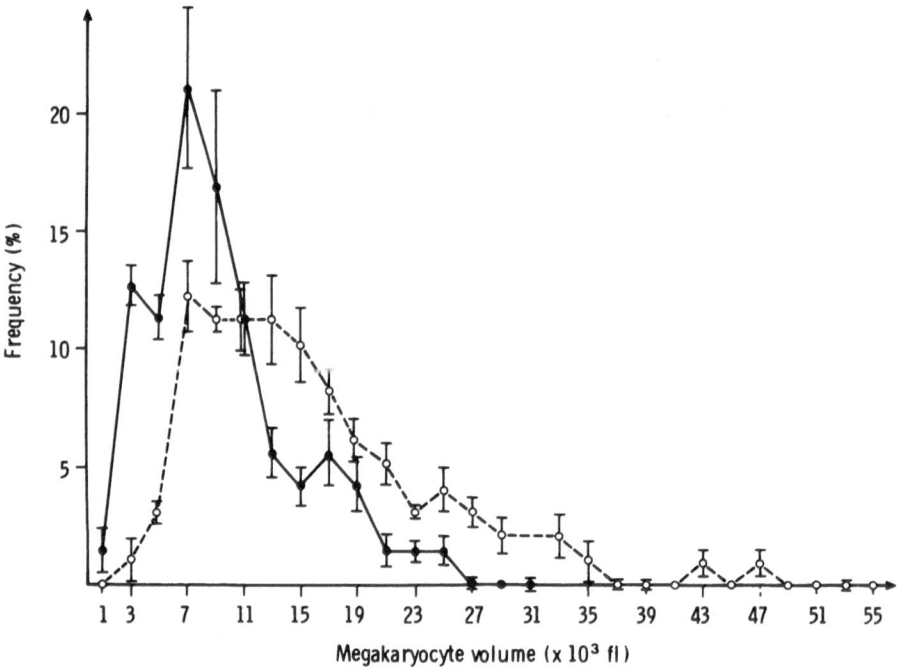

Fig. 7.10. The megakaryocyte volume distributions measured in posterior iliac crest (●——●) and rib marrow (○----○) from the same subjects ($n = 5$, $\bar{x} \pm$ SEM). The planimetric measurements were made by Ann-Marie Gladwin using a Kontron Videoplan Image Analysis system.

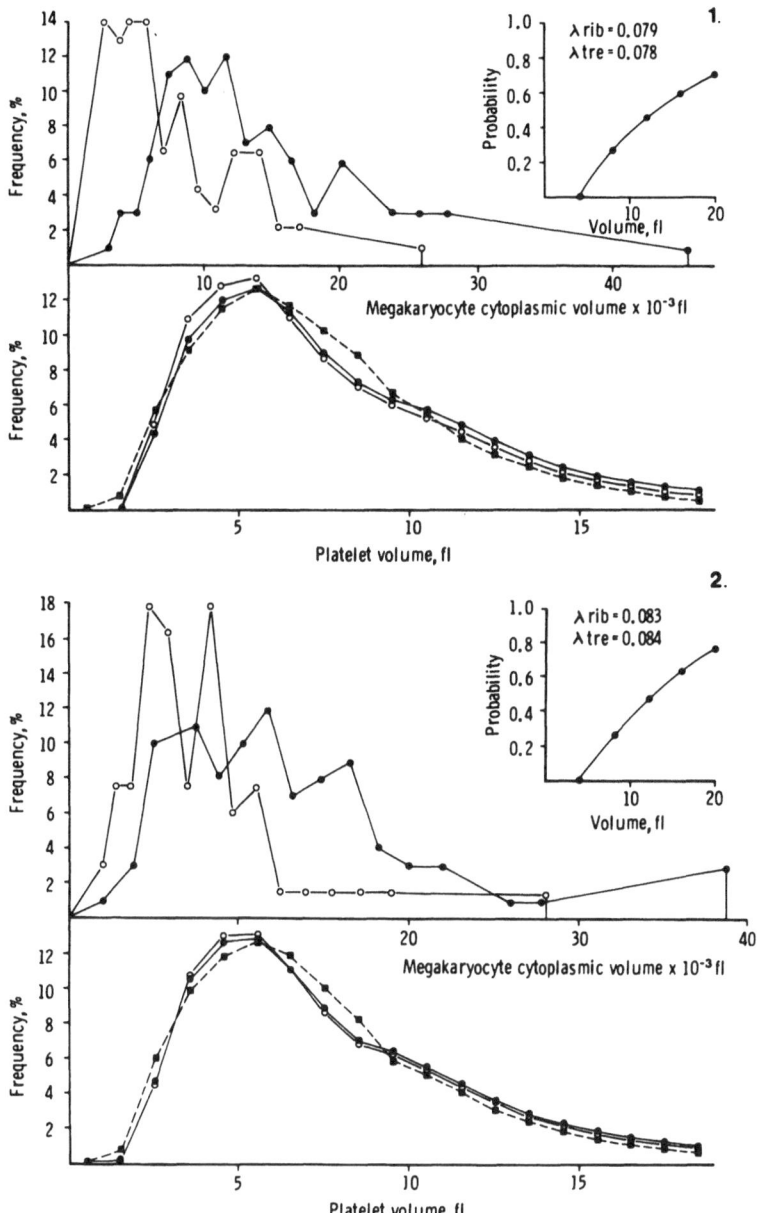

Fig. 7.11. The megakaryocyte cytoplasmic volume distribution associated with two of the subjects shown in Fig. 7.10 taken from posterior iliac crest (PIC) (O——O) and rib (●——●). The distributions are significantly different. If these cytoplasmic volumes are subjected to a sequence of random binary divisions governed by the probability functions shown in the inset then the platelet volume distributions generated from PIC megakaryocytes (O——O) and rib megakaryocytes (●——●) are virtually identical and indistinguishable from the experimentally measured platelet volume distribution (■——■). The probability parameter, λ, and hence the probability function is the same for PIC and rib megakaryocyte cytoplasmic volumes. The experimental results were obtained by Ann-Marie Gladwin and the computer program was written by Peter Harley.

Finally the question arises: are there sufficient circulating MKs to maintain a normal platelet count? Simple calculations based on the MK cytoplasmic size, mean platelet volume, platelet survival and platelet count show that in man 23 MKs/ml of central venous blood are needed to maintain a normal count in steady-state thrombopoiesis (Trowbridge et al. 1984). This is of the same order of magnitude as the 12 MKs/ml of blood reported by Tinggaard Pedersen (1978) and 18 MKs/ml of blood identified by Shoff et al. (1987).

It is worth noting that there is no natural apparatus leading to sequential binary division in the marrow, so that if platelets are produced there it must be by some other mechanism which also leads to the observed heterogeneity in platelet volume.

Conclusions

The conclusions of this article can be summed up by a quotation taken from Julian Huxley (1887–1975): "To speculate without facts is to attempt to enter a house, of which one has not the key, by wandering aimlessly round and round, searching the walls and now and then peering through the window. Facts are the key." Pulmonary platelet production and its relationship to platelet volume hetero-geneity are based on the following facts:

1. MKs and large cytoplasmic fragments leave the bone marrow. Active haemopoietic marrow releases more MKs with cytoplasm than inactive marrow.
2. MKs in central venous blood have significantly more cytoplasm associated with them than the MKs in arterial blood.
3. The lungs act as a filter for MK nuclei and cytoplasm is shed there.
4. The number of pulmonary MKs depends on the central venous blood supply.
5. Volumes which are distributed in an identical fashion to that of platelets can be derived from MK cytoplasmic volume distributions in different mammals by a sequence of random binary divisions. This process provides an explanation for the observed heterogeneity of platelet volume.
6. In man the concentration of MKs in central venous blood is of the same order of magnitude as that concentration needed to maintain a normal platelet count in steady state thrombopoiesis

In contrast, there are no facts, other than subjective judgements, which support bone marrow thrombopoiesis.

References

Aabo K, Hansen KB (1979) New aspects of the morphology of circulating megakaryocytes in rabbits. Acta Path Microbiol Scand (A) 87:173–177

Aschoff L (1893) Uber capillare embolie von mesenkernzellen. Virch Arch Path Anat Physiol Klin Med 134:11–24

Becker RP, De Bruyn PPH (1976) The transmural passage of blood cells into myeloid sinusoids and the entry of platelets into the sinusoidal circulation: a scanning electron microscopic investigation. Am J Anat 145:183–206

Behnke O (1968) An electronmicroscope study of the megakaryocyte of the rat bone marrow. I. Development of the demarcation membrane system and the platelet surface coat. J Ultrastruct Res 24:412–433

Behnke O (1969) An electronmicroscope study of the rat megakaryocyte. II. Some aspects of platelet release and microtubules. J. Ultrastruct Res 26:111–129

Bendix-Hansen K, Aabo K (1981) Distribution of intrapulmonary megakaryocytes. Acta Path Microbiol Scand (A) 89:169–171

Bessman JD, Williams LJ, Gilmer P (1981) Mean platelet volume: the inverse relation of platelet size and count in normal subjects, and an artefact of other particles. Am J Clin Pathol 7:289–299

Breslow A, Kaufman RM, Lawsky AR (1968). The effect of surgery on the concentration of circulating megakaryocytes and platelets. Blood 32:393–401

Breton-Gorius J, Dreyfus B, Sultan C, Basch A, d'Oliveiras JG (1972) Identification of circulating micromegakaryocytes in a case of refractory anaemia: an electron microscopy–cytochemical study. Blood 40:453–463

Breton-Gorius J, Daniel MT, Flandrin G, Dencel K (1973) Fine structure and peroxidase activity of circulating micromegakaryoblasts and platelets in a case of acute myelofibrosis. Br J Haematol 25:331–339

Brill R, Halpern MM (1948) The frequency of megakaryocytes in autopsy sections. Blood 3:286–291

Corash L, Chen HY, Levin J, Baker G, Lu H, Mok Y (1987) Regulation of thrombopoiesis: effects of the degree of thrombopoiesis on megakaryocyte ploidy and platelet volume. Blood 70:177–185

Crosby WH (1976) Normal platelet numbers: pulmonary platelet interactions. Ser Haemat 8:89–97

Dago C, Karpas CM, Dincts L, Tytan A, Oppenheim A (1971) Circulating megakaryocytes: a quantitative observation in normal subjects by age and sex. Acta Cytol 15:410–413.

De Bruyn PPH, Michelson S, Thomas TB (1971) The migration of blood cells of the bone marrow through the sinusoidal wall. J Morph 133:417–438

Efrati P, Rozenszajn L, Shapira E (1961) The morphology of buffy coat from cord blood of normal newborns. Blood 17:497–503

Farr AG, De Bruyn PPH (1975) The mode of lymphocyte migration through post-capillary venule endothelium in lymph node. Am J Anat 143:59–92

Fung YCB, Sobin SS (1969) Theory of sheet flow in the lung. J. Appl Physiol 26:472–488

Gladwin AM, Martin JF, Thorpe JAC, Trowbridge EA (1988) Human megakaryocyte size varies with anatomical site. Br J Haematol 69:445–448

Godwin HA, Ginsburg AD (1974) May Hegglin anomaly: a defect in megakaryocyte fragmentation. Br J Haematol 26:117–128

Haller CJ, Radley JM (1983) Time-lapse cinemicrography and scanning electron microscopy of platelet formation by megakaryocytes. Blood Cells 9:407–418

Hansen KB, Aabo K (1978) Megakaryocytes in pulmonary blood vessels. Acta Pathol Microbiol Scand (A) 86:293–295

Hansen M, Tinggaard Pedersen N (1978) Circulating megakaryocytes in blood from the antecubital vein in healthy adult humans. Scand J Haematol 20:371–376

Hansen KB, Aabo K, Myhre-Jensen O (1979) Response of pulmonary (circulating) megakaryocytes to experimentally induced consumption coagulopathy in rabbits. Acta Path Microbiol Scand (A) 87:165–172

Harker LA (1968) Megakaryocyte quantitation. J Clin Invest 47:452–457

Holme S, Murphy S (1980) Coulter counter and light transmission studies of platelets exposed to low temperature, ADP, EDTA and storage at 22°. J Lab Clin Med 96:481–493

Holme S, Simmonds M, Ballet R, Murphy S (1981) Comparative measurements of platelet size by Coulter counter, microscopy of blood smears, and light-transmission studies: Relationship between platelet size and shape. J Lab Clin Med 97:610–622

Howell WH, Donahue DD (1937) The production of blood platelets in the lungs. J Exp Med 65:177–203

Hume R, West JT, Malmgren RA, Chu EA (1964) Quantitative observations of circulating megakaryocytes in the blood of patients with cancer. N Engl J Med 270:111–117

Jackson CW, Hutson NK, Steward SA et al. (1988) The Wistar Furth rat: an animal model of hereditary macrothrombocytopenia. Blood 71:1676–1686

Kadas L, Szele K (1981) The role of megakaryocytes and tissue mast cells in the respiratory distress syndrome of adults. Acta Morph Acad Sci Hung 29:395–403

Kallinikos-Maniatis A (1969) Megakaryocytes and platelets in central venous and arterial blood. Acta Haematol (Basel) 42:333–335

Kaufman RM, Airo R, Pollack S, Crosby WH (1965a) Circulating megakaryocytes and platelet release in the lung. Blood 26:720–731

Kaufman RM, Airo R, Pollack S, Crosby WH, Doberneck R (1965b) Origin of pulmonary megakaryocytes. Blood 25:767–775

Kinosita R, Ohno S (1961) Biodynamics of thrombopoiesis. In: Johnson SA, Monto RW, Rebuck JW, Horn RC (eds) Blood Platelets. Churchill, London, pp 611–616

Levin J, Bessman JD (1983) The inverse relation between platelet volume and platelet number. J Lab Clin Med 101:295–307

Lichtman MA, Chamberlain JK, Simon W, Santillo PA (1978) Parasinusoidal location of megakaryocytes in marrow: a determinant of platelet release. Am J Haematol 4:303

MacPherson GG (1972) Origin and development of the demarcation system in megakaryocytes of rat bone marrow. J Ultrastruct Res 40:167

Maldonado JE (1974) Dysplastic and circulating megakaryocytes in chronic myeloproliferative diseases. II. Ultrastructure of circulating megakaryocytes. Blood 43:811–820

Martin JF, Trowbridge EA, Salmon GL, Slater DN (1982) The relationship between platelet and megakaryocyte volumes. Thrombosis Res 28:447–459

Martin JF, Plumb J, Kilby RS, Kishk YT (1983) Changes in platelet volume and density in myocardial infarction. Br Med J 287:456–459

Martin JF, Slater DN, Kishk YT, Trowbridge EA (1985) Platelet and megakaryocyte changes in cholesterol-induced experimental atheroscierosis. Arteriosclerosis 5:604–612

Martin JF, Slater DN, Trowbridge EA (1987) Platelet production in the lungs. In: Schuntz-Schumann M, Menz G, Page CP (eds) PAF, platelets, and asthma. Birhanser, Basel, pp 37–57

McDonald TP, Odell TT, Gosslee DG (1964) Platelet size in relation to platelet age. Proc Soc Exp Biol Med 115:684–689

Minot GR (1922) Megacaryocytes in the peripheral circulation. J Exp Med 36:1–7

Muto M (1976) A scanning and transmission electron microscopy study on rat bone marrow sinuses and transmural migration of blood cells. Arch Histol Jpn 39:51

Oelhafen H (1914) Uber Knochenmarkriesenzellen in stromenden Blut. Folia Haematol 18:171–206

Paulus JM, Bury J, Grosdent JC (1979) Control of platelet territory development in megakaryocytes. Blood Cells 5:59–88

Penington DG (1981) Formation of platelets. In: Gordon JL (ed) Platelets in biology and pathology. Elsevier/North-Holland, Amsterdam, Ch 2, pp 19–41

Penington DG, Streatfield K, Roxburgh AE (1976) Megakaryoctyes and the heterogeneity of circulating platelets Br J Haematol 34:639–653

Popescu ER (1974) Letter to the editor. Blood 43:471

Radley JM, Haller CJ (1982) The demarcation membrane system of the megakaryocyte: A misnomer? Blood 60:213–219

Radley JM, Hartshorn MA (1987) Megakaryocyte fragments and the microtubule coil. Blood Cells 12:603–610

Radley JM, Scurfield G (1980) The mechanism of platelet release. Blood 56:996–999

Resl M, Kuna P, Petyrek P (1987) Megakaryocytes in rabbit pulmonary blood vessels. Gen Physiol Biophys 6:383–386

Scheinin TM, Koivuniemi AP (1963) Megakaryocytes in the pulmonary circulation. Blood 22:82–87

Shaklai M, Tavassoli M (1978) Demarcation membrane system in rat megakaryocyte and the mechanism of platelet formation: A membrane reorganization process. J Ultrastruct Res 24:270–285

Sharma GK, Talbot IC (1986) Pulmonary megakaryocytes: 'missing link' between cardiovascular and respiratory disease? J Clin Pathol 39:969–976

Sharnoff JG, Kim ES (1958) Evaluation of pulmonary megakaryocytes. Arch Path 66:176–182

Shoff PK, Kirwin KS, Levine RF (1987) Megakaryocytes in circulating blood. Circulation Suppl 76:1339 (Abstract)

Singhal S, Henderson R, Horsefield K, Harding K, Cumming G (1973) Morphometry of the human pulmonary arterial tree. Circulation Res 33:190–197

Slater DN, Trowbridge EA, Martin JF (1983a) The megakaryocyte in thrombocytopenia: a microscopic study which supports the theory that platelets are produced in the pulmonary circulation. Thromb. Res 31:163–176

Slater DN, Martin JF, Trowbridge EA (1983b) The lung: A platelet factory and megakaryocyte graveyard in health and disease. J Pathol 140:144

Slater DN, Martin JF, Trowbridge EA (1985) The platelet in asthma. Lancet i:110

Suvorov AV, Markosyan RA (1981) Some mechanisms of the effect of EDTA on platelet aggregation. Bull Exp Biol Med 91:651–653

Tavassoli M, Aoki M (1981) Migration of entire megakaryocytes through the marrow–blood barrier. Br J Haematol 48:25–29

Tavassoli M, Crosby WH (1973) Fate of the nucleus of marrow erythroblast. Science 173:912

Tavassoli M, Weiss L (1973) An electron microscopic study of spleen in myelofibrosis with myeloid metaplasia. Blood 42:467

Taylor DL, Candeelis JG, Morre PL, Allen RD (1973) The contractile basis of ameoboid movement: the chemical control of motility in isolated cytoplasm. J Cell Biol 59:378–394

Thiery JP, Bessis M (1956) La genèse des plaquettes sanguines a partir des megacaryocytes observée sur la cellule vivante. R Acad Sci 242:290–292

Thompson CB, Love DG, Quinn PG, Valeri CR (1983) Platelet size does not correlate with platelet age. Blood 62:487–494

Tinggaard Pedersen N (1971) Circulating megakaryocytes in blood from the inferior vena cava in adult rats. Scand J Haematol 8:223–230

Tinggaard Pedersen N (1972) The effect of vinblastine and demecolcine on circulating megakaryocytes in adult rats. Scand J Haematol 9:613–620

Tinggaard Pedersen N (1973) The increase in the number of circulating megakaryocytes and blood platelet in rats after surgery. Scand J Haematol 11:71–77

Tinggaard Pedersen N (1974) The pulmonary vessels as a filter for circulating megakaryocytes in rats. Scand J Haematol 13:225–231

Tinggaard Pedersen N (1978) Occurrence of megakaryocytes in various vessels and their retention in the pulmonary capillaries in man. Scand J Haematol 21:369–375

Tinggaard Pedersen N, Cohn J (1981) Intact megakaryocytes in the venous blood as a marker for thrombopoiesis. Scand J Haematol 27:57–63

Tinggaard Pedersen N, Petersen S (1980) Megakaryocytes in the foetal circulation and in cubital venous blood in the mother before and after delivery. Scand J Haematol 25:5–11

Tinggaard Pedersen N, Laursen B (1983) Megakaryocytes in cubital venous blood in patients with chronic myeloproliferative diseases. Scand J Haematol 30:50–58

Trowbridge EA, Harley PJ (1988) A stochastic model of pulmonary platelet production. IMA J Math Appl Med Biol 5:45–63

Trowbridge EA, Martin JF, Slater DN, Kishk YT, Warren CW, Harley PJ, Woodcock B (1984) The origin of platelet count and volume. Clin Phys Physiol Meas 5:145–170

Trowbridge EA, Reardon DM, Hutchinson D, Pickering C (1985) The routine measurement of platelet volume: a comparison of light-scattering and aperture-impedance technologies. Clin Phys Physiol Meas 6:221–238

Trowbridge EA, Warren CW, Martin JF (1986) Platelet volume heterogeneity in acute thrombocytopenia. Clin Phys Physiol Meas 7:203–210

Trowbridge EA, Reardon DM, Bradey L, Hutchinson D, Warren CW (1989) Automated haematology: Construction of univariate reference ranges for blood cell count and size. Med Lab Sci 76:23–32

Warheit DB, Barnhart MI (1980) Circulating megakaryocytes and the microvasculature of the lung, Scan Electron Micros 3:225–262

Warren CW (1987) The thrombopoietic control system: homeostasis, simulation and perturbation, PhD thesis, University of Sheffield

Wells S, Sissons M, Hasleton PS (1984) Quantitation and pulmonary megakaryocytes: Fibrin thrombi in patients dying from burns. Histopathology 8:517–528

White JG (1983) Time-lapse cinemicrography and scanning electron microscopy of platelet formation by megakaryocytes. Blood Cells 9:419–426

White JG (1987) Megakaryocyte fragments and the microtubule coil: a commentary. Blood Cells 12:611–614

Wright JH (1906) The origin and nature of the blood plates. Boston Med Surg J 154:643–645

Wright JH (1910) The histogenesis of the blood platelets. J Morphol 21:263–278

Yamada E (1957) The fine structure of the megakaryocyte in the mouse spleen. Acta Anat 29:267–290

Zeigler Z, Murphy S, Gardner FH (1978) Microscopic platelet size and morphology in various haematologic disorders. Blood 51:479–486

Zucker MB, Borelli J (1954) Reversible alterations in platelet morphology produced by anticoagulants and by cold. Blood 9:602–608

Zucker-Franklin D, Petursson S (1984) Thrombocytopoiesis: analysis by membrane tracer and freeze-fracture studies on fresh human and cultured mouse megakaryocytes. J Cell Biol 99:390–402

8 The Genesis of Platelet Volume and Density Distributions

J. M. Paulus, M. Sequaris, D. Graas, R. Greimers and J. C. Grosdent

Introduction

Distributions of platelet volumes have been considered to be a meaningful index of platelet heterogeneity since they can be determined with high resolution (McDonald et al. 1964; von Behrens 1975; Paulus 1975; McDonald 1976; Mundschenk et al. 1976; Haynes 1980; Paulus et al. 1986), they are correlated with platelet function (Karpatkin 1969, 1978a; Thompson et al. 1982, 1983a, 1984; Thompson and Jakubowski 1988) and they have clinical significance (Kraytman 1973; Godwin and Ginsburg 1974; Paulus 1975; von Behrens 1975; Paulus and Casals 1978; Zeigler et al. 1978; Levin and Bessman 1983; Bury et al. 1983; Thompson and Jakubowski 1988). However, they are also instructive from the biological point of view because they result from an effective randomizing process which appears in evolution with the emergence of higher orders. Log-normal size distributions may be generated by a limited number of plausible mechanisms (Aitchison and Brown 1957) and they therefore provide insight into the physiology of megakaryocyte terminal maturation. This chapter will summarize the main features of platelet size distributions and discuss the cytological mechanisms which explain their genesis.

Platelet Size Distributions From Normal Subjects Approximate Log-normality

The shape of histograms of platelet size (diameter or surface on smears; or volume in suspensions analysed by microscopy; or volume in suspensions analysed by flow systems based on the Coulter principle) is markedly asymmetrical. However, frequency histograms of log-diameters, log-surfaces or log-volumes can be fitted by Gaussian distributions (McDonald et al. 1964; von Behrens 1975; Paulus 1975; McDonald 1976; Mundschenk et al. 1976; Paulus et al. 1979). The fact that diameters, surfaces and volumes yield the same type of distribution is explained by the so-called reproductive property of the log-normal law, namely that log-normality is conserved when the variable is multiplied by a constant factor and/or elevated at a constant power (Aitchison and Brown 1957). Measurements of platelet dry weights have also yielded log-normal distributions, as have recent histograms of platelet forward and side scatter in flow cytofluorometers (Fig. 8.1).

Deviations from size log-normality have been reported (Dighiero et al. 1980; Threatte et al. 1984; Trowbridge et al. 1984). Some of these deviations were

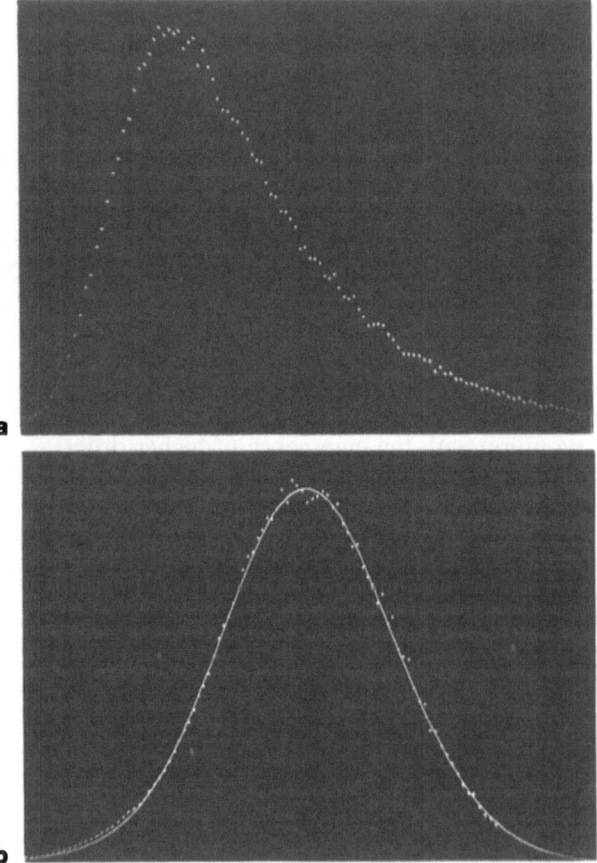

Fig. 8.1. Distributions of 90° light scatter (a) and log 90° light scatter (b) of human platelets. Platelets were separated as a PRP and recorded using a Becton–Dickinson FACS 440 cytofluorometer. Continuous lines superimposed on the data represent the best fit log-normal distributions. Note log-normality of bottom curve.

detected only by using *t* tests, which are notoriously too sensitive when applied to large populations and may indicate significant deviations even when applied to simulated log-normal distributions (Paulus 1974). However, other published curves display a clear discrepancy between calculated log-normal distributions and experimentally obtained histograms (Fig. 8.2; Paulus et al. 1986). The deviation is localized at the right-hand end of the distribution, is small when sized

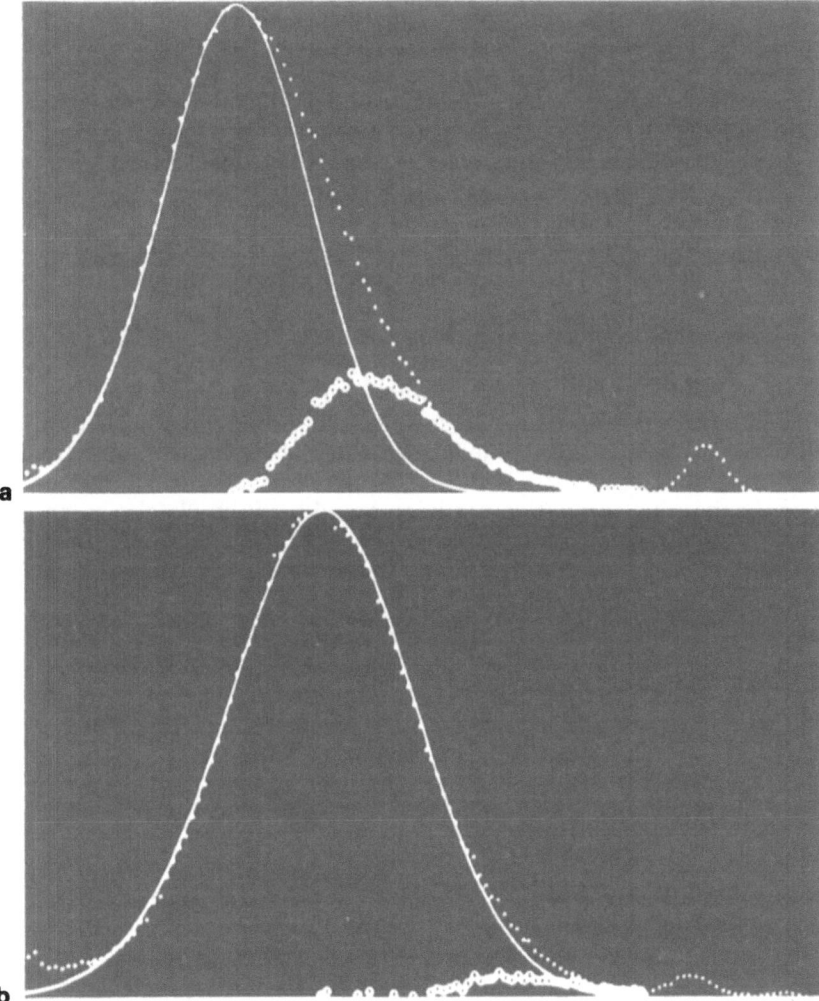

Fig. 8.2. Distributions of platelet log-volumes recorded from ACD-anticoagulated PRP (**a**) and EDTA-anticoagulated PRP (**b**). Both PRPs were prepared from the same patient. As in Fig. 8.1, continuous curves represent the theoretical log-volume distributions. Deviation from log-normality is marked in the top curve but it is much less significant in the bottom curve. The differences between the recorded and theoretical curves are shown as circles. In each curve, the small peak at the right represents the few red cells which remain in PRP after short (25 s) and slow (45 g) centrifugation of whole blood.

platelets are sampled from blood anticoagulated with EDTA and is much more significant when acid–citrate–dextrose (ACD) is used (Fig. 8.2). Because EDTA spheres platelets while ACD preserves their discoid shape, the data suggest that platelet shape plays a role in the deviation from log-normality. In normal humans, the largest platelets tend to be more globular or less discoid than the smallest ones (Chamberlain et al. 1988). In citrated platelet-rich plasma (PRP) platelets from subjects with Mediterranean macrothrombocytopenia (whose mean volume is about twice that of northern Europeans) have a more spherical shape than the smaller population circulating in subjects from northern European origin (von Behrens 1975). Because spherical platelets generate higher-impedence pulses than discoid particles of equal volume, it follows that the size of large platelets is overestimated in counters based on the Coulter principle. By sphering platelets and thus reducing the differences in shape between large and small platelets, EDTA largely eliminates the deviation from log-normality. Use of curve-fitting procedures in 50 reference laboratory personnel showed that only 3.8% of platelets collected in EDTA anticoagulant belonged to a distinct distribution; it is not clear whether this slight discrepancy resulted from residual non-sphericity or whether it was a biological feature of size distributions.

Use of EDTA instead of ACD may have another effect on platelet size. It has been reported that a fraction of recently released platelets are linked together as strings of unfragmented megakaryocyte processes, called proplatelets (Tong et al. 1987). These elements can be demonstrated in ACD blood and increase in percentage following antiplatelet serum-induced thrombocytopenia. Use of EDTA disrupts these processes and yields single-cell suspensions, an effect which may help attenuate the deviation from log-normality observed in samples treated with ACD or citrate.

In normal subjects a correlation has been found between platelet mean log-volume and standard deviation of log-volumes. Coefficients of 0.22 ($p<0.001$) were recorded in 980 consecutive size distributions analysed with a Coulter F instrument (having no hydrodynamic focusing system). Using an Ultraflo 100 equipped with the latter feature (Haynes 1980), an even higher correlation was obtained in 50 reference subjects ($r=0.60$; $p<0.001$; Fig. 8.3). The significance of this correlation will be discussed later.

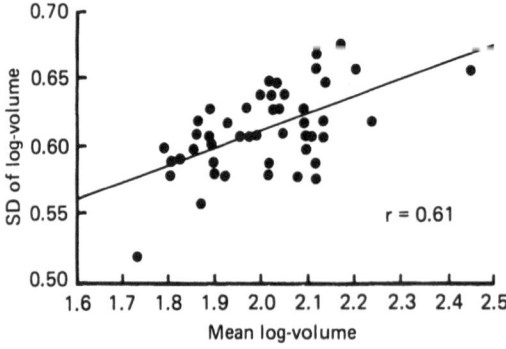

Fig. 8.3. Correlation between mean and standard deviation of log-volumes in 50 reference subjects, based on determinations made on PRPs anticoagulated with EDTA, using an Ultraflo 100 and a logarithmic amplifier from Becton–Dickinson (Haynes 1980).

Circulating Platelet Populations of Widely Different Age Distributions Approximate Log-normality

Because it was initially believed that platelet size was determined by platelet ageing in circulation and that young platelets were larger than old ones (Karpatkin 1969), log-normality was assessed on smeared platelet populations whose mean age varied from 0.5 days (as in idiopathic thrombocytopenic purpura) to about 4.0 days, the reference value for normal subjects (Paulus 1974). Mean age was determined as the area underlying the normalized population survival curve obtained after autologous transfusion of [^{51}Cr]chromate labelled platelets (Paulus 1974, 1975). These experiments indicated that log-normality was present as early as 0.5 days after platelet release, suggesting first that the shape of platelet size distributions was generated during thrombopoiesis or shortly thereafter, and second that ageing in circulation did not alter log-normality. In fact, simulation studies have demonstrated that a number of conceivable ageing processes involving a reduction in platelet volume with platelet age would not cause significant deviations from log-normality (Esch 1983). Thus, any reduction in size due to ageing in circulation would not generate log-normality, neither would it alter the log-normal shape of size distributions of newly born platelets.

Platelet Volume Can Be Regulated

Following platelet depletion, the newly released platelets have been found to be normal in size at 4 hours (Harker 1974) but increased in size at 6 hours (Trowbridge and Martin 1984), 8 hours (Corash et al. 1987) and 12 hours (Odell et al. 1976). The stimulus to release these platelets must have hit mature, non-DNA-synthesizing megakaryocytes since no change in the ploidy histogram is present at these times. Others changes in platelet characteristics continue to occur after 12 hours, including the appearance of irregular-shaped, beaded fragments (Kraytman 1973; Tong et al. 1987), and of reticulated platelets containing RNA (Ingram and Coopersmith 1969) and ribosomes (Ts'Ao 1971).

After administration of graded doses of thrombopoietin, an increased rate of appearance of [^{35}S]sulphate or [^{75}Se]selenomethionine in platelets occurs first, followed by macrothrombocytosis and elevation in platelet count (McDonald 1976). Both in platelet-depleted rats (McDonald et al. 1964) and in human platelet hyperdestruction (Paulus 1975), platelet volume distributions remain essentially log-normal, although the presence of mixed populations introduces uncertainty in cases where non-steady state exists.

Platelet Volume Is Inversely Correlated to Platelet Count

This relation, which has been found in many conditions (von Behrens 1972; O'Brien and Jamieson 1974; Paulus 1974, 1975; Zeigler et al. 1978; Levin and

Bessman 1983), probably does not reflect mutual regulation of size and count but rather appears as a corollary of the fragmentation process (see later) which generates platelets. High platelet counts and relatively small platelet volumes are likely to result from intense megakaryocyte fragmentation. The converse occurs in some normal northern Europeans with relatively low platelet counts and high platelet volumes as well as in Mediterranean macrothrombocytopenia (von Behrens 1972, 1975; Paulus and Casals 1978), in the May–Hegglin anomaly (Godwin and Ginsburg 1974), Bernard–Soulier syndrome, Epstein's syndrome, Fechtner's syndrome and in the Wistar Furth rat (Jackson et al. 1988).

Platelet Volume and Density Are Partially Correlated

Platelet density distributions markedly differ from platelet volume distributions. Firstly, platelet density is very homogeneous. From published data (Martin et al. 1983; Savage et al. 1986) the coefficient of variation of platelet density in a given individual is less than 1% (to be compared to 50% for the coefficient of variation of platelet volumes). Secondly, platelet density distributions are essentially Gaussian (Martin et al. 1983; Savage et al. 1986). In fact normality and log-normality cannot be discriminated in such homogeneous distributions. Platelet density is determined by platelet organelle concentration (Corash et al. 1977, 1984; van Oost et al. 1984, Duyvené de Wit et al. 1987; Chamberlain et al. 1988). Although concentrations of organelles would be expected to follow Poisson distributions, and asymmetrical distributions have been recorded for dense granule contents (Costa et al. 1977), it is likely that organelle contents per unit volume are large enough to approximate closely to Gaussian distributions. In humans, platelet density was found by some authors to decrease during ageing in circulation (Karpatkin 1969; Corash et al. 1978; Rand et al. 1981), a finding compatible with the finding that haemostatic encounters may degranulate platelets without affecting their ability to circulate (Reimers et al. 1976). However, others have found that platelet density increases (Mezzano et al. 1984, 1987; Savage et al. 1986) or remains constant (Leone et al. 1979; Boneu et al. 1982) with platelet ageing. There is also evidence that the effect of ageing on density depends on the species (Thompson and Jakubowski 1988). The mean life-span of the densest and lightest platelets is identical (Savage et al. 1986).

Whatever the relationship between platelet ageing and density, the mean platelet volume of platelet subpopulations separated in density gradients increases with density (Corash et al. 1977; Martin et al. 1983; Savage et al. 1986; Duyvené de Wit et al. 1987; Chamberlain et al. 1988), although in each density layer platelets display the same wide, asymmetrical distribution of volumes as in total blood (Corash et al. 1977; Martin et al. 1983). Platelet subpopulations separated in function of size by counterflow elutriation show a rather small increase in density with mean volume (Thompson et al. 1982) and those separated as a function of forward scatter show no dependence of density on size (Martin et al. 1983). These data suggest that one or several factors, possibly linked to granule intracytoplasmic transport and distribution, have a common effect on platelet size and density but that these two parameters are otherwise determined independently. Another conclusion which can be drawn from the considerable difference in the coefficient of variation between platelet volumes and densities is that platelet volume should prove the more rewarding as a clinical and biological index of platelet heterogeneity.

Platelet Function Is Linked to Platelet Size and Density

It has been a frequent observation that platelet metabolic and functional activity increases when platelet subpopulations of increasing size and density are studied. It is noteworthy that this relationship often holds when activity is calculated per unit volume or weight of platelets (Karpatkin 1969; Thompson et al. 1982; Corash et al. 1984; Thompson and Jakubowski 1988). This applies also to granule concentration (Corash et al. 1977, 1984; Thompson et al. 1982; Duyvené de Wit et al. 1987; Chamberlain et al. 1988). Except in one study (Thompson et al. 1983b), large dense platelets have been shown to have greater specific activity 24 hours after [^{75}Se]selenomethionine (Karpatkin 1978b), [^{35}S]sulphate (Rand et al. 1981) or [^{3}H]amino acid (Corash and Shafer, 1982) administration than light small ones. These repeated observations suggest that presumptive platelet fields within megakaryocytes are heterogeneous, so that fields destined to become large dense platelets are endowed with both the greatest concentration of organelles and the greatest growth potential.

Megakaryocyte Ploidy Heterogeneity Cannot Explain Log-normality

When it became apparent that platelet volume distributions were determined by thrombopoietic processes it was suggested that the heterogeneity in megakaryocyte ploidy could influence platelet size. This suggestion was made first from studies of various dysthrombocytopoieses in which 2–4N, small mature megakaryocytes released platelets of heterogeneous size and content (Paulus et al. 1974) and then from morphometric studies of normal megakaryocytes (Penington et al. 1976). However, because platelet-producing megakaryocytes fall into sharply delineated ploidy classes, i.e. 4N, 8N, 16N, 32N or 64N (with little or no biological dispersion in DNA content within each class), it was readily apparent that ploidy heterogeneity alone could not generate the smooth, continuous log-normal distribution of platelet sizes.

A correlation has been noted between average megakaryocyte ploidy and platelet size (Bessman 1984). However, correlation does not imply causal relationship. As indicated earlier, thrombopoietic stimulation induces macrothrombocytosis (Odell et al. 1976; Corash et al. 1987) and an increased number of megakaryocyte endoduplications (Harker and Finch 1969; Odell et al. 1976; Corash et al. 1987). That megakaryocyte ploidy does not determine platelet size has been shown by combined temporal studies of size and ploidy following platelet depletion (Corash et al. 1987). In conditions where changes in the ploidy histogram occurred, they could only be detected about half a day after large stress platelets appeared. When platelet depletion was moderate, platelet size increased, while the ploidy histogram was not modified (Corash et al. 1987). Correlation between platelet size and ploidy in human diseases is best explained by the fact that thrombopoietic stimulation is often associated with an elevation of both parameters. Thus megakaryocyte ploidy cannot by considered a significant determinant of platelet size.

Fragmentation and Growth of Megakaryocyte Cytoplasm Are Major Determinants of Platelet Size

Since neither a decrease in size of platelets with ageing (if it exists) nor megakaryocyte ploidy heterogeneity can account for platelet log-normality, other thrombopoietic processes must be involved. The role of fragmentation mechanisms has been stressed by some authors (Paulus 1975; von Behrens 1972; Trowbridge et al. 1984), because: (a) fragmentation must occur for megakaryocyte cytoplasms, which have volumes of several thousand cubic micrometres (Harker and Finch 1969) to be able to release platelets having volumes of 1–40 μm^3; (b) breakage processes are a well-known cause of log-normality in biology as well as other fields (Aitchison and Brown 1957); and (c) fragmentation processes account for the inverse relationship between size and volumes, as discussed earlier. However, the exact mechanism and time of the fragmentation process deserves discussion. Although the development of the open canalicular system has suggested a multi-step fragmentation resulting in progressive delineation of platelet territories (Paulus 1975; Paulus et al. 1979), the role of this membrane system is now questioned. At platelet release, megakaryocytes extend thread-like processes into the sinusoids and these processes undergo attenuation and stricture. The open canalicular system may thus be a pre-formed invaginated reserve of membrane with which the processes surround themselves when they protrude into the sinusoids (Radley and Haller 1982). The actual fragmentation may then take place at platelet release and be mediated by the formation of the microtubule ring (Leven and Yee 1987). However, what determines the location of stricture in the processes and when it is determined is unclear. Interestingly, in the Wistar Furth rat, which has a hereditary macrothrombocytopenia analogous in many respects to Mediterranean macrothrombocytopenia, abnormalities in the maturation of the open canalicular system have been demonstrated (Jackson et al. 1988). These anomalies have also been found in macrothrombocytosis associated with leukaemias (Paulus 1974). Furthermore the most dense platelets, which have the highest granule concentration (Corash et al. 1977, 1984; van Oost et al. 1984; Duyvené de Wit et al. 1987; Chamberlain et al. 1988), tend to be the largest ones (Corash et al. 1977; Martin et al. 1983; Savage et al. 1986; Duyvené de Wit et al. 1987; Chamberlain et al. 1988). There may thus be unknown factors, acting before platelet release, which determine the location of the stricture and, as a result, the size of the platelet fragment.

Although a number of characteristics of platelet size distributions can be explained by fragmentation processes, other features cannot be interpreted solely on this basis. Total megakaryocyte cytoplasmic volume increases with maturation time, both before and after cessation of polyploidization (Ebbe et al. 1968). Cytoplasmic growth is stimulated by platelet depletion, which results in further cytoplasmic enlargement occurring within each ploidy class (Odell et al. 1976; Ebbe et al. 1988). The stimulation of cytoplasmic growth appears to be translated as increased platelet size, since low doses of thrombopoietin result in elevated levels of [^{35}S]sulphate and [^{75}Se]selenomethionine in platelets, while higher doses induce in addition macrothrombocytosis (McDonald 1976). A final reason to believe that growth plays a role in determining platelet size, namely the fact that large dense platelets have a greater functional and metabolic activity *per unit volume or weight* than light small ones, has been discussed above. It seems difficult to interpret these findings in the light of fragmentation processes only: it must be the case that, on average, large platelets have undergone during their formation within megakaryocytes a more intense growth than small ones.

Growth, like fragmentation processes, has often provided the explanation for log-normality in biological systems (Aitchison and Brown 1957). The active synthesis of platelet components which takes place in normal megakaryocytopoiesis and is amplified in stimulated conditions is unlikely to be uniform throughout the cytoplasm of megakaryocytic cells. Instead random spatial variations must occur, involving the incorporation of amino acids into proteins, the transport and distribution in the cytoplasm of newly formed granules and a number of other synthetic processes. This random dispersion of growth activity may ultimately be reflected in the functional and size heterogeneity of platelets.

An early scheme depicting the combined effects of fragmentation and growth on platelet volume distribution has been presented in mathematical form (Paulus 1975) and is shown graphically in Fig. 8.4. This scheme assumed that fragmentation was effected by the demarcation ("open canalicular") system. Since recent observations cast some doubt on the role of the open canalicular system and instead suggest that the actual fragmentation occurs in the cytoplasmic processes protruding through the vessel wall, the scheme of Fig. 8.4 may need to be adapted. There is no difficulty in this, however. The mathematical explanation does not require that the percentage volume changes associated with growth and fragmentation be constant at each maturation step. As pointed out by Aitchison and Brown (1957), the notion of temporal succession is not essential. As far as fragmentation is concerned, this notion can well be replaced by that of a rapid, nearly simultaneous division of the cytoplasmic processes, provided that the final platelet volume results from the multiplicative effects of elementary causes operating at random.

In log-normal distributions, the mean and SD of log-volumes, unlike the mean and SD of volumes, are a priori independent parameters. However, using a system equipped with hydrodynamic focusing and a logarithmic amplifier, a significant correlation between the former two parameters was found (Fig. 8.3), confirming earlier results recorded with a less advanced instrumentation (Paulus et al. 1979). The observation suggests two mutually non-exclusive explanations, namely that when fragmentation is reduced, or when growth is stimulated, these processes become more erratic, resulting in correlated increases in mean and SD of log-volumes.

Trowbridge and co-workers (1984) have proposed a modified model of the

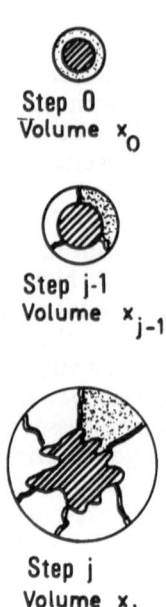

Step 0
Volume x_0

Step j-1
Volume x_{j-1}

Step j
Volume x_j

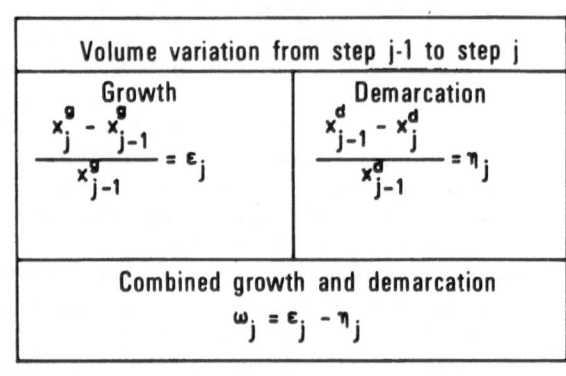

Volume variation from step j-1 to step j	
Growth	Demarcation
$$\dfrac{x_j^g - x_{j-1}^g}{x_{j-1}^g} = \epsilon_j$$	$$\dfrac{x_{j-1}^d - x_j^d}{x_{j-1}^d} = \eta_j$$
Combined growth and demarcation	
$$\omega_j = \epsilon_j - \eta_j$$	

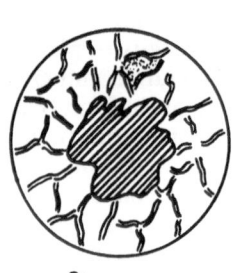

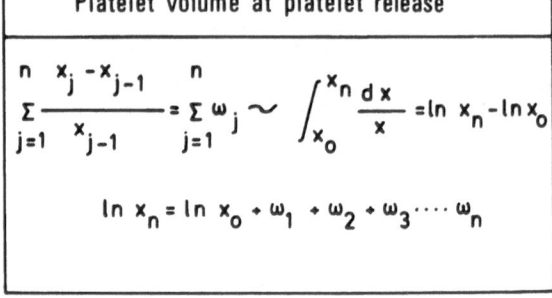

Platelet volume at platelet release

$$\sum_{j=1}^{n} \frac{x_j - x_{j-1}}{x_{j-1}} = \sum_{j=1}^{n} \omega_j \sim \int_{x_0}^{x_n} \frac{dx}{x} = \ln x_n - \ln x_0$$

$$\ln x_n = \ln x_0 + \omega_1 + \omega_2 + \omega_3 \cdots \omega_n$$

Step n .
(platelet release)
Volume x_n

Fig. 8.4. Explanation of the genesis of log-normality of platelet volume, based on the model published by Paulus (1975), in which random variations of percentage changes in growth and delineation of presumptive platelet fields determine platelet volume distribution. Platelet volume at platelet release qualis $\ln x_0$ (log volume of initial cytoplasm of diploid precursor) plus a series of aleatory terms representing the series of percentage changes in presumptive fields. By the central limit theorem, $\ln x_n$ must be normally distributed and x_n log-normally distributed. A slightly modified scheme is described in the text.

genesis of platelet size distribution based on fragmentation processes. Apart from the organ location of platelet release, which is not relevant to the present discussion, their model differs from the one proposed in this chapter in being based solely on binary fragmentation, rather than growth and *n*-ary fragmentation of megakaryocyte cytoplasm. Their model is a particular case of that shown here. Although both models can explain the genesis of platelet log-normal size distributions, we feel that the restriction implied in a binary mechanism is both unverified and unnecessary and that megakaryocyte cytoplasmic growth must be taken into account to explain fully the genesis of platelet volume distributions.

References

Aitchison J, Brown JAC (1957) The lognormal distribution with special reference to its use in economics. Cambridge Univ Press

Bessman JD (1984) The relation of megakaryocyte ploidy to platelet volume. Am J Hematol 16:161–170

Boneu B, Vigoni F, Boneu A, Caranobe C, Sie P (1982) Further studies on the relationship between platelet buoyant density and platelet age. Am J Hematol 13:239–246

Bury J, Casals FJ, Dive G, Grosdent JC, Monfort F, Paulus JM (1983) Platelet macrocytosis and anisocytosis: a retrospective study of 30,000 platelet size distributions. In: Reicher V, Barclay JE (eds) Innovative technology in automated haematology for improved patient care. Technicon International Division, Garges-les-Gonesse, pp. 77–89

Chamberlain KG, Froebel M, MacPherson J, Penington DG (1988) Morphometric analysis of density subpopulations of human platelets. Thrombos Haemost 60:44–49

Corash L, Shafer B (1982) Use of asplenic rabbits to demonstrate that platelet age and density are related. Blood 60:166–171

Corash L, Tan H, Gralnick HR (1977) Heterogeneity of human blood platelet subpopulations. I. Relationship between buoyant density, cell volume and ultrastructure. Blood 49:71–87

Corash L, Shafer B, Perlow M (1978) Heterogeneity of human whole blood platelet subpopulations. II. Use of a subhuman primate model to analyze the relationship between density and platelet age. Blood 52:726–734

Corash L, Costa JL, Shafer B, Donlon JA, Murphy D (1984) Heterogeneity of human blood platelet subpopulations. III. Density-dependent differences in subcellular constituents. Blood 64:185–193

Corash L, Chen HY, Levin J, Baker G, Lu H, Mok Y (1987) Regulation of thrombopoiesis: effects of the degree of thrombocytopenia on megakaryocyte ploidy and platelet volume. Blood 70:177–185

Costa JL, Detwiler TC, Feinman RD, Murphy DL, Patlak CS, Pettigrew KD (1977) Quantitative evaluation of the loss of human platelet dense bodies following stimulation by thrombin or A 23187. J Physiol 264:297–306

Dighiero G, Lesty C, Leporrier M, Couty MC (1980) Computer analysis of platelet volumes. Blood Cells 6:365–370

Duyvené de Wit LJ, Badenhorst PN, Heynes AduP (1987) Ultrastructural morphometric observations on serial sectioned human blood platelet subpopulations. Eur J Cell Biol 43:408–411

Ebbe S, Stohlman F Jr, Overcash J, Donovan J, Howard D (1968) Megakaryocyte size in thrombocytopenic and normal rats. Blood 32:383–392

Ebbe S, Yee T, Carpenter D, Phalen E (1988) Megakaryocytes increase in size within ploidy groups in response to the stimulus of thrombocytopenia. Exp Hematol 16:55–61

Esch L (1983) Modèles stochastiques de la thrombocytopoièse. PhD thesis, Faculty of Sciences, University of Liege, Belgium

Godwin HA, Ginsburg AD (1974) May–Hegglin anomaly: a defect in megakaryocyte fragmentation? Br J Haematol 26:117–128

Harker LA (1974) Control of platelet production. Ann Rev Med 25:383–400

Harker LA, Finch CA (1969) Thrombokinetics in man. J Clin Invest 48:963–974

Haynes JL (1980) High resolution particle analysis: Its application to platelet counting and suggestions for further application in blood cell analysis. Blood Cells 6:201–213

Ingram M, Coopersmith A (1969) Reticulated platelets following acute blood loss. Br J Haematol 17:225–229

Jackson CW, Hutson NK, Steward SA, Ashmun RA, Davis DS, Edwards HH, Rehg JE, Dockter ME (1988) The Wistar-Furth rat: an animal model of hereditary macrothrombocytopenia. Blood 71:1676–1686

Karpatkin S (1969) Heterogeneity of human platelets. I. Metabolic and kinetic evidence suggestive of young and old platelets. J Clin Invest 48:1073–1082

Karpatkin S (1978a) Heterogeneity of human platelets. VI. Correlation of platelet function with platelet volume. Blood 51:307–316

Karpatkin S (1978b) Heterogeneity of rabbit platelets. VI. Further resolution of changes in platelet density volume and radioactivity following cohort labelling with ^{75}Se-selenomethionine. Br J Haematol 39:459–469

Kraytman M (1973) Platelet size in thrombocytopenias and thrombocytosis of various origins. Blood 41:587–598

Leone G, Agonstini A, Decrescenzo A, Bizzi B (1979) Platelet heterogeneity. Relationship between buoyant density, size, lipid, peroxidation and platelet age. Scand J Haematol 23:204–210

Levin J, Bessman JD (1983) The inverse relation between platelet volume and platelet number: abnormalities in hematologic disease and evidence that platelet size does not correlate with platelet age. J Lab Clin Med 101:295–307

Leven R, Yee MK (1987) Megakaryocyte morphogenesis stimulated in vitro by whole and partially fractionated thrombocytopenic plasma: a model system for the study of platelet formation. Blood 69:1046–1052

Martin JF, Shaw T, Heggie J, Penington DG (1983) Measurement of the density of human platelets and its relationship to volume, Br J Haematol 54:337–352

McDonald TP (1976) A comparison of platelet size, platelet count and platelet ^{35}S incorporation as assays for thrombopoietin. Br J Haematol 34:257–267

McDonald TP, Odell TT Jr, Gosslee DG (1964) Platelet size in relation to platelet age. Proc Soc Exp Biol Med 115:684–689

Mezzano D, Aranda E, Rodriguez S, Foradori A, Lira P (1984) Increase in density and accumulation of serotonin by human aging platelets. Am J Hematol 17:11–21

Mezzano D, Hwang KL, Catalano P, Aster RH (1987) Evidence that platelet buoyant density, but not size, correlates with platelet age in man. Am J Hematol 11:61–76

Mundschenk DD, Connelly DP, White JG, Brunning RD (1976) An improved technique for the electronic measurement of platelet size and shape. J Lab Clin Med 88:301–315

O'Brien JR, Jamieson S (1974) A relationship between platelet volume and platelet number. Thromb Diath Haemorrh 31:363–365

Odell TT Jr, Murphy JR, Jackson CW (1976) Stimulation of megakaryocytopoiesis by acute thrombocytopenia in rats. Blood 48:765–775

Paulus JM (1974) Production et destruction des plaquettes sanguines. Masson, Paris

Paulus JM (1975) Platelet size in man. Blood 46:321–336

Paulus JM, Casals FJ (1978) Platelet formation in Mediterranean macrothrombocytosis. Nv Rev Frans Hematol 20:151–154

Paulus JM, Breton-Gorius J, Kinet-Denoel C, Boniver C (1974) Megakaryocyte ultrastructure and ploidy in human macrothrombocytosis. In: Baldini MG, Ebbe S (eds) Platelets: production, function, transfusion and storage. Grune & Stratton, New York, pp 131–141

Paulus JM, Bury J, Grosdent JC (1979) Control of platelet territory development in megakaryocytes. Blood Cells 5:59–88

Paulus JM, Esch L, Grosdent JC, Goddet JC (1986) Deviation from lognormality in platelet volume distributions: inferences about the mechanism of thrombopoiesis. In: Levine RF, Williams N, Levin J, Evatt B (eds) Megakaryocyte development and function. Liss, New York. pp 417–426

Penington DG, Streatfield K, Roxburgh AE (1976) Megakaryocytes and the heterogeneity of circulating platelets. Br J Haematol 34:639–653

Radley JM, Haller CJ (1982) The demarcation membrane system of the megakaryocyte: a misnomer? Blood 60:213–219

Rand ML, Greenberg JP, Packham MA, Mustard JF (1981) Density subpopulations of rabbit platelets: size, protein and sialic acid content, and specific radioactivity changes following labeling with ^{35}S-sulfate in vivo. Blood 57:741–746

Reimers HJ, Kinlough-Rathbone RL, Cazenave JP et al. (1976) In vitro and in vivo functions of thrombin-treated platelets. Thromb Haemost 35:151–166

Savage B, McFadden PR, Hanson SR, Harker LA (1986) The relation of platelet density to platelet age: survival of low- and high-density [111]Indium-labeled platelets in baboons. Blood 68:386–393

Thompson CB, Jakubowski JA (1988) Review: the pathophysiology and clinical relevance of platelet heterogeneity. Blood 72:1–8

Thompson CB, Eaton KA, Princiotta SM, Rushin CA, Valeri CR (1982) Size-dependent platelets subpopulations: relationship of platelet volume to ultrastructure, enzymatic activity and function. Br J Haematol 50:509–519

Thompson CB, Jakubowski JA, Quinn PG, Deykin D, Valeri CR (1983a) Platelet size as a determinant of platelet function. J Lab Clin Med 101:205–213

Thompson CB, Love DG, Quinn PG, Valeri CR (1983b) Platelet size does not correlate with platelet age. Blood 62:487–494

Thompson CB, Jakubowski JA, Quinn PG, Deykin D, Valeri CR (1984) Platelet size and age determine platelet function independently. Blood 63:1372–1375

Threatte GA, Adrados C, Ebbe S, Brecher G (1984) Mean platelet volume: the need for a reference method. Am J Clin Pathol 81:769–772

Tong M, Seth P, Penington DG (1987) Proplatelets and stress platelets. Blood 69:522–528

Trowbridge EA, Martin JF (1984) An analysis of the platelet and polyploid megakaryocyte response to acute thrombocytopenia and its biological implications. Clin Phys Physiol Meas 5:263–277

Trowbridge EA, Martin JF, Slater DN et al. (1984) The origin of platelet count and volume. Clin Phys Physiol Meas 5:145–170

Ts'Ao C (1971) Rough endoplasmic reticulum and ribosomes in blood platelets. Scand J Haematol 8:134–140

van Oost BA, Timmermans APM, Sixma JJ (1984) Evidence that platelet density depends on the alpha-granule content in platelets. Blood 63:482–485

von Behrens WE (1972) Evidence of phylogenetic canalisation of the circulating platelet mass in man. Thromb Diath Haemorrh 27: 159–172

von Behrens WE (1975) Mediterranean macrothrombocytopenia. Blood 46:199–208

Zeigler Z, Murphy S, Gardner FH (1978) Microscopic platelet size and morphology in various hematologic disorders. Blood 51:479–486

Discussion (Chapters 7 and 8)

The following is a discussion of the contributions forming Chapters 7 and 8.

Bessman: I would like to ask Dr Trowbridge two questions. The first is related to the platelet volume distribution histograms showing the stippled area around it that is the 95% confidence limits for the 13 subjects. Most published reports of normal subjects show that the range for platelet count is from 150 to 400×10^9 platelets/l blood, while there is a range of normal mean platelet volume from 7.5 to 11 fl. If one takes this into account I think one would find there is a substantially greater variation in the normal histogram, always being log-normal one understands, than the very small stippled area.

The other question that I had agrees with what Dr Paulus said. It would seem unlikely that the megakaryocytes trapped in the pulmonary bifurcation, which by the way are not perfect bifurcations if one looks at the numbers you have got on your chart, fall on a point and are split like a log with a wedge. That seems less likely than the megakaryocyte trying to get into an aperture that is a little bit too big for it so that a small amount is shaved off. Alternatively, the megakaryocyte will find itself in a shearing situation like the one Brian Bull described for red cells. There certainly was not binary fission in that case.

Trowbridge: In answer to the question about the platelet volume distribution, I think that the question is nit-picking in the sense that we are demonstrating that there is a massive difference between animal and human platelet volume distributions. The fact that I have taken 13 men whose counts may be very much the same and therefore have obtained an average distribution for which I have very tight confidence limits is irrelevant relative to the totally different rat platelet volume distribution that is there. Rat and man do not have the same mean platelet volume or heterogeneity. The rat platelet volume distribution is not log-Gaussian, nor is the rabbit platelet volume distribution. They are positively skewed but you can show that they are not log-Gaussian. In many pathological states in human beings the distributions are not log-Gaussian, so I think that the question is not that important in that it does not solve the main problem.

In reply to the second question, for a cytoplasmic volume which is of the order of 20 000 fl I showed the size of vessel that it can pass through without deformation. It will block at the next bifurcation that it comes to, it cannot possibly get through, it may squeeze a bit down one side, and Sharnoff has actually shown pictures of that happening. We have also got a picture published of a megakaryocyte astride a bifurcation. If it is a dichotomous branch then the most natural division is binary. Also the whole process is so incredibly simple. In addition, you only have to change the stochastic parameters slightly to explain all the features we have been talking about today. You can explain Dr Jackson's platelet volume distributions and the differences in size. He has a different demarcation membrane system in one strain of rats, and this is where I agree with Dr Paulus. The demarcation membrane system is probably important for the fragmentation process but I would disagree with him on his mechanism. There is a lot of evidence which indicates that the demarcation membrane system, as such, disappears in the pseudopodia that the megakaryocyte throws out. What I am interested in is the real mechanism behind platelet production, rather than talking about demarcation membrane system and then platelets, because that leaves a big chunk missing there. There is no quantitative evidence that the demarcation membrane system delineates platelet territories. There is a lot of evidence from freeze–fracture studies, and there is evidence from Radley with his vincristine and temperature effects that the demarcation membrane system does not actually delineate platelet territories. When the particles get smaller later on and we have the system where there are avascular posts asymmetrically placed, then it is more difficult to be absolutely certain what is happening, but I would say the closest that we can get at the moment to actually looking into the lungs is to use a computer to simulate what we think is happening. That is a reasonable way of trying to see what is happening. We have got the numbers. We start off with the megakaryocytes, we measure the platelets and we finish the simulation with those volumes to identify the mechanism. Nobody else has come up with a quantitative mechanism which allows you to go from the megakaryocytes to the platelets. Now if somebody does that and then they tell me what the biological mechanism is behind it, it also has to be a candidate. At the moment, the binary division mechanism quantitatively is the only candidate. Dr Paulus's model says it is log-Gaussian. I do not disagree with that, but there are no numbers in it, it is not quantitative.

Born: It is very ingenious. However, there are a number of things that worry me. If you think of a sequence of binary division in the pulmonary circulation, it surely implies that each binary division occurs because of the squeezing and blocking effect? Because they cannot go down through the microcirculation then it must depend on the force that is applied to this cell. Would you agree with that, there has to be a force? If the megakaryocyte blocks the vessel it is not even a shear force, it is pushing force. There is no instance to my knowledge and I do know something about this because I have been working with a flow kineticist for 15 years, in which, in fact, despite many people claiming the contrary, it has never been shown that cells are destroyed anywhere in the circulation. I will modify that slightly, by the shear forces in the circulation. Now the sharpest shear forces in the circulation occur in the heart, round the valves, where they are of the order of up to 500–600 dynes/cm^2. In low shear situations, as in the microvessels of the lungs, it seems to me from the strength of the cells they may not break. You are quite right in that one does not know about the physical strength, but it worries me. Now there is another argument; the blood on average takes 2 seconds to go through the lung. That is a short time. You have given the number of total bifurcations that exist in such a system, but I wonder whether when you actually look at the microcirculation you could break up a megakaryocyte into a thousand or thereabout platelets in that 2 seconds. If you do not do that you must come out of the pulmonary venous side with variously distributed nuclei still containing cytoplasm of various sizes. If I have understood it correctly the evidence is, and I am sure you are right, the megakaryocyte nuclei have their cytoplasm only in central venous blood on the incoming side. That may be so, but the rigorous proof would be to show that in fact there is then some kind of stepwise distribution of cytoplasm associated with the cells in the arterial circulation. That must be very difficult to do, but perhaps it could be done experimentally. I have no difficulty in the megakaryocytes producing platelets in the lungs, but I have difficulty with the binary division. It is much easier to see that the megakaryocyte somehow attaches itself here and there in the pulmonary circulation and goes through its last few minutes or maybe hours of maturation there and then breaks up. There is one further point; Kinosita and Ohno are supposed to have filmed the process. I have a copy of this film but cannot find it anywhere. He put a window into the bone marrow of a rabbit and filmed this process.

There is one last point that I would like to put to everybody. When the platelets are fully formed they have got the most wonderful surface receptors, such as 5-HT receptors and vasopressin receptors. Now how do they get there? Are they performed? If it is the breaking up with the canaliculi and so on then presumably one could envisage that the receptors have been pre-synthesized and are swimming around in that megakaryocyte and then concentrate on the membranes when they form. On your system it must be somehow that these receptors plus all other surface constituents must be there.

Trowbridge: Are you saying that you do not feel that there is a mechanism for a binary division? If you are talking about how many dichotomous branches there are and the fact that production takes 2 seconds, you must realize that the blood is spreading out right through the pulmonary circulation. I do not see why you have any difficulty about the cytoplasm coming down through the circulation and as it does so it breaks into two and again it breaks into two, and then again in two and so on.

Born: If you consider the flow through the pulmonary capillaries, the number of divisions that, for example, a red cell meets in its way through this circulation is about half a dozen or a dozen, and then it is already in the venules.

Trowbridge: That is not what Singhal et al. show. They show that there are 17 Strahler orders to the precapillary arteriole level and then you have to go down into the microcirculation. So you have many more sites for binary division than you are suggesting.

Martin: Can I just support Dr Trowbridge, not that he needs much support. Professor Born, those of us who are separating megakaryocytes by elutriation, have come to realize that they are immensely fragile cells. We have to go to great lengths in pretreating them with prostacyclin and other things to stop them breaking up during elutriation. Secondly, I think I would envisage this, not as a lump of cytoplasm smashing up like a Yorkshire pudding, but almost as a sort of toilet paper effect. The demarcation membrane system is there and you can imagine it ripping, as along the perforations in toilet paper, and easily separating into two pieces. If that happens then all your receptors are still there pre-formed on those surfaces, there is no problem about that.

I think there is a philosophical problem here. It is difficult to accept a physical process producing the distribution of size of a biological unit. That seems to be your difficulty. However, we are dealing with a unique process in biology. Platelets are only found in mammals, not elsewhere. In mammals all other cells are produced by mitosis. We have to invoke some unique mechanism. I realize Dr

Paulus's hypothesis is also unique, but, I think Dr Trowbridge's mechanism should stimulate everybody to produce a quantitative answer. I think his solution must be a candidate for the production process because it creates the correct numbers. As he says in other mechanisms, for example in Dr Paulus's process, the platelet territories need to be measured to show they give the predetermined volume distribution.

Jackson: Three short comments. First, I would agree with Dr Martin that mature megakaryocytes are very fragile. We also do these isolations and most of the mature megakaryocytes are already coming apart by the time you get them suspended. The second point is related to the binary fission. How does one explain the larger platelets shortly after acute thrombocytopenia? That is my biggest problem. I do not have a problem that platelets are created in the lungs or wherever, but how does binary fission account for that larger size?

Trowbridge: We would suggest that there is an increased protein synthesis, which goes along with what has been said before, in acute thrombocytopenia induced by anti-platelet serum. The quality of the cytoplasm, in some way, is changed. You can show this in the computer simulation. Dr Warren has taken megakaryocytes observed immediately after the anti-platelet serum injection and these have been fragmented under the sequence of binary divisions. You only need to change the number of binary divisions, ever so slightly, and it gives you your increased mean platelet volume and change in heterogeneity. Let me give you some very simple numbers. If you have 1024 platelets per megakaryocyte, i.e. 2^{10}, that is 10 binary divisions of the megakaryocytes on average to produce the platelets. If you change that to $2^{9.7}$, you will account for the mean platelet volume that you get after thrombocytopenia. So the change in protein synthesis and the quality of the cytoplasm and the sort of things that you are seeing by electrophoresis, where proteins have been shown to be missing, as well as different demarcation membrane systems, changes the fragmentation pattern slightly and accounts for the larger volumes. It also happens in essential thrombocythaemia, and in the May–Hegglin syndrome, and it also accounts for the differences in rat and human platelet volume distributions. That would be our explanation.

Corash: Can you just answer one question? In Shirley Ebbe's work with the SL, SLD and WWF animals, which I think people would agree have macro-megakaryocytosis, I do not know of any information that supports that they have an abnormal pulmonary circulation, yet they have normal sized platelets. How does that fit?

Trowbridge: You do not have to have an abnormal pulmonary circulation. You do not have to have an abnormal demarcation membrane system. As long as there are changes in the protein constituents within the cytoplasm, for example. Cholesterol is an example. In rabbits fed on a high-cholesterol diet, the megakaryocytes take up the cholesterol. If one asks the question, what is the value of the probability parameter λ I referred to, then for the five cholesterol-fed animals the value of λ comes out exactly the same for each animal; and significantly different from the five values of λ you obtain from the control animals on a normal diet. So all you have is a change in the protein within the megakaryocyte which changes the fragmentation pattern very slightly. I am not talking about big changes but small ones. So Shirley Ebbe can have these large megakaryocytes. What I would say is that if you search carefully you will find that there is no difference in those megakaryocytes, apart from size, from normal ones, which allows the platelet volume to be produced in the same way as normal animals. If you take megakaryocytes that are found in the rib and megakaryocytes that are in the iliac crest of the same human subject the probability parameter for production is exactly the same for the two sites, even though the megakaryocytes are larger in the rib than in the iliac crest marrow.

Born: Why don't you do the following experiment? Megakaryocytes can now be obtained in culture in large amounts. Why don't you measure their fragility under shear forces? We do it all the time with other cells: I would like to be convinced that they are fragile in the sense that you mean.

Paulus: I disagree with what has been said on two points. First, it has been said that there are many cases when you do not have log-normal volume distributions and it is true that some deviations from log-normality occur (see Chap. 8). I think that most of these cases are technical. When you are dealing with small animals you may not amplify sufficiently. The platelets are smaller and when you do not amplify sufficiently you distort the curve. That would occur with the Coulter counter systems. We have seen that repeatedly. Also in human pathology we have looked for strong deviation from log-normality. We have seen none. The most important deviation that you see is due to the shape factor, that I have mentioned in my chapter. So I think log-normality is a rather constant law and attention should always be paid to technical factors. Also logarithmic amplifiers can be very misleading and can make big distortions if they have not been checked.

Secondly, Dr Trowbridge has said that nothing is quantitative in the model I presented. There is no difficulty in making it quantitative. The variables are the volume of the diploid cell, which is starting polyploidization. You can measure the volume and take the logarithm of it. Then take the logarithm of platelet size at platelet production. You can get that data too. Then you can specify the number of steps. I have said 2000, but it depends on what you use as a time unit. If you take a time unit which is twice as long you will have 1000 steps. You can specify that and have a completely quantitative model. In addition, Dr Trowbridge speaks of the probability of division. Where does that come from? That is a number that you can adapt to any situation. It demonstrates nothing. It is quantitative but purely speculative.

Mustard: Can we change the subject slightly? We have had a paper by Dr Thompson which argued about platelet mass having a large influence on what was produced, and another by Dr Jackson showing a group of rats with a low platelet count, but they actually had large platelets. This suggests that you might be getting into this mass control of megakaryocyte function. I thought it would be useful to have some discussion about that aspect. In terms of the discussion we have been having, surely it creates an interesting experimental situation. I do not know how you can exploit it. You have rats with a congenital abnormality, in which they produce large platelets, but a smaller number of platelets than normal rats. It might be interesting to test those megakaryocytes in a pulmonary circulation.

The question I want to ask in terms of the debate we have been having is: can this theory of pulmonary platelet production be tested experimentally? As Professor Born was saying, you could culture megakaryocytes, put them into a system and pump them through a pulmonary circulation to see what comes out. If that has been done, it would be rather exciting to know about. I have another question about your theory of platelet production in the pulmonary circulation.

What is the distribution of the megakaryocytes in the flowing blood that hits the bifurcation? Only a minority may have the opportunity to interact with a bifurcation. We should have some direct testing of the hypothesis rather than debating. I wondered if the rat model could be exploited, but I wanted to be sure that I had understood the two earlier speakers correctly.

Thompson: I want to comment on the aspects of platelet mass. A lot of the credit must be given to Alex Nakeff for the instigation of that work. He compared a variety of species on a normagram. The species themselves ensured that, in fact, you could find an argument for mass over mammalian development based simply on the mean platelet volume and the platelet count of individual species. We have certainly been able to see that in primates. Different primate species have, on average, a different mean platelet volume, but they also have a concordant change in platelet count, such that they would be regulating along the same line. I think the direct testing of that hypothesis within a given species, say man – Mediterranean macrothrombocytopenia would be an example – is important. You would do what Dr Mustard suggested, using the megakaryocytes from the two different rats to investigate whether or not the pulmonary circulation is sufficient to create that event or whether you need, as I think Dr Paulus has suggested, a growth phase which is regulated in the marrow itself. This would be a different effect. You could test the pulmonary circulation against bone marrow megakaryocytes by doing switching experiments.

Martin: We have looked at the determinants of bleeding time in three situations and found it to be platelet mass on each occasion, when we have performed multivariate analysis. We studied asthmatics as well as vascular disease and their respective control groups. This again supports the idea that platelet mass may be the determinant of platelet production.

Dickinson: If one studied patients with right to left shunts we should find considerably more, in proportion, of megakaryocytes in arterial blood. Conversely, if one studies patients with left and right shunts, whose blood goes through the pulmonary circuit, two or three times, we should have considerably reduced numbers. Do you know whether that is actually the case?

Trowbridge: I said in my lecture that Tinggaard Pedersen had investigated small children with right to left shunts. He found megakaryocytes with cytoplasm in the arterial system. That answers the first part. If the platelets are produced in the way that we are suggesting, by one passage through the lungs, then the fact that they go through a second time will not make any difference, because the microtubular system in the platelet will already be there and you will not get any further fragmentation.

Jackson: I wish to respond to Dr Mustard's question. Our reciprocal bone marrow transplantation study in the rats showed that the platelet size was determined by the marrow donor.

9 Platelet Heterogeneity in Vascular Disease

J. F. Martin

Introduction

Obstruction of the myocardial and cerebral circulation is the commonest cause of death in industrialized society. There is much evidence that these diseases are related to physical obstruction initiated by platelets themselves, or due to spasm induced by platelet secretory products. Although platelet changes per se are difficult to separate from the effects of atherosclerosis, intrinsic changes in platelets are likely to be a cause of arterial obstruction.

Alterations in platelet size and density have been described in arterial disease (Trowbridge et al, 1984a; Martin et al. 1983a; Cameron et al. 1983; Kishk et al. 1985). If these occur as a consequence of change in the circulation, the manipulation of the megakaryocyte and its control system would probably be of limited importance in preventing arterial occlusion. However, if changes in density and size, both in normal physiology and in the presence of vascular disease, occur because of changes in thrombopoiesis, then both megakaryocytes and platelet production offer new therapeutic targets for the prevention of arterial disease.

The Origin of Platelet Heterogeneity

Although the subject of this chapter is pathological manifestations of platelet heterogeneity, it is relevant to start by explaining some evidence concerning the physiological origin of heterogeneity, since this author believes that in man the origin of the heterogeneity of circulating platelets is in thrombopoiesis, as proposed by Penington et al. (1976), and that the same is true for most pathological states where changes in platelet heterogeneity are seen.

Convincing evidence that platelet density does not change with platelet age comes from an experiment which used young male monkeys and validated continuous linear gradients to measure density (Martin and Penington 1983). A truly representative population of platelets was radiolabelled with chromium and re-injected into the primates. Five days later the density distribution of the labelled platelets was again measured. There was no movement from heavy to light platelets in the 12 monkeys used; the density of the platelet subfractions was as it was when they had been injected five days previously. This is an analogous study to that of Thompson and colleagues (1983), who separated platelets by size, labelled and then re-injected them. No change in size with platelet age was found. These two results, using validated methodology, would have been expected because of the relationship between platelet size and density (Figs 9.1 and 9.2).

These results are at variance with those of Corash and colleagues (1978) who, using a related species of monkey, interpreted their results to show that platelet density decreased with platelet age. The difference in these two results probably lies with the differing methodology used.

It is of interest that those authors who conclude that platelet density decreases with age have used discontinuous arabinogalactan gradients (Corash et al. 1977; Corash et al. 1978; Rand et al. 1981), whereas those who find no decrease in density with age use continuous linear gradients of Percoll (Martin and Penington 1983; Savage et al. 1986). It is theoretically more difficult to measure the true density of the platelet in a discontinuous gradient. The platelet will move in the force field, generated by rotation, towards its isopycnic point, but in its journey it will also have to deal with the interface forces between layers of the gradient. These combined forces will determine the final position of the cell in the gradient.

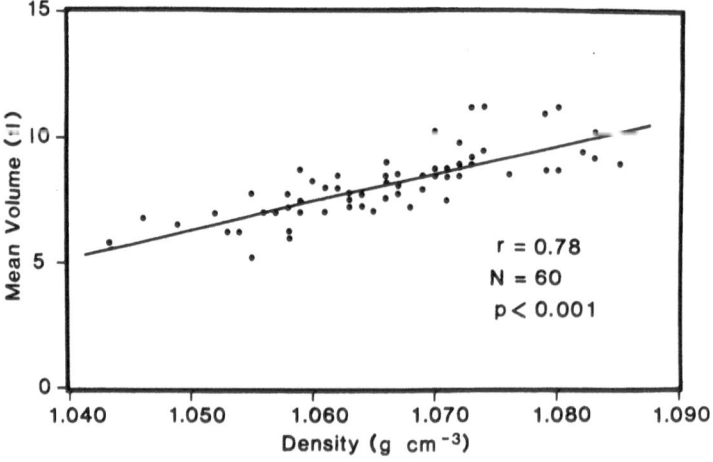

Fig. 9.1. The relationship between mean platelet volume and mean density. The data were derived by analysis of platelet populations from six normal males (Martin et al. 1983b).

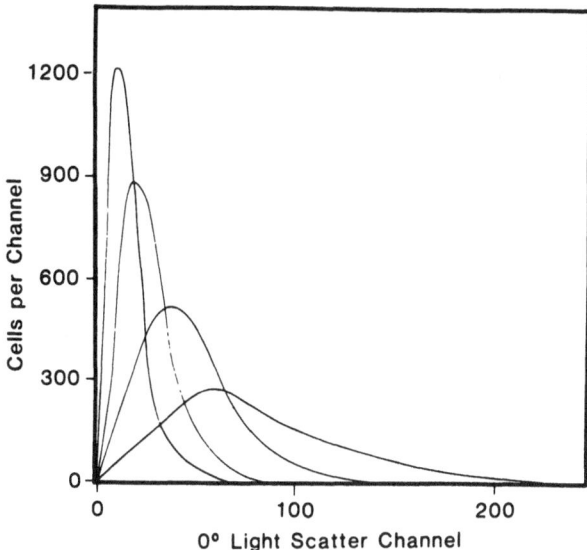

Fig. 9.2. Frequency distribution of cell size (light scattering) in the four fractions of glutaraldehyde-fixed platelets separated into volume subpopulations by cell sorter. The modal densities of these four populations, in order of increasing volume were: 1.070, 1.070, 1.071 and 1.072 g/cm^3 (Martin et al. 1983b)

The combination of forces may be reproducible on rebanding but they do not necessarily give a measure of the true density of the cell (Martin and Trowbridge 1982). If the discontinuous gradient gives a combination of density and cellular resistance to passing through interfaces then such a combination of density and artefact may be reproducible between experiments and between laboratories. Even the continuous Percoll gradients used by Packham and colleagues (Evans et al. 1985) are less than ideal since they are non-linear, causing platelet crowding at higher and lower densities.

The continuous gradients used by Martin and colleagues (Martin and Penington 1983; Martin et al. 1983b) were validated by finding the minimum conditions under which platelets did not descend further in the gradient. Under the protection of prostaglandin E_1 (PGE$_1$) the secretion of granule contents did not occur (Martin et al. 1983b). Furthermore, when the platelets from a single interface of a discontinuous arabinogalactan gradient were rebanded in a continuous linear gradient of either Percoll or arabinogalactan, those platelets were seen to be from a range of densities that spanned the adjacent interfaces of the original gradient. Probably some platelets had become lighter by undergoing secretion of granules but others had been held up at densities lighter than their true density by interface forces (Martin et al. 1983b).

A further problem in comparing the studies of Corash et al. (1978) with those of Martin and Penington (1983) is the number of animals used. The latter authors used 12 monkeys, whereas Corash et al. used only three.

It is becoming accepted that the primary determinant of platelet density heterogeneity is thrombopoiesis. A major problem to be resolved is how much change in platelet density occurs in animals that have abnormal blood vessels. It is theoretically possible that platelet activation might occur due to lack of prostacyclin and nitric oxide production from endothelial cells, or damage to endothelial cells themselves, leading to loss of granule contents from platelets that otherwise remain viable. Furthermore, turbulence may cause non-fatal platelet–platelet collision, causing loss of granule contents. Since granules are the heaviest organelles within the platelet these events might lead to decrease in density with platelet age in vascular disease.

However, these are theoretical possibilities only. There is no evidence in man that a decrease in platelet density occurs because of changes in the blood vessel wall. In fact, evidence against the proposition exists. Martin et al. (1983a) measured the density of platelets from men suffering from myocardial infarction and from control subjects. Blood was taken within 12 hours of the onset of chest pain. The control subjects were young non-smokers with normal ECG. The average mean density was significantly greater in patients than in control subjects (Fig. 9.3). The presence of vascular disease in man is difficult to ascertain without invasive techniques. One exception is myocardial infarction, which is indicated in man by ECG changes and alterations in levels of creatine phosphokinase. Myocardial infarction is nearly always associated with atherosclerosis. In such patients much of the cardiac output would be passing through vessels with abnormal endothelium and with flow abnormalities. If platelets decreased in density with age in the circulation in man then this would be *par excellence* the

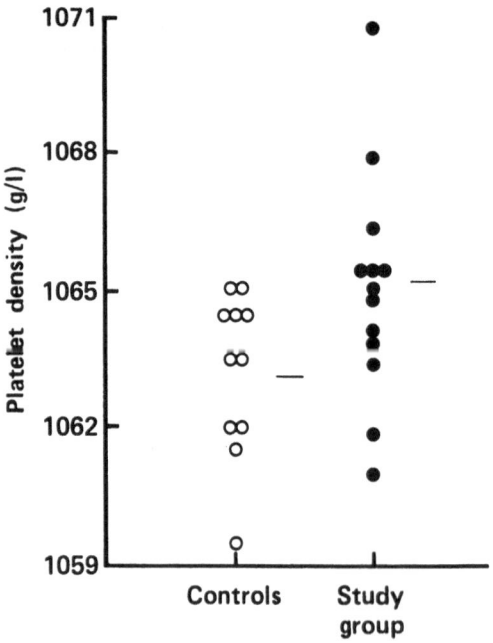

Fig. 9.3. Modal platelet density in 13 patients with acute myocardial infarction (●, measured within 12 hours of the onset of chest pain) and in 11 controls (○). The mean density is higher in the acute myocardial infarction group ($p < 0.05$, Mann–Whitney U test) (Martin et al. 1983a).

situation under which it would occur. However, the platelets in myocardial infarction were, in fact, denser. Although the platelets were bigger than those from control subjects, this did not affect the measurement of platelet density since equilibrium conditions were achieved. The platelets measured represented 97% of the circulating population.

Therefore platelets in human vascular disease are denser than normal. If the theory that platelets decrease their density with age were correct then one might have expected them to have been lighter than controls. It might be counter-argued that in myocardial infarction platelets were even denser at thrombopoiesis than their mean model density when sampled. This is possible (evidence will be offered later that thrombopoiesis is altered in vascular disease), but the fact that platelets are denser in established atherosclerosis questions whether in man platelets change their density as they circulate under any circumstances.

Further evidence that platelet density in man does not change with ageing in the circulation comes from a study of platelet heterogeneity in idiopathic thrombocytopenic purpura. Illes and colleagues (1987) measured platelet density in such patients where the mean platelet age can be assumed to be young, and compared them to normal subjects. There was no difference in platelet density between the two groups.

Cyclophosphamide can destroy megakaryocytes in the bone marrow, leaving the circulating platelets to decrease in number until, on the final day of platelet survival time, the only circulating platelets are aged platelets. Lack of platelet production after cyclophosphamide administration can be verified by lack of blood radioactivity after intravenous labelled selenomethionine. Such a study in the rat demonstrated that platelet volume did not decrease with platelet age (Eason et al. 1988). This is further evidence supporting the conclusion of Thompson et al. (1983) that platelets do not change their volume as they age in the circulation.

The bulk of the evidence, both here and elsewhere in this book, is that platelets do not change their volume as they circulate. Although the studies were done in several mammalian species they are probably applicable to man. It is highly unlikely that a property so fundamental as platelet heterogeneity should have its origin through differing mechanisms in different mammalian species. Platelets do not occur in non-mammalian orders but are found in all mammals (Parmley 1988). The production of platelets from a polyploid megakaryocyte is related to the nature of being a mammal. Platelet volume distribution tends towards the log-normal in all mammals studied, including man. Even though there may be biochemical and antigenic differences between some species it is not tenable that the origin of platelet heterogeneity in man is different from the origin in other mammals. It is therefore likely that differences in platelet volume between individuals within a species occur because of random variation or because of pathological differences in thrombopoiesis. It is also probable that differences in platelet volume occur at thrombopoiesis. Even if one held that differences in platelet volume distribution occurred during circulation this view could not explain the observed pathological changes in man. It will be shown that platelets in vascular disease are larger than controls, whereas application of the theories of Karpatkin (1969a, b) and Corash and colleagues (1977, 1978) that volume changes occur in the circulation would predict smaller platelets. The weight of evidence is that changes in the volume and density of platelets occurring in disease states in man arise within megakaryocytes or at thrombopoiesis.

Normal Physiological Response to Change in Platelet Destruction

A constant number of circulating platelets is maintained by the number of platelets destroyed being matched by the number of platelets produced in unit time. Why platelet number is maintained above those numbers needed for haemostasis is not clear, although the role of the platelet in maintaining the integrity of the vessel wall is probably partly responsible. Mean platelet volume is maintained at constant levels within an individual (von Behrens 1972; Martin et al. 1983a) and is inversely related to platelet count (O'Brien 1974; Bessman et al. 1981). Increased platelet destruction rate can occur through bleeding, thrombosis or immune-mediated removal from the circulation. In these situations haemorrhage with a low platelet count could be fatal. The response to this challenge must be mediated by circulating chemical messengers. Although much has been postulated about "thrombopoietin", a controlling hormone, little experimental evidence exists as to the nature of the hormone. However, there are several animal experiments that indicate how haemostatic potential is restored after increased platelet destruction and there is sufficient evidence to postulate the overall system.

When platelets are destroyed by anti-platelet antibody to less than 90% of the normal count then the first change observed is a change in platelet volume. This is seen in the rat 2 hours after injection of anti-platelet antibody, rising to 65% above normal volume at 6 hours (Trowbridge et al. 1986). In the mouse, Corash and colleagues (1987) have seen that platelets have increased volume at 8 hours after platelet destruction. It is unlikely that these large platelets are released from the splenic pool, as presumably the platelets are destroyed in that part of the circulation as elsewhere. The same response also occurs in man without the presence of anti-platelet antibody. Fig. 9.4 shows the response of platelet volume and count to loss of platelets from the circulation in the extra-corporeal circulation used in cardio-pulmonary bypass at heart valve replacement. Mean platelet count had dropped following operation, but average mean platelet volume was unchanged. The platelet volume only increased subsequent to the drop in platelet count (Martin et al. 1987). The animal model described above therefore appears to be a model of the situation in man.

Since there are now strong arguments that platelet volume heterogeneity does not arise through platelet ageing in the circulation (Thompson et al. 1983) it is likely that platelet volume changes after platelet destruction occur because of changes in thrombopoiesis. These may be a consequence of changed megakaryocytes or of an alteration in the way platelets are produced from megakaryocytes. Large platelets are produced after increased platelet destruction and smaller ones following increased platelet production (Martin et al. 1987) (Fig. 9.4).

Larger platelets have increased haemostatic ability and are therefore probably part of the response to stop potential life-threatening haemorrhage. When platelets were destroyed in a rabbit model the response in platelet volume was similar to that described above in the mouse and rat (Martin et al. 1982; Martin et al. 1983c). The ability of these large platelets to produce thromboxane A_2 (a vasoconstrictor and pro-aggregatory metabolite of arachidonic acid) was measured after stimulation with three agonists, each of which produced more

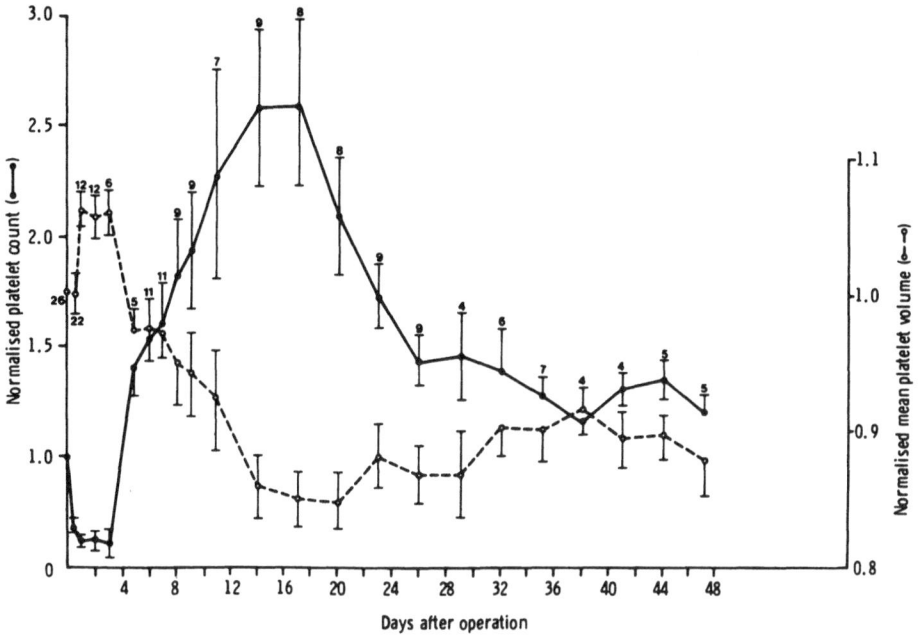

Fig. 9.4. The changes in platelet count (●) and mean volume (○) following cardiopulmonary bypass surgery. The numbers above each value indicate the number of patients studied at each interval (mean ± 1 SD). The fall in mean platelet volume during the rapid rise in platelet production argues against the proposition that all new platelets are necessarily small (Martin et al. 1987).

thromboxane A_2 per platelet in the large platelets than in platelets from control animals which had not undergone change in destruction rate. Even when the thromboxane A_2 production was expressed as picomoles per femtolitre of platelet there was still increased production, suggesting either that the megakaryocyte cytoplasm from which the large platelets were produced was more reactive than the control cytoplasm or that the way they were produced from megakaryocyte cytoplasm had made them more reactive (Martin et al. 1983c). When bleeding time was determined and the results normalized for platelet size, the large platelets reduced bleeding time more than platelets from the control animals (Martin et al. 1983c). Again this indicates that they are functionally more competent per unit volume of cytoplasm. It should be noted that large platelets in the tail of the log-normal volume distribution from an individual are not necessarily more reactive per unit volume than smaller ones from the same distribution in that individual. However, a shift in the volume distribution to the right, either sequentially within an individual or between individuals, does produce more reactive platelets.

In order to study the relationships between platelets and megakaryocytes the equilibrium of platelet production and destruction rates can be disturbed by a single acute intervention as above or by a slow prolonged intervention. Metcalfe et al. (1984) studied rats kept in a hypoxic chamber for 36 days. Thrombocytopenia developed gradually over that period. At the same time there was an increase in platelet volume and a concomitant slow change in the ploidy of the bone marrow megakaryocytes. The control modal ploidy was 16N. This gradually increased until there were equal numbers of 16N and 32N megakaryocytes on day 21 of hypoxia. At the end of 36 days of study the modal ploidy was 32N. Although it is possible that the hypoxia itself affected bone marrow ploidy, it is more likely that ploidy changed in response to a chronic increase in platelet destruction rate, since platelet count dropped continuously over the study period. It may be concluded that megakaryocyte ploidy can change slowly and continuously following a prolonged stimulus.

It is argued strongly elsewhere in this book that platelet volume heterogeneity does not change as platelets circulate. It is therefore highly likely that a change to large, more reactive platelets after platelet destruction occurs because megakaryocytes have changed or because platelets fragment differently from unchanged megakaryocytes. Further evidence that the large circulating platelets following platelet destruction arise at thrombopoiesis comes from an examination of their volume distribution curve. The argument that platelet volume heterogeneity arose through ageing was based upon the theory that a differential rate of ageing in the circulation would produce a skewed volume distribution of the total circulating cell population of all ages (Karpatkin 1969a). However, when the volume distribution of the large platelets produced shortly after platelet production was examined it was found already to be skewed, tending to the log-normal (Paulus 1975). This is further evidence that platelet volume heterogeneity arises at thrombopoiesis.

Megakaryocyte size and ploidy have been examined after platelet destruction in rat, mouse and rabbit (Warren 1987; Corash et al. 1987; Martin et al. 1982; Martin et al. 1983c). However, these experiments have limitations in relating megakaryocyte changes to circulating platelet volume heterogeneity changes. First, even the most mature megakaryocytes will give rise only to future platelets, and not to those whose volume distribution is measured at the time of sacrifice of an experimental animal. Therefore, even if Levine's Stage III and IV megakaryocytes alone are measured (1982), it is not possible to say with certainty what platelet volume they will produce. This is further complicated by the fact that the platelet volume distribution after perturbation is the product of previously circulating platelets and new entrants into the circulation. The mean volume of new entrants may alter with unit time.

Furthermore, in quantification of the ploidy distribution in the bone marrow, we have a "snapshot" of a dynamic situation, with several variables contributing to the measured distribution. These are: (1) rate of entry of megakaryoblasts into the polyploid compartment; (2) rate of movement of a megakaryocyte to its final polyploid destination; (3) rate of maturing of cytoplasm; and (4) rate of megakaryocyte release from the bone marrow (if circulating megakaryocytes produce platelets). Any one of these factors may be influenced by perturbation of equilibrium, and so influence the ploidy distribution measured in the marrow.

There is now increasing evidence that it is circulating megakaryocytes which produce platelets in the pulmonary circulation (Tinggaard-Pedersen 1978; Tinggaard-Pedersen and Cohn 1981; Trowbridge et al. 1982; Trowbridge et al. 1984b; Slater et al. 1983; Shoff et al. 1987). Therefore, in order to investigate the relationship between megakaryocytes and platelets it would be appropriate to relate megakaryocytes from the pulmonary artery to platelet parameters in steady-state thrombopoiesis. However, if the same megakaryocyte parameters are measured in test and control animals, evidence may be provided in support of platelet changes arising at thrombopoiesis. In measuring megakaryocyte changes after thrombopoiesis different anatomical sources of megakaryocytes, different preparation methods, different ways of measuring ploidy and size, different time intervals after thrombocytopenia and different levels of thrombocytopenia have been used between authors and between experiments. Thus the interpretation of results is different. However, there are certain consistent changes observable in the bone marrow. The earliest platelet size change was measured at 2 hours after platelet destruction (Trowbridge et al. 1986). At that time there was no change observed in bone marrow megakaryocytes. Corash and colleagues (1987) have measured platelet volume at 8 hours and found it to be increased in the mouse. Both these groups measured megakaryocyte size and ploidy in the same experiment and found it to be unchanged at times when the platelet volume had changed (Corash et al. 1987; Warren 1987). The measuring of the relationship between bone marrow megakaryocytes and circulating platelets has been criticized above; however, a lack of change in bone marrow megakaryocytes is more likely to have meaning than a change. The change in platelet volume after thrombocytopenia is unlikely to be artefactual since it occurs when different methods of platelet destruction are used. If unchanged bone marrow megakaryocytes produce the large newly circulating megakaryocytes then the way in which megakaryocyte cytoplasm becomes platelets must be altered so that it fragments into fewer, yet larger, platelets. Presumably this rapid change is under hormonal control.

There must, therefore, be a mechanism which is responsive to loss of platelets from the circulation. The nature of this mechanism is unknown. A signalling system must then be involved in increasing platelet count and increasing platelet size. It has been discussed above that platelet volume in the circulation can change within a few hours before a change in megakaryocyte ploidy occurs in the marrow. This implies that a hormone probably acts on a receptor on the plasma membrane of megakaryocytes determining that the platelets produced from that megakaryocyte will be larger than if the receptors were not activated. Ploidy change occurs later in the bone marrow and is probably associated with the production of more megakaryocyte cytoplasm to produce more platelets. The control of the ploidy is probably independent of the control of that megakaryocyte change that influences platelet volume (Martin 1989).

The Control of Platelet Production

The regulation of platelet count and volume (and possibly reactivity) must be via a chemical messenger system which presumably alters the number of megakaryocytes, their ploidy, cytoplasmic and membrane qualities. Such a system must have a sensor that detects a change in a parameter related to circulating platelets. Although a hormone "thrombopoietin" has been postulated (Levin et al. 1982; McDonald et al. 1974) and a number of cytokines have been shown to affect or alter megakaryocytes in culture (Williams et al. 1989), there is no convincing evidence of how the system works. Changes in platelet heterogeneity in vascular disease are described in this chapter. Overactivity and underactivity of hormonal control gives pathological changes in other organs; it is therefore possible that change in the control of thrombopoiesis may be a cause of change in platelet heterogeneity in disease, or at least may mediate it.

Because platelet destruction is associated with increase in megakaryocyte ploidy (Penington and Olsen 1970; Odell et al. 1976; Martin et al. 1982, 1983c; Corash et al. 1987) and platelet hypertransfusion with decreases in ploidy (Penington and Olsen 1970; Harker 1968), it could be concluded that ploidy change is a mechanism by which circulating platelet counts may be adjusted, probably to adjust to haemostatic needs. Fig. 9.5 proposes the putative relationships, based upon many pieces of evidence in the literature, between change in platelet destruction rate and bleeding time. It presupposes that change in platelet destruction rate is the event that signals changing haemostatic need and that, in response, change in bleeding time is the ultimate physiological manifestation of the changes in cellular haemostasis.

Let it be supposed that platelet destruction rate can increase either acutely and severely or slowly and slightly (this second example being a special case of the equilibrium situation). When platelet count is decreased acutely platelet thromboxane A_2 production increases per unit volume of platelet cytoplasm (Martin et al. 1983c). This implies a preceding change in megakaryocyte cytoplasmic reactivity, occurring within the 24 hours following platelet destruction. These platelets reduced bleeding time more than controls per unit volume of cytoplasm (Martin et al. 1983c).

A further result of the change in platelet count is a rapid increase in platelet volume. Corash and co-workers (1987) found this to occur firstly at 8 hours after thrombocytopenia in the mouse, before any change in megakaryocyte ploidy. Trowbridge et al. (1986) have confirmed these results in the rat, where mean platelet volume was significantly increased at 2 hours, rising to 65% above normal at 6 hours, yet significant increases in megakaryocyte ploidy did not occur until 3 days after platelet depletion (Warren 1987). If this is not the result of liberation of platelets from the splenic pool, it implies rapid change in fragmentation of megakaryocyte cytoplasm to produce larger platelets as discussed above (represented as in Fig. 9.5). The change in mean bone marrow megakaryocyte ploidy is

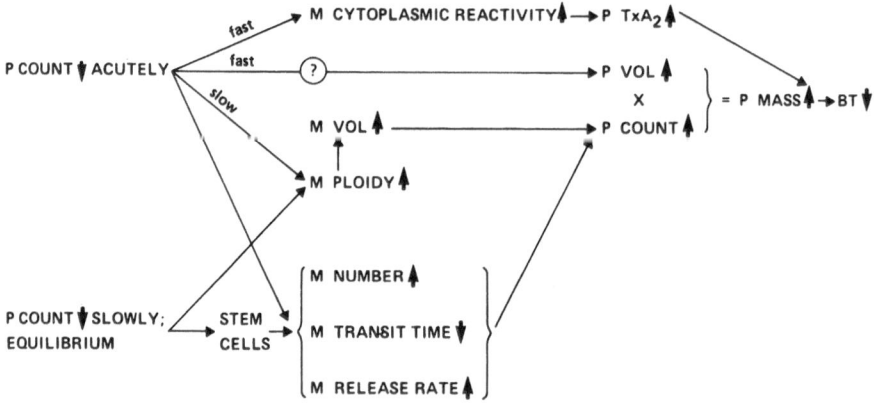

Fig. 9.5. A proposal for the system of relationships between change in platelet destruction rate, alteration in megakaryocyte variables, change in platelet mass and bleeding time. The relationships are all supported by evidence in the literature (see text). P, platelet; M, megakaryocyte; TxA$_2$, thromboxane A$_2$; BT, bleeding time; vol, volume; ↑, increased; ↓, decreased; →, an association (Martin 1989).

slow, first becoming significant after 3 days, and is associated with an increase in megakaryocyte cytoplasmic volume (Warren 1987). Such a change is associated with a sustained increase in platelet volume when platelets are continuously destroyed to reveal the size of the newly produced platelets (Martin et al. 1982). In contrast, when newly produced platelets are mixing with previously circulating platelets, the net result is a decrease in platelet volume, although megakaryocyte ploidy in the bone marrow is increasing (Warren 1987). However, an increase in ploidy appears to be associated consistently with an increase in platelet count (Harker 1968; Penington and Olsen 1970; Odell et al. 1976; Martin et al. 1983c; Warren 1987). The product of platelet count and mean platelet volume is platelet mass, which itself is the primary determinant of changes in bleeding time (Szczeklik et al. 1986; Milner and Martin 1985).

Fig. 9.5 also demonstrates the relationship in thrombokinetic equilibrium, or in states of slow chronic change. Kristensen et al. (1988a) have shown that in man, under normal conditions, there is a significant negative correlation between megakaryocyte ploidy and bleeding time. However, platelet volume was not related to megakaryocyte ploidy in these normal individuals in steady-state platelet production. If change in megakaryocyte ploidy is induced without change in destruction rate, by injection of vincristine, then a thrombocytosis occurs without a change in platelet volume (Martin et al. 1981).

When rats were kept in a hypoxic chamber, platelet count decreased slowly through 36 days of study as platelet volume increased slowly. Over the same period megakaryocyte modal ploidy increased gradually, moving from a control modal value of 16N to one of 32N after 36 days (Metcalfe et al. 1984). Thus, as has been said, a continuing slow change in ploidy may be associated with a slow change in platelet volume. However, once the system is stimulated acutely, no such relationship is perceivable.

Furthermore, there is evidence that megakaryocyte number is increased (Penington and Olsen 1970; Rolovic et al. 1970; Odell et al. 1969; Bentfield-Barker and Bainton 1977) and bone marrow transit time decreased (Ebbe et al. 1968) after acute depletion of platelets. Both these events would elevate platelet count, as would an increase in megakaryocyte release rate (assuming that platelets are produced from circulating megakaryocytes). It has also been argued that in equilibrium there is a stem cell relationship to platelet count, operating via megakaryocyte number (Milner et al. 1987).

The putative relationship between change in platelet destruction rate and change in bleeding time as shown in Fig. 9.5 is, at best, an underestimation of the relationships involved. Therefore, it is perhaps simplistic to suppose that only one hormone, thrombopoietin, should be involved in the control of such a system.

It can therefore be concluded that increase in megakaryocyte ploidy occurs consistently in association with increase in platelet production rate. Increase in platelet size in the circulation is found only with or following increased platelet destruction rate. These two events, possibly controlled independently, may be chronologically associated or may occur independently.

Platelet Volume in Myocardial Infarction

The study described earlier demonstrating that platelet density was increased in acute myocardial infarction also showed that platelet volume was increased at the same time (Martin et al. 1983a). This was confirmed by Cameron and colleagues (1983) and the results repeated in a larger study (Kishk et al. 1985). The concomitant increase in both platelet density and volume in myocardial infarction accords with the relationship between the two in normal subjects (Fig. 9.1). Myocardial infarction is, in the majority of cases, associated with thrombus in the coronary artery related to atherosclerosis that may have fissured (Davies and Thomas, 1984). The first cellular change leading to arterial thrombus is platelet aggregation. Aspirin, which decreases platelet aggregability, has been shown to decrease the incidence of myocardial infarction (Veterans Administration Co-operative Study 1983). Large platelets are more reactive than small platelets (Martin et al. 1983c; Karpatkin 1969a, b; Thompson et al. 1982). It is therefore reasonable to assume that if large platelets are present in the circulation before myocardial infarction in a proportion of patients, then in these patients the large platelets may be causally linked to the occurrence of thrombus in the coronary artery, no matter what other prothrombotic events might determine the timing of thrombus formation.

Fig. 9.6 shows platelet count and mean platelet volume from patients with myocardial infarction in a well-controlled study. Patients had platelet volume and

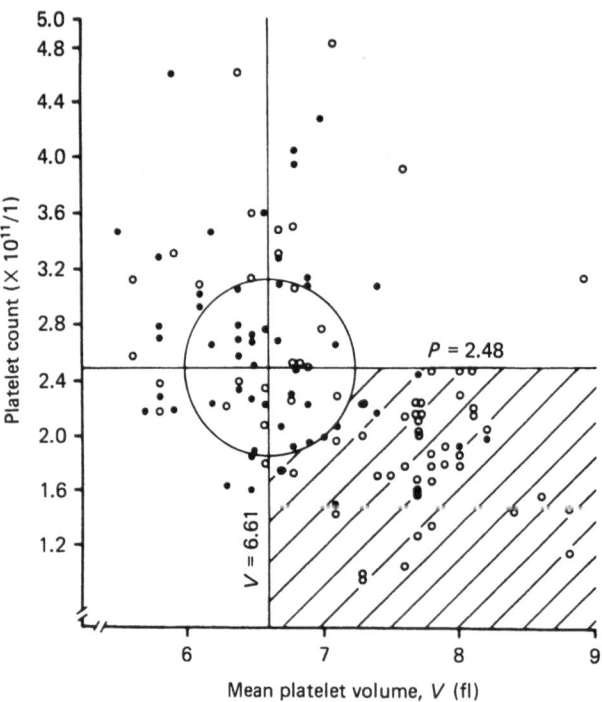

Fig. 9.6. Scattergram of the platelet count, P, and mean platelet volume, V, of patients with acute myocardial infarction (O) and those with chest pain and no myocardial infarction (●). The *hatched area* represents the indented quadrant in which are found high mean platelet volume and low platelet count. This region contains significantly more of the acute myocardial infarction group (62%, $p<0.001$) compared with the control group (13%). Since the control group had ischaemic heart disease and chest pain but no infarction the study was controlled for occlusion of the coronary artery (Kishk et al. 1985).

count measured blindly in a coronary care unit within 24 hours of the onset of chest pain. Myocardial infarction was diagnosed according to World Health Organization criteria. The controls were those patients who had chest pain but no infarction at the time of the study. However, they all had past evidence of ischaemic heart disease. Therefore the study was controlled for the occurrence of clot in the coronary artery in the presence of vascular disease. Sixty-two per cent of the patients with myocardial infarction ($p<0.01$) lie in the area of low platelet count and high platelet volume (Kishk et al. 1985). Since the platelets were studied within 24 hours of the onset of chest pain and platelet life-span in man is approximately 10 days, it is probable that the large platelets were circulating before the infarction occurred.

In acute myocardial infarction not only is the average mean platelet volume increased but the whole of the platelet volume distribution is shifted to the right (Trowbridge and Martin 1987) (Fig. 9.7). If the platelet volume distribution curve has its origin in thrombopoiesis, then this implies a change in megakaryocytes in myocardial infarction. Furthermore, the models described above indicate that low platelet count and large platelet volume may follow acute platelet destruction (Martin et al. 1982) or chronic slow platelet destruction (Metcalfe et al. 1984). In both these cases there is a change to larger higher ploidy megakaryocytes, although the large platelets following acute destruction occur before megakaryocyte changes (Corash et al. 1987; Warren 1987).

When bone marrow biopsy was carried out on patients following myocardial infarction it was found that the megakaryocytes were indeed bigger than the controls with chest pain and no myocardial infarction (Trowbridge et al. 1984a) (Table 9.1). Although mean ploidy was not significantly different, there was an

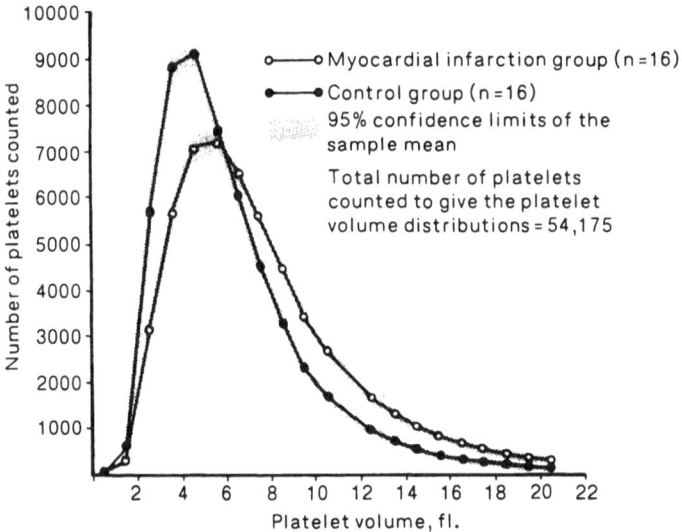

Fig. 9.7. The average platelet volume distribution of patients with acute myocardial infarction (○) and the control group (●) of patients with chest pain but no infarction. There is an increased number of larger platelets in the tail of the platelet volume distribution associated with acute myocardial infarction. As discussed in the text such large platelets are more reactive than the smaller ones in the tail of the control distribution (Trowbridge and Martin 1987).

increase in the frequency of high-ploidy megakaryocytes. However, since there is a relationship between megakaryocyte volume and ploidy within an anatomical area (Penington and Olsen 1970; Gladwin et al. 1988), it is likely that mean ploidy would also be increased if a larger number of patients were studied. The megakaryocytes were studied after the infarction and it could be argued that the changes were a result of the acute event itself. However, a second study, also summarized in Table 9.1, investigated megakaryocyte volume in autopsy-proven sudden unexpected cardiac death (Trowbridge et al. 1984a). The conditions of this study precluded the study of ploidy. The controls were age-matched men who had suffered sudden traumatic death and had no evidence of vascular disease at autopsy. Bone marrow biopsy was taken within 3 hours of death in both groups. The size of the megakaryocytes was significantly larger in the sudden cardiac death group, and not significantly different from the myocardial infarction group described above. The importance of this study is that the larger megakaryocytes were present at the time of sudden cardiac death and therefore could not have been an effect of the acute event.

Table 9.1. Mean bone marrow megakaryocyte volume and range in men having suffered acute myocardial and in control subjects admitted to the same coronary care unit with chest pain but no infarction

| | Megakaryocyte volume (fl) | |
	Mean	Range
Myocardial infarction ($n=7$)	13 879	1672–46 779
	(±2188)	(±1077 ±3578)
Controls ($n=6$)	10 033	896–23 949
	(±404)	(±186 ±938)
Sudden cardiac death ($n=11$)	12 030	938–40 358
	(±404)	(±187 ±1747)
Controls ($n=11$)	8973	835–23 559
	(±321)	(±244 ±2082)

The mean volume and range of megakaryocytes are larger in myocardial infarction. When the same values were measured in men suffering sudden unexpected cardiac death compared to age- and sex-matched controls having suffered sudden unnatural death with no evidence of coronary artery disease at autopsy, similar significant differences were seen between the two groups. Furthermore, there is no significant difference in megakaryocyte volume between the myocardial infarction group and the sudden cardiac death group. The presence of large megakaryocytes in the bone marrow are a risk factor for myocardial infarction and sudden unexpected cardiac death (Trowbridge et al. 1984a).

There are four possible reasons why megakaryocytes may be larger in myocardial infarction and sudden cardiac death: (1) they may be congenitally large; (2) they may be virally transformed cells; (3) they may be the consequence of an abnormality of the control system of platelet production; or (4) they may be the consequence of a period of increased platelet destruction before the infarction. The latter seems the most appropriate explanation. If so, it is not possible to say whether an increase in platelet destruction rate would occur for hours, days or months before infarction. Myocardial infarction itself might have a variety of causes, only one of which is related to changes in megakaryocytes and platelet heterogeneity; however, in the autopsy study and clinical study above, all patients with infarct or sudden death had larger mean megakaryocyte size than controls.

If the proposed model of the relationships involved in the control of platelet production described in Fig. 9.5 is applied to myocardial infarction then the presence of large (possibly high-ploidy) megakaryocytes in conjunction with a low platelet count and a high platelet volume in myocardial infarction gives rise to the following hypothesis. The large megakaryocytes are associated with an increase in platelet production rate. The large platelets occur secondarily to an increased, continuing, platelet destruction rate. Therefore the two independent control mechanisms proposed earlier would both be activated, probably secondarily to an increased platelet destruction rate before the infarct occurs.

The Bleeding Time in Myocardial Infarction

Bleeding time was first shown to be related to platelet count by Duke in 1912. Using a sensitive method (Mielke 1984), Szczeklik and colleagues (1986) took these observations further by showing that platelet mass (count × volume) was the primary determinant of bleeding time in normal subjects. Therefore larger platelets in man would be expected to give a shorter bleeding time (for a given platelet count). In the animal models described above large platelets produced after increased platelet destruction were not only more biochemically reactive (Thompson et al. 1982; Karpatkin 1969a, b; Martin et al. 1983c) but also reduced bleeding time more per unit volume than controls (Martin et al. 1983c).

Since the average mean platelet volume is increased in myocardial infarction the bleeding time in that disease has been studied by Milner and Martin (1985). Fig. 9.8 shows that the mean bleeding time in myocardial infarction is shortened compared to controls similar to those used above. Multivariate analysis showed that the primary determinant of the bleeding time in myocardial infarction was platelet mass (count × volume), as it is in normal subjects.

This same cohort of patients was studied again two years later by Kristensen and colleagues (1988b). It was found that the significant shortening in bleeding time had been normalized. However, Fig. 9.8 shows that the patients who had myocardial infarction two years earlier may still have a shortened bleeding time. A later study confirmed the shortened bleeding time in myocardial infarction but found that patients with unstable angina did not have shortened bleeding time compared to those with non-cardiac chest pain (Kristensen et al. 1989a). Using aspirin as a probe for cyclo-oxygenase activity it was found that the bleeding time in myocardial infarction lengthened significantly more than in control subjects or those with unstable angina after aspirin administration. However, the bleeding time in myocardial infarction still remained significantly shorter than in the other two groups. This remaining shortening was related to circulating adrenaline levels, which were increased only in the myocardial infarction group. It is therefore proposed that the shortened bleeding time in myocardial infarction has two components: one related to increased adrenaline levels and probably secondary to the infarction, and one related to increased cyclo-oxygenase activity in platelets, possibly preceding the infarction. However, the shortening of bleeding time before infarction still requires demonstration.

It is also of interest that bleeding time was found to be inversely related to megakaryocyte size and ploidy in normal subjects (Fig. 9.9). The shortened bleeding time, large platelets and large megakaryocytes as contributors to myocardial infarction are therefore compatible with several pieces of independent evidence.

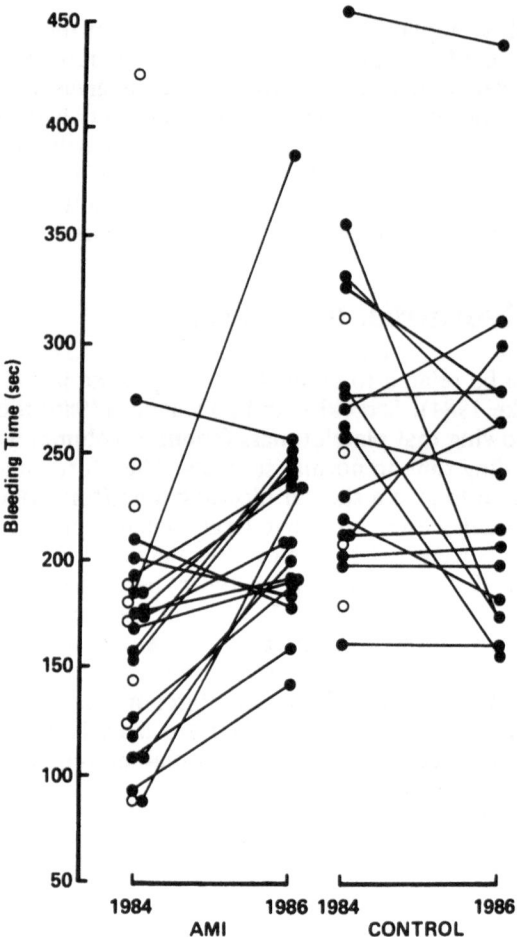

Fig. 9.8.   Bleeding times (s) in 18 patients with definite acute myocardial infarction (AMI), by WHO criteria, and in 16 patients admitted to the same coronary care unit with chest pain but no definite myocardial infarction (control), at the time of admission (1984) and at follow-up 2 years later (1986). The bleeding time was significantly shorter in the AMI group at the time of admission. It was also significantly prolonged in the AMI group 2 years later compared with the earlier values obtained during the acute myocardial infarction ($p < 0.01$). Although in 1986 there was no significant difference between the two groups the bleeding time in the AMI group was still shorter; (O), values for patients who died before follow-up (Kristensen et al. 1988).

Platelet Volume and Megakaryocytes in Animal Models of Vascular Disease

Further evidence that megakaryocyte and platelet heterogeneity might be altered in vascular disease comes from rabbit and guinea-pig models (Martin et al. 1985; Schick and Schick 1985; Dupont et al. 1987; Kristensen et al. 1988c). Increased cholesterol is a major risk factor for death from myocardial infarction (Castelli et

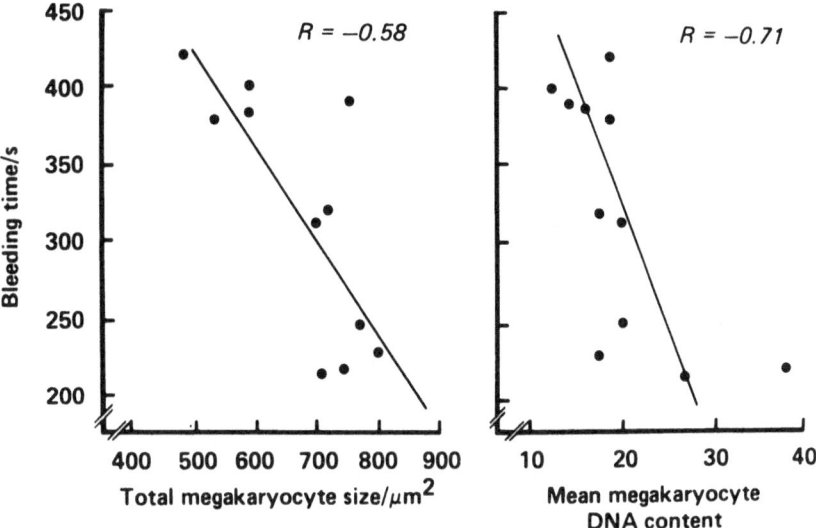

Fig. 9.9. Scattergrams illustrating the significant inverse relationship between the bleeding time and total megakaryocyte size ($p<0.05$) and between the bleeding time and mean megakaryocyte DNA content ($p<0.05$) in 11 human subjects with normal thrombopoiesis. The megakaryocyte measurements were done blindly by different investigators (Kristensen et al. 1988a).

al. 1986). It is not taken up by circulating platelets, but by megakaryocytes which then incorporate it into future platelets (Schick and Schick 1985). When rabbits are fed a high-cholesterol diet for 12 weeks their aortae become atheromatous and their megakaryocytes are found to be increased in size and ploidy (Martin et al. 1985). However, the platelets produced from these megakaryocytes do not follow the pattern that has evolved in this chapter: they are smaller than controls. The picture is further complicated by the fact that after 6 days of low-cholesterol diet rabbit megakaryocytes are smaller than controls (Kristensen et al. 1988c). A different model was used by Dupont, who fed rabbits a high-cholesterol diet for 12 weeks followed by a normal diet. The megakaryocytes were then found to be smaller than controls (Dupont et al. 1987). Clearly high-cholesterol diet does have an effect on megakaryocytes. It is, however, a dynamic effect with time, possibly explained by the dual effect of the direct effect of cholesterol on the megakaryocyte itself and the indirect effect on megakaryocytes of the platelet interaction with the vessel wall in vascular disease. There may also be species differences since Schick and Schick (1985) found megakaryocytes to increase in size after short-term cholesterol diet in the guinea-pig, using similar conditions to Kristensen et al. (1988c) in the rabbit who found them to be smaller. It does appear, however, that platelet destruction enhances atherosclerosis at the same time as megakaryocyte ploidy and size are increased (Kristensen et al. 1989b). Litter-mate rabbits divided into three groups were either fed normal diet (one group) or high-cholesterol diet for 6 weeks (two groups). Seven days before sacrifice one group on the high-cholesterol diet was given a control injection of serum alone and the other an injection of anti-platelet serum, which produced an immediate thrombocytopenia followed by a thrombocytosis. It is difficult to measure platelet volume in the presence of high serum cholesterol, but control experiments indicated that such thrombocytopenia would be associated with the production of large platelets. Megakaryocyte size and DNA were significantly increased when measured on the fourth day after the induction of thrombocytopenia. The striking result in this study is that the mean percentage of the aorta which had become atheromatous was nil in the normal-diet group, 42% in the high-cholesterol group given an injection of control serum and 97% in the group on high-cholesterol diet that underwent platelet destruction and change to larger, higher-ploidy megakaryocytes (Fig. 9.10). Accelerated atherogenesis probably does not result from endothelial damage by the anti-platelet antibody since Evans blue staining of endothelium showed no difference between the three groups. A possible explanation is that change to large and high-ploidy megakaryocytes, producing initially large, and later more, platelets is atherogenic. Activated megakaryocytes may produce increased amounts of platelet-derived growth factor.

Although there is a lack of consistency between animal models of atherogenesis when megakaryocytes are studied, there is agreement that bone marrow megakaryocyte distribution is altered. Whether megakaryocyte involvement in vascular disease is cause, effect or an association remains to be established. It is of great interest, however, that megakaryocyte changes and alterations in platelet volume heterogeneity occur both in human and animal vascular disease.

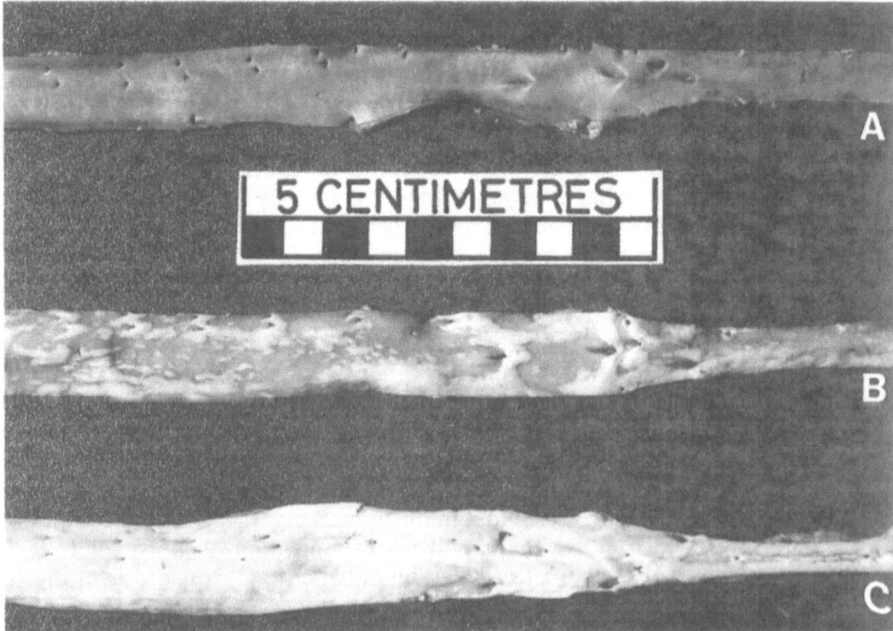

Fig. 9.10.   Aortae from (A) a rabbit fed a normal diet, (B) a rabbit fed a cholesterol-enriched diet for 12 weeks and injected with control serum one week before sacrifice, and (C) from a rabbit fed cholesterol-enriched diet for 12 weeks and injected with anti-platelet antibody one week before sacrifice. The rabbits were siblings. One representative aorta is shown for each group ($n=5$). The anti-platelet antibody has caused rapid acceleration of atheroma over the 7 days. The possible explanations are discussed in the text (Kristensen et al. 1989b).

Conclusions

Platelet heterogeneity is altered in human vascular disease. These changes may play an important part in both atherogenesis and thrombosis. Platelet destruction, either acutely or slowly, can alter megakaryocyte ploidy to produce more platelets. Platelet volume changes after platelet destruction are independent of changes in megakaryocyte ploidy and are probably under separate control. Megakaryocytes are larger in myocardial infarction and sudden cardiac death. Platelets with altered size and density, produced from activated megakaryocytes, may contribute to coronary artery thrombosis.

Although there is still some opinion in this book that platelet density may decrease with age, the main discussion is what percentage change in platelet density that might be, especially when platelets interact with damaged endothelium. The finding of increased platelet density in myocardial infarction argues against any change in platelet density with age in vascular disease in man.

References

Bentfeld-Barker ME, Bainton DF (1977) Ultrastructure of rat megakaryocytes after prolonged thrombocytopenia. J Ultrastruct Res 61:201–214

Bessman JD, Williams LJ, Gilmer PR (1981) The inverse relation of platelet size and count in normal subjects, and an artifact of other particles. Am J Clin Path 76:289–293

Cameron HA, Philips R, Ibbotson RM, Carson PHM (1983) Platelet size in myocardial infarction. Br Med J 287:449–457

Castelli WP, Garrison RJ, Wilson PWF, Abbott RD, Kalousian S, Kannel WB (1986) Incidence of coronary heart disease and lipoprotein cholesterol levels: The Framingham Study. J Am Med Assoc 256:2835–2838

Corash L, Tan H, Gralnick HR, Shafer B (1977) Heterogeneity of whole human blood platelet subpopulations: I. Relationship between buoyant density, cell volume and ultrastructure. Blood 49:71–87

Corash L, Shafer BI, Perlow M (1978) Heterogeneity of whole human blood platelet subpopulations. II. Use of a subhuman primate to analyse the relationship between density and platelet age. Blood 52:726–734

Corash L, Chen HY, Levin J et al. (1987) Regulation of thrombopoiesis: Effects of the degree of thrombocytopenia on megakaryocyte ploidy and platelet volume. Blood 70:177–185

Davies MJ, Thomas A (1984) Thrombosis and acute coronary artery lesions in sudden cardiac ischaemic death. New Eng J Med 310:1137–1140

Duke WW (1912) The pathogenesis of purpuras haemorrhagicae with especial reference to the part played by blood platelets. Arch Int Med 10:445–469

Dupont H, Dupont MA, Larrue J, Boisseau ML, Bricaud H (1987) Megakaryopoiesis disturbances in atherosclerotic rabbits. Atherosclerosis 63:15–26

Eason CT, Pattison A, Howells DD, Bonner FW, Martin JF (1988) The effects of amrinone, cyclophosphamide and anti-platelet serum on platelet production in the Gunn rat. J Appl Toxicol 8:29–34

Ebbe S, Stohlman F, Donovan J, Overcash J (1968) Megakaryocyte maturation rate in thrombocytopenic rats. Blood 32:787–795

Evans RM, Packham MA, Rand ML et al. (1985) Platelet buoyant density: Similar results by centrifugation on discontinuous Stractan and continuous Percoll gradients. Thromb Haemost 54:243

Gladwin AM, Martin JF, Thorpe JAC, Trowbridge EA (1988) Human megakaryocyte size varies with anatomical site. Br J Haematol 69:445–448

Harker LA (1968) Kinetics of thrombopoiesis. J Clin Invest 47: 458–465

Illes I, Pfueller SL, Hussein S, Chesterman CN, Martin JF (1987) Platelets in ideopathic thrombocytopenic purpura are increased in size but not in density. Br J Haematol 67:173–176

Karpatkin S (1969a) Heterogeneity of human platelets. I. Metabolic and kinetic evidence suggestive of young adult platelets. J Clin Invest 48:1073–1082

Karpatkin S (1969b) Heterogeneity of human platelets. II. Functional evidence suggestive of young and old platelets. J Clin Invest 48:1083–1087

Kishk YT, Trowbridge EA, Martin JF (1985) Platelet volume sub-populations in myocardial infarction: an investigation of their homogeneity for smoking, infarct size and site. Clin Sci 68:419–425

Kristensen SD, Bath PMW, Martin JF (1988a) The bleeding time is inversely related to megakaryocyte nuclear DNA content and size in man. Thromb Haemostas 59:357–359

Kristensen SD, Milner PC, Martin JF (1988b) Bleeding time and platelet volume in acute myocardial infarction: a 2 year follow-up study. Thromb Haemost 59:353–356

Kristensen SD, Roberts KM, Lawry J, Martin JF (1988c) Megakaryocyte and vascular changes in rabbits on a short-term high cholesterol diet. Atherosclerosis 71:121–130

Kristensen SD, Bath P, Martin JF (1989a) Differences in bleeding time, aspirin resistivity and adrenaline between acute myocardial infarction and unstable angina. Cardiovasc Res (in press)

Kristensen SD, Roberts KM, Kishk YT, Martin JF (1989b) Platelet destruction increases megakaryocyte size and DNA content while enhancing atherosclerosis in the hypercholesterolaemic rabbit. Eur J Clin Invest (in press)

Levin J, Levin FC, Hull DF III, Penington DG (1982) The effects of thrombopoietin on megakaryocyte–CFC_1 megakaryocytes and thrombopoiesis: with studies of ploidy and platelet size. Blood 60:989–998

Levine RF, Hazzard KC, Lamberg JD (1982) The significance of megakaryocyte size. Blood 60:1122–1130

Martin JF (1989) The relationship between megakaryocyte ploidy and platelet volume: Commentary. Blood Cells 15:108–117

Martin JF, Penington DG (1983) The relationship between the age and density of circulating ^{51}Cr-labelled platelets in the sub-human primate. Thromb Res 30:157–164

Martin JF, Trowbridge EA (1982) Theoretical requirements for the density separation of platelets with comparison of continuous and discontinuous gradients. Thromb Res 27:513–522

Martin JF, Francis P, Lee L, Shaw T, Macpherson J, Penington DG (1981) Differences in the volume of stress platelets and vincristine stimulated platelets. Thromb Haemost 46:410

Martin JF, Trowbridge EA, Salmon GL, Slater DN (1982) The relationship between platelets and megakaryocyte volume. Thromb Res 28:447–459

Martin JF, Plumb J, Kilby RS, Kishk YT (1983a) Changes in platelet volume and density in myocardial infarction. Br Med J 287:449–457

Martin JF, Shaw T, Heggie J, Penington DG (1983b) Measurement of the density of human platelets and its relationship to volume. Br J Haematol 54:337–352

Martin JF, Trowbridge EA, Salmon G, Plumb J (1983c) The biological significance of platelet volume: its relationship to bleeding time, platelet thromboxane B_2 production and megakaryocyte nuclear DNA concentration. Thromb Res 32:443–460

Martin JF, Slater DN, Kishk YT, Trowbridge EA (1985) Platelet and megakaryocyte changes in cholesterol-induced experimental atherosclerosis. Atherosclerosis 5:604–612

Martin JF, Daniel TD, Trowbridge EA (1987) Acute and chronic changes in platelet volume and count after cardiopulmonary bypass induced thrombocytopenia in man. Thromb Haemost 57:55–58

McDonald TP, Cottrell M, Clift R, Lane K (1974) Purification and assay of thrombopoietin. Exp Haematol 2:355–361

Metcalfe BC, Warren CW, Slater DN, Trowbridge EA, Martin JF, Barer GR (1984) Changes in platelets and megakaryocyte in simulated high altitude. Clin Sci 6:76P (Abstract)

Mielke CH (1984) Measurement of the bleeding time. Thromb Haemostas 52:210–211

Milner PC, Martin JF (1985) Shortened bleeding time in acute myocardial infarction and its relation to platelet mass. Br Med J 290:1767–1770

Milner PC, Johl S, Martin JF (1987) Platelet count is positively correlated with white cell count and red cell count. Haemostasis 17:211–216

O'Brien JR (1974) A relationship between platelet volume and platelet number. Thromb Diath Haemorrh 31:363–365

Odell TT, Jackson CW, Friday TJ, Charsha DE (1969) Effects of thrombocytopenia on megakaryocytopoiesis. Br J Haematol 17:91–101

Odell TT, Murphy JR, Jackson CW (1976) Stimulation of megakaryocytopoiesis by acute thrombocytopenia in rats. Blood 48:765–775

Parmley RT (1988) Mammals. In: Rowley AF, Ratcliffe NA (eds) Vertebrate blood cells. Cambridge University Press, Cambridge, New York; New Rochelle, Melbourne, Sydney, pp 337–424

Paulus JM (1975) Platelet size in man. Blood 46:321–336

Penington DG, Olsen TE (1970) Megakaryocytes in states of altered platelet production: cell numbers, size and DNA content. Br J Haematol 18:447–463

Penington DG, Lee NYL, Roxburgh AE, McGready JR (1976) Platelet density and size: the interpretation of heterogeneity. Br J Haematol 34:365–376

Rand ML, Greenberg JP, Packham MA, Mustard JF (1981) Density subpopulations of rabbit platelets: size, protein and sialic acid content, and specific radioactivity changes following labelling with ^{35}S-sulfate in vivo. Blood 57:741–746

Rolovic Z, Baldini M, Dameshek W (1970) Megakaryocytopoiesis in experimentally induced immune thrombocytopenia. Blood 35:173–188

Savage B, McFadden PR, Hanson SR, Harker LA (1986) The relation of platelet density to platelet age: survival of low- and high-density ^{111}Indium-labelled platelets in baboons. Blood 68:386–393

Schick BP, Schick PK (1985) The effect of hypercholesterolemia on guinea pig platelets, erythrocytes and megakaryocytes. Biochim Biophys Acta 833:291–302

Shoff PK, Kirwin KS, Levine RF (1987) Megakaryocytes in circulating blood. Circulation 76:1339

Slater DN, Trowbridge EA, Martin JF (1983) The megakaryocyte and thrombocytopenia: A microscopic study which supports the theory that platelets are produced in the pulmonary circulation. Thromb Res 31:163–176

Szczeklik A, Milner PL, Birch J, Watkins J, Martin JF (1986) Prolonged bleeding time, reduced platelet aggregation, altered PAF–Acether sensitivity and increased platelet mass are a trait of asthma and hay fever. Thromb Haemost 56:283–287

Thompson CB, Eaton KA, Princiotta SM, Rushin CA, Valeri CR (1982) Size dependent platelet subpopulations: relationship of platelet volume to ultra structure, enzymatic activity and function. Br J Haematol 50:509–519

Thompson CB, Love DG, Quinn PG, Valeri CR (1983) Platelet size does not correlate with platelet age. Blood 62:487–494

Tinggaard-Pedersen N (1978) Occurrence of megakaryocytes in various vessels and their retention in the pulmonary capillaries in man. Scand J Haematol 21:369–375

Tinggaard-Pedersen N, Cohn J (1981) Intact megakaryocytes in various vessels and their retention in the pulmonary capillaries in man. Scand J Haematol 27:57–63

Trowbridge EA, Martin JF (1987) The platelet volume distribution: a signature of the prethrombotic state in coronary heart disease? Thromb Haemost 58:714–717

Trowbridge EA, Martin JF, Slater DN (1982) Evidence for a theory of physical fragmentation of megakaryocytes implying that all platelets are produced in the pulmonary circulation. Thromb Res 28:461–475

Trowbridge EA, Slater DN, Kishk YT, Woodcock BW, Martin JF (1984a) Platelet production in myocardial infarction and sudden cardiac death. Thromb Haemostas 52:167–171

Trowbridge EA, Martin JF, Slater DN et al. (1984b) The origin of platelet count and volume. Clin Phys Physiol Meas 5:145–170

Trowbridge EA, Warren CW, Martin JF (1986) Platelet volume heterogeneity in acute thrombocytopenia. Clin Phys Physiol Meas 7:203–210

Veterans Administration Co-operative Study (1983) Protective effects of aspirin against acute myocardial infarction and death with unstable angina. N Engl J Med 309:396–402

von Behrens WE (1972) Evidence of phylogenetic canalization of the circulating mass in man. Thromb Diath Haemorrh 27:163–169

Warren CW (1987) The thrombopoietic control system: homeostasis, simulation and perturbation. PhD thesis, University of Sheffield

Williams N, Jackson H, Walker F, Oon SH (1989) Multiple levels of regulation of megakaryocytopoiesis. Blood Cells 15:123–133

Technical Questions

Corash: You have given us a series of different types of experiments to support a theoretical construction. Now you are attaching a lot of significance to haemostasis, as judged by the bleeding time. I do not know of any test, at least in our Institution, with which we have more difficulty in terms of reproducibility than the bleeding time. I am very concerned that you have taken a test, with a high degree of variability, that is not well characterized in the data that you have shown us and are attaching a lot of significance to it. That troubles me a lot. Especially, when I think back to that old linear relationship between platelet count and bleeding time published by Harker in the *New England Journal of Medicine* in 1971. We now know that there are people with fairly severe thrombocytopenia who can maintain normal bleeding times. Clearly they have great perturbations in their megakaryocyte mass if we believe Harker's data. I do not know how to fit all that together.

Martin: I am not putting great emphasis on bleeding time. You could leave bleeding time off my diagram and leave it at platelet mass and things would still work. I introduced bleeding time several times throughout my lecture, because we had measured it and the statistics associated with that measurement were good. Kristensen, for example, looked at 11 patients with DNA versus bleeding time. If we had a large coefficient of variation of those measurements then we would not have got the linearity of the relationship. You have to admit that.

Corash: I do not think the correlation coefficient of 0.7 associated with those subjects is that fantastic.

Martin: It is not fantastic, but is biologically acceptable in 11 patients. I bring up bleeding time in this environment to try and be provocative – to try and look at the end physiological manifestation of our discussions to see if it can be fitted in. If you go back to our paper on asthma, platelet mass and bleeding time, we looked at a large number of patients and the statistics there were very tight. If you consider the 50 patients we have investigated after myocardial infarction at King's College Hospital, the bleeding time statistics are again very tight. There is now good evidence that the determinant of that parameter is good. I would agree the bleeding time has a large coefficient of variation. I repeat, the mechanism would work if we left it at platelet mass, or even if we left it at the product of platelet volume and count, but bleeding time, probably is the only physiological manifestation of what we have been talking about that we have got at the moment. It is certainly better than platelet aggregation, I am afraid, Professor Born.

10   The Heterogeneity of Platelets

J. D. Bessman

In this chapter I will attempt to reconcile the existing data on such variables as platelet size, age, survival, cytoplasmic demarcations and megakaryocyte heterogeneity in order to construct a coherent whole.

First, to introduce mean platelet volume (MPV), I will discuss the disc-to-sphere shape change induced by ethylene diamine tetra-acetic acid (EDTA). This is the anticoagulant that is generally used for blood collection, and that is used in the data to be shown. However, the distinctions that will be made for MPV among patient groups are equally valid if acid–citrate–dextrose (ACD) anticoagulant is used to avoid the shape change. The absolute scale of MPV differs, but the distinctions remain (Table 10.1). While EDTA causes an apparent change in MPV, the platelets that are smallest to begin with are smallest after EDTA exposure: all patients' MPV values change about 15% after EDTA exposure. Therefore, the well known disc-to-sphere "artefact" introduced by EDTA is a constant. Different MPV values are caused by different thrombopoietic conditions as discussed below, not by differing EDTA effect.

The relation between platelet count and platelet size (MPV) is inversely but non-linearly related, as published by several groups from 1981 onwards (Bessman

Table 10.1.   Comparison of mean platelet volume in EDTA and ACD anticoagulant

		None	Anticoagulant	
			ACD, 30 min	EDTA, 30 min
Nominal MPV	6.0	5.2±0.3	5.4±0.2	5.8±0.3
(see legend)	7.5	6.8±0.4	6.8±0.4	7.4±0.2
	9.0	7.9±0.3	8.0±0.7	8.7±0.6
	10.5	9.1±0.6	9.3±0.5	10.8±0.6
	12.0	10.4±0.4	10.7±0.4	12.1±0.5

Subjects with normal platelet counts were selected for their mean platelet volume (MPV) in a routinely run automated blood count: this was considered the "nominal platelet size". Five subjects were in each MPV group. A second blood specimen then was drawn and either anticoagulated for 30 minutes and then measured, or the un-anticoagulated blood measured within 90 seconds of venipuncture. All measurements were done with a Coulter Counter model S-Plus IV (Coulter, Hialeah, Florida). The data show that ACD anticoagulation changes the measured MPV little versus no anticoagulant. EDTA anticoagulant does cause an approximate 15% increase in measured MPV; however, the hierarchy of platelet size is not affected, since all platelet sizes increase by the same proportion.

et al. 1981; Giles 1981; Rowan and Fraser 1982; Levin and Bessman 1983). Above a platelet count of 350–400 × 10^9/l, an asymptote seems to be reached for the MPV. This is shown in a large group of normal subjects (Fig. 10.1). Using the relation of MPV and platelet count in normal subjects as a background, we can distinguish between different types of abnormal subjects. Those with an intact bone marrow and a normal platelet count will have an MPV that matches what is found in normal subjects with the same platelet counts. Such patient groups include those with diabetes, or atherosclerotic heart disease. When the platelet count is low, but the marrow is intrinsically normal and trying to compensate, the MPV rises as platelet count falls. An example of this situation is immune thrombocytopenia. When the platelet count is high but the bone marrow is intrinsically normal, the MPV is approximately the same as in normal subjects with the highest normal platelet counts. An example of this situation is reactive thrombocytosis. In both these abnormal cases, the relation between the MPV value and the platelet count extends the inverse non-linear relation that is seen in normal subjects (Table 10.2).

The same relation of the MPV and platelet count that is characteristic of groups of subjects is true in a given individual whose thrombopoietic status changes. Single individuals recovering from acute idiopathic thrombocytopenic purpura (ITP) have the same inverse, non-linear relation of platelet count and MPV. As they recover into the normal range of platelet count, their MPV value again is the same as in normal subjects with the same platelet count. These data indicate that the bone marrow compensates in ITP, to adjust thrombopoiesis to any given

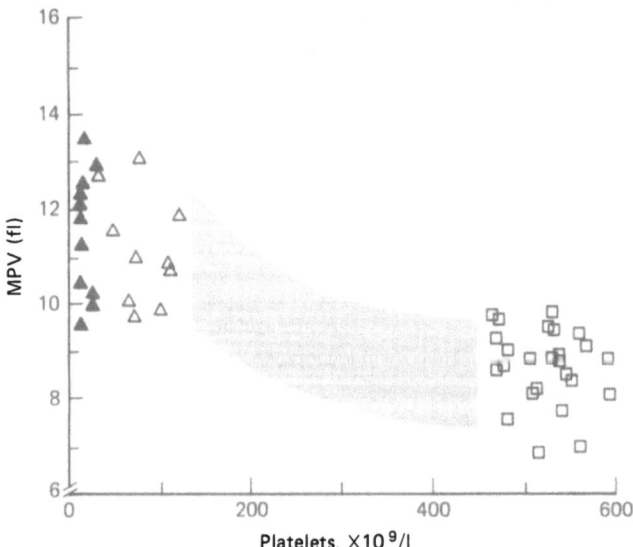

Fig. 10.1.   Relation of platelet number and size. The *shaded area* represents the central 95% of data in 6000 normal subjects (compare Table 10.2). Contrasted are 3 groups of patients. The *open triangles* represent patients with chronic, partially compensated immune thrombocytopenia (ITP). The *closed triangles* represent patients with the acute presentation of ITP. The *open squares* represent patients with mild reactive thrombocytosis (platelets 450–599 × 10^9/l). In these groups, as in normals, it is presumed that there is no intrinsic abnormality of the bone marrow, but hyperproduction due to external stimuli. The data show an inverse, but non-linear relation between platelet count and MPV.

Table 10.2. Relation of platelet count and size in normal subjects

Mean platelet volume (fl) vs. Platelet count, ×10^9/l

MPV (fl)	130–149	150–169	170–189	190–209	210–229	230–249	250–269	270–289	290–309	310–329	330–349	350–369	370–389	390–409	410–429
13.0+	1	0	1												
12.5–12.9	0	1	0		1										
12.0–12.4	0	1	1	0	0			1	1						
11.5–11.9	1	2	1	1	0	0	1	1	0	0	1	1			
11.0–11.4	3	1	2	3	2	2	0	0	2	2	0	1			
10.5–10.9	5	9	5	15	7	1	4	4	0	3	6	2	0	1	
10.0–10.4	11	12	24	21	11	27	15	6	3	7	5	3	1	1	1
9.5–9.9	3	16	18	30	32	36	26	39	17	19	29	18	6	1	
9.0–9.4	6	8	9	17	37	39	57	64	56	36	45	19	9	7	4
8.5–8.9			3	8	14	35	54	70	73	74	57	53	14	16	7
8.0–8.4	1		2	1	8	19	22	28	28	25	26	30	21	15	4
7.5–7.9					1	3	8	13	11	16	9	19	15	10	6
7.0–7.4							1	4	3	1	0	5	3	9	1
6.5–6.9							1	2	0	1	0	2	2	3	1
6.0–6.4													1	1	

Table 10.3. Hypothetical relation of platelet age to platelet size

Day	Platelets (× 10^9/l)	MPV (fl)	Minimum number of "new" platelets	MPV of "old" platelets a	b	MPV of "new" platelets a	b
4	10	13.3	–	–	–	–	–
5	21	12.9	11	13.3	12.1	12.6	13.6
6	56	12.1	35	12.9	11.6	10.7	12.4
7	180	10.7	124	12.1	10.9	10.1	10.6
8	294	9.6	114	10.7	9.6	7.9	9.6
9	415	8.7	121	9.6	8.6	6.5	8.9

As noted in the text, the following assumptions are made: (1) all platelets survive at least 4 days when they are released between days 4 and 8 and, (2) MPV changes as follows as platelets age in the circulation:
(a) No change with age
(b) After the first day, an average 10% shrinkage
Columns a and b above use these assumptions respectively. If the residual "old" platelets are the indicated size, what size must the newly produced platelets be to yield the known MPV for all platelets on that day?
The data show that newly produced platelets are smaller and smaller as the platelet count rises, whether it be assumed that platelets shrink in the circulation or not. This suggests that the size of "young" platelets depends more on the degree of thrombopoietic stimulation than on the platelet's age.
Prednisone was given for 10 days.

degree of thrombocytopenia. An individual case is shown in more detail in Table 10.3. As the platelet count after therapy rises, the MPV falls; as the patients suffers a relapse, the platelet count falls and the MPV rises (Levin and Bessman 1983).

The data of this individual can be shown in a different way (Fig. 10.2). The serial values of platelet count and MPV are shown against the nomogram of normal values. At first the platelet count was very low and the MPV was high. As the patient initially recovered, the platelet values entered the nomogram of normals. As the patient then relapsed, the platelet changes reversed those seen during recovery (not shown). Again, the non-linear inverse relation is preserved in both phases of the illness.

A different relation is apparent in individuals with bone marrow suppression, such as is seen in patients receiving cytotoxic chemotherapy. In such cases, as the bone marrow is suppressed, both the platelet count and the MPV fall. After a nadir is reached, the first sign of recovery is the change in the MPV. The MPV rapidly rises, to indicate the return of megakaryocytes capable of thrombopoiesis compensating for peripheral thrombocytopenia. After the MPV rises, the platelet count rises. As the platelet count reaches a normal value, MPV also is normal (Bessman 1982). Similar data can be seen in patients with septic thrombocytopenia. The degree to which the MPV falls, rather than rises, as the platelet count falls, indicates the degree to which the bone marrow is suppressed during sepsis. A low MPV also distinguishes bone marrow suppression from peripheral destruction of platelets in these individuals (Bessman and Gardner 1983).

The initial rise in MPV after hyperacute platelet destruction is slight. Our data in patients with septic thrombocytopenia suggest the change that develops within 1 day after acute platelet loss is 5%–10% (Bessman and Gardner 1983). This corresponds well with the published data of Martin et al. (1987) in patients after cardiopulmonary bypass. Note that in these patients the marrow must compensate for sudden thrombocytopenia. About 3 days are needed for the megakaryocyte to proceed from ploidization to platelets in the periphery. Therefore, the

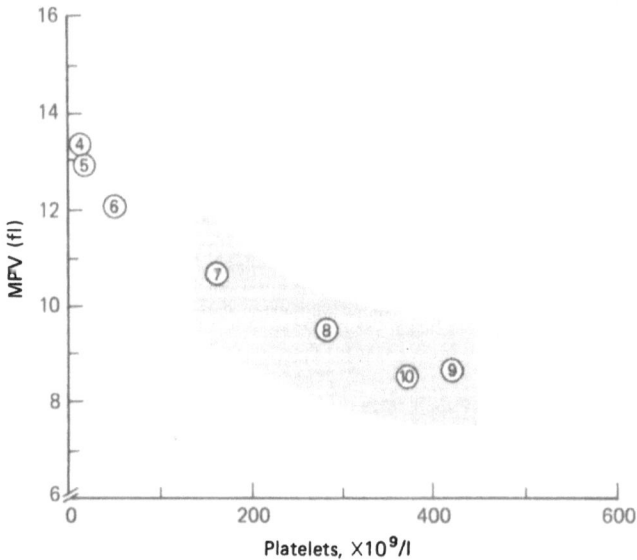

Fig. 10.2. Sequential platelet data in a patient recovering from ITP. The *shaded area* represents the central 95% of data in normal subjects. The numbers indicate the day of prednisone therapy (See Table 10.3). As the platelet count rose, the MPV fell, analogous to the relation in groups of patients shown in Fig. 10.1.

initial new platelets will be from megakaryocytes that have been stimulated only briefly. Patients with ITP, in contrast, have been thrombocytopenic for weeks at a minimum. Their megakaryocytes are therefore fully stimulated by thrombocytopenia, and as we have seen, their MPV is far larger.

Parenthetically, the same relation between peripheral cell mass and change in cell size is seen in red cells. Individuals with haemolytic anaemia have both high reticulocyte counts and abnormally large erythrocytes. Individuals with haemolysis which is compensated to such an extent that there is no anaemia do not have macrocytosis (Bessman 1986). The mere presence of rapid cell turnover is not enough: cytopenia seems to be necessary to produce feedback that alters the size of cell formation.

The question of the relation of platelet age to MPV is an important one. Table 10.4 shows the progressive platelet count and MPV in an individual's recovery from ITP. As is typical, the platelet count rises rapidly, and the MPV falls. What size are the newly formed platelets? Let us make several somewhat arbitrary assumptions:

1. The increment of platelet count from one day to the next represents newly formed or "young" platelets. No existing platelets are lost, and no existing platelet breaks into pieces measurable as platelets.

2. The existing platelets do not shrink in the circulation as they age. We can alternatively posit that they do shrink by 10% or 20%. It is assumed that all "old" platelets shrink by an equal proportion.

We can then calculate the number of "young" and "old" platelets each day, as well as what their respective MPVs must be. Regardless of whether it be assumed that platelets do shrink in the circulation or do not, one fact is apparent. As the platelet count rises, newly formed platelets must each day be smaller than the newly formed platelets on the previous day. It does not appear that fine-tuning the two assumptions will change this.

Thus, young platelets can be of various sizes. In ITP, platelets are not large because they are young: they are large because they are young *and* the patient has peripheral thrombocytopenia. Again, this has a parallel in erythropoiesis. In haemolytic anaemia, the reticulocytes are large; in haemolysis without anaemia, they are not (Bessman 1986).

The relation of megakaryocyte ploidy to MPV and platelet count suggests that megakaryocytopoiesis changes before MPV. Individuals receiving cytotoxic chemotherapy have a fall in platelet count, MPV and megakaryocyte ploidy, roughly simultaneously. However, during recovery the megakaryocyte ploidy rose about 1 day before the platelet count (Bessman 1982). Our unpublished data have shown that after marrow suppression megakaryocyte colony-forming units (CFU) rise about 1 day before megakaryocyte ploidy rises. This relation can also be inferred from the studies of Yeager et al. (1982). In other human subjects with steady-state instead of changing thrombopoiesis, we have shown that there is a direct relation between megakaryocyte ploidy and MPV (Bessman 1984). Furthermore, in the groups in which platelet count and MPV follow the nomogram for compensated or normal bone marrow, the same relation is seen between megakaryocyte ploidy and platelet count. However, in patients with suppressed marrow, there is an abnormal relation between megakaryocyte ploidy and platelet count (Bessman 1984).

Fig. 10.3 summarizes these data in a hypothetical scheme of platelet production

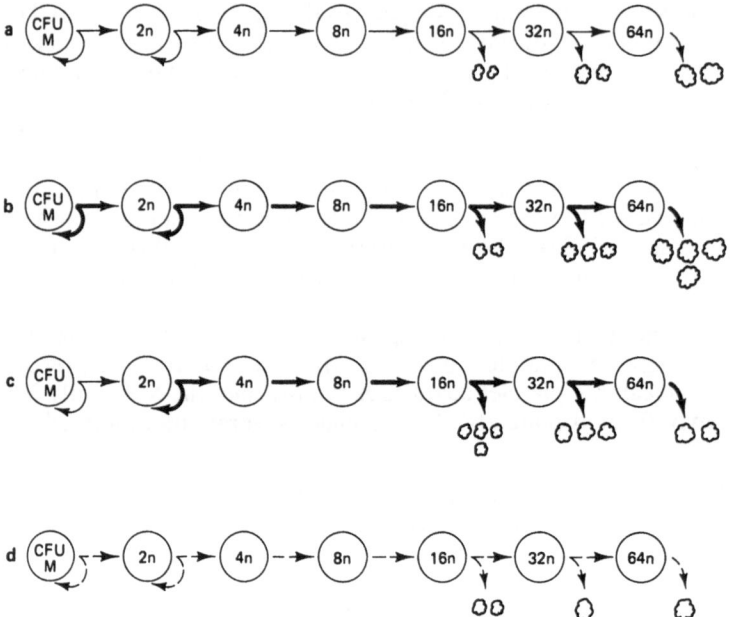

Fig. 10.3. Diagram of possible alterations in thrombopoiesis. **a** Normal. Progenitors (CFU M) and possibly the 2N megakaryocytes proliferate; megakaryocytes mature by endoreduplication, with 16N, 32N and 64N classes producing most of the platelets. Higher-ploidy megakaryocytes make larger platelets. **b** ITP. There is increased proliferation and CFU M, and increased ploidy (*heavy arrows*). Platelet production by higher-ploidy megakaryocytes is relatively increased (*heavy arrows*, more platelets). **c** Reactive thrombocytosis. CFU M are normal; megakaryocytes are increased, ploidy is decreased. Platelet production is from an increased number of megakaryocytes, so platelet number is increased. A higher proportion are smaller platelets from lower-ploidy cells. **d** Hypoproliferative thrombocytopenia (e.g. aplastic anaemia, drug toxicity). CFU M may be reduced; proliferation and endoreduplication are impaired (*dashed lines*). A reduced number of megakaryocytes produce a reduced number of platelets; higher-ploidy megakaryocytes, and so the larger platelets, are especially reduced.

(Bessman 1984). Megakaryocytes become committed, endoreduplicate, and produce platelets at several ploidy classes. The higher the ploidy class, the larger, *on average*, the platelet that is produced. ITP causes an increase in all stages of thrombopoiesis, but with preferential increase of higher-ploidy megakaryocytes and hence larger platelets. Reactive thrombocytosis is a lesser stimulus: CFU and endoreduplication change little, though the total number of platelets does. The average megakaryocyte ploidy is the same as or slightly lower than these values in normal subjects, and likewise MPV is the same, or slightly lower than in normal subjects. In contrast, marrow suppression reduces all aspects of thrombopoiesis, but especially reduced are the higher-ploidy megakaryocytes. The MPV is abnormally low (Bessman and Gardner 1985). Each of the alterations shown in this scheme is supported by published data. However, this does not exclude an additional contribution to platelet size made by in-circulation shrinkage.

As Table 10.4 shows, platelet size heterogeneity is far greater than lymphocyte or red cell heterogeneity. We must conclude that there is a need for what is a very large range of platelet size, although it is not yet known what physiological

Table 10.4. Heterogeneity of cell size

Cell	CV of size distribution
Erythrocyte	0.118–0.149
Lymphocyte	0.073–0.114
Neutrophil	0.145–0.290
Platelet	0.643–1.386

Observations in 75 normal subjects.

function requires this range. We have measured platelet volume heterogeneity as platelet distribution width (PDW) (Bessman et al. 1982). There is a direct but non-linear relation between MPV and PDW. This is also true in individuals with changing platelet counts and MPV values.

Patients with myelodysplastic syndrome often have thrombocytosis. While they do not usually have abnormal MPV, their PDW is typically abnormally large (Bessman et al. 1982). Their megakaryocyte ploidy is normal. Fig. 10.3 shows these data in a manner to parallel other platelet disorders. The MPV and the megakaryocyte ploidy are normal, but at any given ploidy class abnormally heterogeneous platelets are being made.

The several factors affecting heterogeneity of platelet size can be summarized by paraphrasing a British statesman quoting a British author: Some platelets are born small: they are the smallest among the heterogeneity intrinsic to the demarcation process (see Chap. 8); some platelets achieve smallness: as platelets shrink to whatever degree they do over time in the circulation, the oldest are smaller than they were when younger (see Chaps. 1 and 2); and some platelets have smallness thrust upon them: they are the progeny of the smallest-ploidy megakaryocytes to demarcate into platelets (see Chaps. 6, 9 and 10).

References

Bessman JD (1982) Prediction of platelet production during recovery from acute leukemia. Am J Hem 13:219–227
Bessman JD (1984) The relation of megakaryocyte ploidy to platelet size. Am J Hem 16:161–170
Bessman JD (1986) Automated blood counts and differentials. Johns Hopkins, Baltimore.
Bessman JD, Gardner FH (1983) Platelet size in thrombocytopenia due to sepsis. Surg Gynecol Obstet 156:177–180
Bessman JD, Gardner FH (1985) Persistence of abnormal red cell and platelet phenotype during recovery from aplastic anemia. Arch Int Med 145:293–296
Bessman JD, Williams LJ, Gilmer PR (1981) Mean platelet volume. Am J Clin Path 76:289–293
Bessman JD, Williams LJ, Gilmer PR (1982) Platelet size in health and hematologic disease. Am J Clin Path 78:150–153
Giles C (1981) The platelet count and mean platelet volume. Br J Haem 48:31–38
Levin J, Bessman JD (1983) The inverse relationship between platelet volume and platelet number. J Lab Med 101:295–307
Martin JF, Daniel TD, Trowbridge EA (1987) Acute and chronic changes in platelet volume and count after cardiopulmonary bypass induced thrombocytopenia in man. Thromb Haemost 57:55–58
Rowan RM, Fraser C (1982) Platelet size distribution analysis. In: van Assendelft DW and England JM (eds) Advances in haematologic methods: the blood count. CRC Press, Boca Raton
Yeager AM, Levin FC, Levin J (1982) Effects of cyclophosphamide on murine bone marrow and

splenic megakaryocyte CFC, granulocyte–macrophage CFC, and peripheral blood cell levels. J Cell Physiol 112:222–228

Technical Questions

Trowbridge: In your nomagram the assumption that has been made is that the groups can be divided into different platelet counts and then you take the number of people in those different groups and form 2 standard deviations based on the mean platelet volume. Is that the way it was done?

Bessman: Correct.

Trowbridge: If you perform the analysis the other way around and take the mean platelet volumes and work out 2 standard deviations for the platelet counts associated with the same mean platelet volume you get a different nomagram. That is the first thing. Secondly, by taking standard deviations the assumption that is being made is that the distribution is Gaussian for each of those segments. Since you only have small numbers (27, 17, 15, 11) at the ends of the nomagram, one cannot be sure that they are Gaussian distributions. If you perform the analysis for a large group of people – we used over 700 blood donors – and you consider the mean platelet volumes and platelet counts separately one finds that you have a bivariate Gaussian distribution, which gives you reference ranges associated with ellipses. These are not very far away from your nomagram, but it cuts off at both ends. I am suggesting that the statistics are producing the non-linearity you show because of the lack of subjects studied at the lower platelet counts.

Bessman: Let me answer those points one by one. First, I cannot possibly disagree with you that your study of 700 patients is bigger than ours of 683. Second, however, if you consider 3000 patients that we studied in a different article, that we did not divide up in this way, but simply printed the scattergram, and the several thousand Martin Rowan has published as well as the several hundred that Giles and Inglis have published and superimpose them they are all the same. That is just on a Coulter-type instrument. However, there have been data that have not been published in peer review, but rather in trade journals for Technicon, as well as data by Lippi and Capolleti on this point for the Technicon instrument, which uses a different principle, but shows the same superimposed features – not only inverse but non-linear. Do not forget these are only normal subjects. If we include the general run of a hospital population, as we have done in other articles, then we are not limited to the small number of people who are inevitably going to be normal and have a platelet count over 350×10^9 platelets/l blood. In addition, we will not be limited by small numbers that have only the lowest possible normal platelet count, we will have a large number of people with hyperdestructive thrombocytopenia. So I would not rely on the precise statistics of 683, but the aggregate statistics of almost 10 000 will give you the same data and will also give you the valuable groups at the far reaches of the platelet count spectrum. Yes, this is less than convincing taken by itself.

Trowbridge: I am not arguing about the numbers. I am arguing about the way you have analysed the data. We have looked at Technicon data and the difference between those data and Coulter is really marked. What I am saying is if you take a haematological normal population you should stick to that population and then in pathological states create another area for that group. So really, the argument about the high platelet count end of the spectrum does not apply. I am not arguing about whether it is 10 000, 700 or 600 subjects. What I am saying is that you have got no evidence that you can take the platelet counts and then create 2 standard deviations unless you have a Gaussian distribution for each of those subgroups.

Bessman: Actually I do. This is the graph I have for my 683 subjects. It was one year's data. Now we have ten year's worth of data. I have the aggregate data that I would be glad to send you.

Paulus: In your diagram that shows the relationship between mean platelet volume and platelet distribution width these two variables are bound to be correlated. You have put two variables on the graph that depend on the same thing. To be more specific, the standard deviation of volume depends on the mean log-volume and the standard deviation of log-volume. The mean platelet volume also depends on these two variables. So there is an intrinsic correlation. It is as though you were correlating the haematocrit with the number of red cells. Do you see what I mean?

Bessman: No, I do not see. Wait, let me respond to that, because we have been through the same thing with red cells. That is, it is possible to have the same thing with red cells. That is, it is possible to have the same red cell distribution width, the same coefficient of variation, of red cell size, whether the subject has heterozygous thalassaemia, with mean red cell size of 70 fl, or has aplastic anaemia, with a mean red cell size of 140 fl. The standard deviation will change, the mean will change, but the coefficient of variation will not. For platelets the platelet distribution width is not a coefficient of variation. Am I right?

Paulus: That is right. In the arithmetic distribution of volumes, the width depends on the SD of volumes, while in the distribution of log-volumes it represents the SD of log-volumes. If the mean and SD of log-volumes of a platelet sample are represented by μ and σ respectively, the relevant mathematical formulae are as follows:

$$\text{Mean volume (MPV)} = \exp(\mu + 0.5\,\sigma^2)$$
$$\text{Median volume} = \exp(\mu)$$
$$\text{Modal volume} = \exp(\mu - \sigma^2)$$
$$\text{CV of volume} = \exp(\sigma^2 - 1)^{1/2}$$
$$\text{SD of volume} = \text{MPV.CV}$$

Bessman: So one might ask what would happen to the coefficient of variation rather than the platelet distribution width, which is essentially the standard deviation. That is where the non-linearity of that relation comes in, such that the coefficient of variation, itself, would not be constant, but rather it would go up as the mean platelet volume went up.

Paulus: I think the correct plot would relate either the mean unit SD of *log-volumes* or the *median* and coefficient of variation of volumes. These two couples of variables do not have *intrinsic* correlation.

General Discussion

Corash: Dr Bessman, you are making a very strong pitch for different ploidy classes producing different sizes of platelets, if I understand your model, with the little platelets falling off the ends of the different sizes of megakaryocytes. In the animal models of acute thrombocytopenia, when you evaluate the ploidy shift at 48 hours you see an enormous change in ploidy class distribution. By that stage and afterwards platelet volume is going in the opposite direction of what your model would imply. So I think you have to keep in mind that there is a major inconsistency there. I do not know how to resolve it, but I am just posing it as an observation. Perhaps platelet volume and ploidy are very much dissociated. So we have to think in terms of a new model.

Bessman: Well, you are very kind to suggest I think of a new model, but let me try mine on for a while [laughter]. First, I think we have to recognize that there seems to be different data in humans, rats and mice. The different data came out in various different ways. It would appear that the ploidy, the mean ploidy of the megakaryocyte, is different in humans than in the murine model. Now if that is just changing the baseline, but everything else follows the same, then that should not make any difference. In any event, that is one way in which they are different. In fact, it tends to go along in another way, and that is, as you say, there has been a fair amount of data suggesting that there is an acute and large change in platelet size in acutely thrombocytopenic animals. The same acute change in size has not been demonstrated in thrombocytopenic people. The studies shown by Dr Martin on cardiac bypass are a case in point beside mine. He showed a 6% change, that is true, but that is not in the same zip-code as the change that has been reported again and again in animals. So it is hard for me to be sure that we have exactly the same system. You may say that megakaryocytes are the same the world over. You can equally take this model and say each class of megakaryocyte does not produce a different size of platelet. You can say that there are the various types of megakaryocytes, but that they are programmed differently, depending on the humoral stimulation, and so any ploidy class of megakaryocyte can make any size platelet. There is a fair amount of data against that too, but the truth may be somewhere in between. The part of the model that stipulates that megakaryocytes produce a specific size of platelet certainly is more questionable in animals than it is in humans.

Thompson: I just want to clarify one pont, to make sure I understand your explanation for why the mean platelet volume goes down in the chemotherapy patients after day 10, between day 10 and 15. I know you see a decrease in the mean ploidy, but then again there is probably not an effective chemotherapy as we have seen from the bone marrow transplant data in the poster today. What is the explanation in your model for why the platelet volumes goes down?

Bessman: Multivariate. First, you have to assume that some platelets are being made, because these patients do not become absolutely thrombocytopenic within the life-span of the platelet. Their platelet count does go down, but if their marrow was just ablated immediately their platelet count should be zero in 7 or 8 days and it is not. Hence, there is some residual platelet production, presumably, although I cannot prove it, from marrow that is damaged, to one degree or another, as time goes on, from the chemotherapy. I cannot tell you very quantitatively what is the ploidy of that marrow because we have only so much data in that area. Further, you could argue that those platelets that are in the circulation are, to a substantial degree, the residual platelets and they are ageing and getting smaller, if you like. So both of those explanations are possible. It is also possible that there is no ploidy change at all in the marrow, but that in a general megaloblastic way the demarcation in the individual megakaryocyte has in some way been altered. That then produces smaller platelets or produces platelets that are susceptible to shrinkage when they get out into the peripheral blood. I cannot choose among those and I certainly cannot say one versus the other, nor can I give relative importance to the several choices.

Thompson: What are your data to substantiate that the platelets can get smaller as they circulate?

Bessman: I have no data at all to substantiate that they can. I am trying to accommodate all camps. That is by no means a condition of any of this. I am saying that if they become smaller in the circulation it does not negate other factors.

11 Summing Up: Platelet Heterogeneity: Biology and Pathology

J. F. Mustard

The key question of the chapters in this book focused on the source of platelet heterogeneity. The debate could be considered to be between those who believe that the production of platelets from megakaryocytes is the primary determinant of heterogeneity and those who believe that exposure of platelets to stimuli during their circulation in the blood contributes to platelet heterogeneity.

There is little doubt that platelets produced from megakaryocytes are heterogeneous in size and density. What is less clear is whether platelets that are freshly produced from the megakaryocytes are substantially different in terms of function from older platelets, and whether among the freshly produced platelets, those that are larger, or more dense, respond more effectively to aggregating and release-inducing agents than smaller, less dense platelets.

Although the data from human and sub-human primates are controversial, the data from other animals (rabbits, rats, dogs) seem to indicate that as platelets circulate they tend to become less dense. Among the convincing pieces of evidence about platelet density changes with age in the circulation are the observations in rabbits that after injection of the most dense subpopulation of labelled platelets, radioactivity gradually appears in the least dense platelets, whereas after infusion of the least dense subpopulation of labelled platelets, scarcely any label appears in the most dense platelets (Corash et al. 1978; Rand 1983). The results of the human studies and some of the primate studies are more difficult to interpret because consideration was not given to the effect of sequestration in the spleen of larger, most dense platelets. In the studies in which it has been claimed that there is no difference in survival between the most dense and least dense platelets when they are infused into primates, the survival curves do appear to indicate that the larger, most dense platelets are sequestered in the spleen and subsequently released (Mezzano et al. 1981). If this point were taken into account, the evidence would be entirely compatible with the larger, most dense platelets having a longer survival time than the least dense platelets.

There is evidence showing that when baboon platelets are separated by size, the smaller platelets have a shorter survival than the larger platelets (Thompson et al. 1983b). There is also some indication that the smaller platelets may function less effectively than the larger platelets (Karpatkin 1978; Martin et al. 1983b;

Thompson et al. 1984), although again this is inconclusive and is beset by the problem of whether this may be an effect of age rather than an effect of size. Thompson et al. (1984) have concluded that size and age are independent, but that both are related to platelet function.

If platelets are separated on the basis of density and then their size is determined, there is considerable overlap in platelet size in the least dense fraction and the most dense fraction (Karpatkin and Charmatz 1969; Corash et al. 1977; Rand et al. 1981; Martin et al. 1983a). Thus there are large, least dense platelets and small, most dense platelets and platelets cannot be differentiated into density subpopulations that contain only large or small platelets. Although I am not aware of any evidence on this point, it seems likely that if platelets are separated on the basis of their size, the density distributions of the large and small platelets will also overlap. Because sharply differentiated populations cannot be obtained by the techniques of separation on the basis of size or density, modification of platelet size or density after the platelets have been released from the megakaryocytes may produce only a modest change in these characteristics of the total platelet population and it may be difficult to detect this change unless one can identify a group of platelets that have been stimulated.

The question of how platelet size and density are changed in the circulation is undoubtedly related to the functions of platelets. One of their critical roles is the maintenance of the integrity of the vessel wall, but this process is poorly understood, although we believe that it differs from the reactions in which platelets take part in the formation of haemostatic plugs and arterial thrombi, which have been moderately well studied. A lack of platelets has been shown experimentally to increase the permeability of the vessel wall, and to lead to loss of the integrity of the endothelium and the escape of red blood cells into subendothelial spaces in the microcirculation (Aursnes 1974). Severely thrombo-cytopenic animals or humans frequently bleed to death. Platelets have been shown to maintain the vascular integrity of perfused organs and prevent the oedema that develops if a perfusing fluid without platelets is used (Gimbrone et al. 1969; Dodds et al. 1973). If we knew how platelets contribute to maintaining the integrity of the vessel wall, we might be able to determine whether this process itself would modify their properties. It seems reasonable to speculate that however the platelets contribute to the integrity of the vessel wall, the process is not an all-or-nothing reaction. The platelets that take part in it will probably return to the circulation if, indeed, direct interaction of platelets with the vessel wall does occur.

We do have substantial evidence about the changes in platelet density, and possibly size, that would result from the adhesion of platelets to severely damaged vessel walls and during the platelet-to-platelet interactions that can occur as a consequence of these reactions. However, under some circumstances, platelets may react with a vessel wall that shows only minimal signs of alteration. In early studies we demonstrated that platelets and platelet-fibrin thrombi could be found on the surface of the aortae of normal, young animals and in the arteries of young humans killed in accidents; these deposits occurred at sites where atherosclerotic lesions typically develop (Jørgensen et al. 1972). More recently, Spurlock and Chandler (1987) have been doing an extensive scanning electro-scopic study of the surface of the aorta and coronary arteries of people who have died suddenly in accidents. Again, they have found platelets and platelet thrombi on the surface of these large arteries, even in children.

Next I shall examine and review the existing evidence concerning the changes in the properties of platelets that can occur when they interact with a damaged vessel wall or with each other.

First, let us consider the stimuli that cause platelets to stick to each other and to release their granule contents. ADP causes an increase in the size of rabbit platelets as measured by changes in light transmission in an aggregometer cuvette as well as in a Coulter counter Channelyzer; this ADP-induced change in platelet size is reversible (Packham et al. 1985). In contrast, the decrease in the density of rabbit platelets that ADP causes does persist. Thrombin, which causes platelet aggregation and the release of the contents of platelet granules, produces a marked shift of platelets from the most dense fraction into the least dense fraction (Cieslar et al. 1979; van Oost et al. 1983). Plasmin, even in low concentrations which induce very little release of granule contents, also causes a shift in platelets from the most dense fraction to the least dense fraction (Guccione et al. 1985). These observations are relevant to the question of whether platelets with decreased density due to encounters with aggregating and release-inducing agents can persist in the circulation. Although ADP, thrombin, and probably thromboxane A_2, decrease platelet density, these agonists do not shorten platelet survival (Reimers et al. 1976; Packham et al. 1980). Thus, upon the return to the circulation of platelets that have been incorporated into reversible thrombi under the influence of these aggregating agents, the platelets would circulate for a normal period of time, but with decreased density. In contrast, platelets that have been exposed to plasmin in sufficiently high concentrations to cleave membrane glycoproteins would be expected to be rapidly cleared from the circulation, and therefore it would not be possible to detect that their density had also been decreased.

I would next like to review some data obtained from rats and rabbits with indwelling aortic catheters that damage the vessel wall and, in rabbits, cause the formation of thrombi. In rats, catheter-induced vessel injury results in platelet accumulation on the subendothelial surface, but thrombi do not form (Winocour et al. 1983a). After platelets have adhered to the damaged vessel wall, their release from it probably requires cleavage of the platelet membrane glycoproteins or the adhesive proteins involved in their attachment to the damaged wall. One possibility is that plasmin is activated at the injury site and frees the adherent platelets. To test this theory, we examined the effect of ε-aminocaproic acid (EACA) on platelet survival in rats with indwelling aortic catheters (Table 11.1)

Table 11.1. Effect of EACA on platelet survival in rats with indwelling aortic catheters or sham operations

Treatment	Platelet survival mean ± SEM (h)	Significance of difference between means
Placebo + sham operation (9)	70.5±4.4	
Placebo + aortic catheter (10)	38.6±1.9	$p<0.001$
EACA + aortic catheter (9)	53.8±3.8	$p<0.01$
EACA + sham operation (9)	78.9±4.9	$p<0.001$

EACA was given orally 3 hours before insertion of the catheter, at the time of its insertion and at 4-hour intervals thereafter. The numbers in parentheses are the number of rats in each group. The significance of the difference between means was calculated by Student's t test.
Reproduced from *The Journal of Clinical Investigation*, 1983, 71:159–164 by copyright permission of the American Society for Clinical Investigation.

(Winocour et al. 1983b). EACA inhibits fibrinolysis by inhibiting the action of plasmin and in these experiments we found that administration of EACA did indeed lengthen platelet survival. This observation is compatible with the concept that plasmin (and possibly other proteolytic enzymes such as leukocyte elastase) does influence the turnover of platelets on the damaged vessel wall of the rat. Since in rats with an indwelling aortic catheter, shortened platelet survival is associated with an increased proportion of the most dense platelets and a decreased platelet count (Winocour et al. 1983a), it may be that the reduced platelet count stimulates the marrow to produce new platelets that are more dense. The platelets from rats that have had the catheters in place for 6 days survive much longer than the platelets from sham-operated rats when the platelets are injected into the circulation of normal rats, indicating that there is a higher proportion of young platelets in the circulation (Winocour et al. 1983a).

In contrast to the situation in the rat, thrombi form around indwelling aortic catheters in rabbits. If platelets that have been stimulated by agents that cause platelet aggregation and the release of granule contents escape from the thrombi and return to the circulation, one would expect an increased proportion of platelets that are less dense, and this is indeed what is observed (Somers 1984). Even though new platelets are being produced at this time (as evidenced by the fact that platelets taken from rabbits with indwelling aortic catheters have a prolonged survival when injected into normal rabbits (Somers 1984)), because of the stimulation the platelets receive in the thrombus, the density of the circulating platelets is decreased.

The observations from these in vivo experiments with rats and rabbits indicate that platelets are involved in "battles" in the circulation, but the changes in density and size are not readily predictable because of the diversity of the reactions in which platelets may take part.

Several of the contributors to this book have emphasized the point that the techniques used in handling platelets in the laboratory can influence their size and density. Because the distribution curves of size and density overlap to such great extents, the choice of the cut-off points can greatly enhance or blur the differences between most dense and least dense platelets or between large and small platelets. The solutions used in isolating platelets and preparing them for centrifugation on the gradients can affect their properties. For example, a number of investigators have used prostaglandin E_1 to inhibit activation of platelets during their preparation and centrifugation on density gradients. However, prostaglandin E_1 and other agents that increase the concentration of cyclic AMP in platelets have been shown to increase the size and decrease the density of rabbit platelets (Packham et al. 1985). Since these agents inhibit the release of granule contents, they must decrease platelet density and increase size by promoting the uptake of water by the platelets.

There is an additional problem with human platelets and some non-human primate platelets. When platelets from these species are brought into close contact with each other by stirring or centrifugation in a medium with a low concentration of Ca^{2+}, the arachidonate pathway leading to the formation of thromboxane A_2 may be activated (Packham et al. 1987). Thromboxane A_2 causes the release of the contents of the platelet granules and hence will decrease platelet density. Thus any handling procedure in which human or subhuman primate platelets in a medium with a low concentrations of Ca^{2+} are brought into close contact with each other introduces the risk of activating the platelets, with a resultant decrease in density. Platelets from rabbits, rats and some dogs do not respond in this way to close platelet-to-platelet contact (Packham and Mustard 1984), so this potential problem does not arise in work with platelets from these species. Aspirin and other non-steroidal anti-inflammatory drugs prevent the formation of thromboxane A_2 and hence block its effects on platelets (Packham et al. 1987).

I have been speculating that a similar process of activation of human platelets may occur under the high shear conditions at stenoses in coronary arteries that are associated with unstable angina, because aspirin has been shown to have a major beneficial effect in carefully selected male patients with this condition (Lewis et al. 1983; Cairns et al. 1985). It is my prediction that platelets that have been activated in stenosed vessels will circulate with decreased density, and perhaps an increased size. Although this type of activation is most readily demonstrated in vitro in media with unphysiologically low concentrations of Ca^{2+}, it is my suspicion that such a process may be activated in vivo if shear forces are very high, as they are at stenoses.

Although there may be species differences, human platelets must encounter the same hazards that rat and rabbit platelets encounter in the circulation. It is certainly established that exposure of human platelets to an artificial surface during cardiopulmonary bypass decreases platelet density (van Oost et al. 1983).

Bone Marrow and Thrombopoiesis

It is clear from published evidence that animals and humans with a low platelet count tend to have platelets with increased size (O'Brien and Jamieson 1974; Thompson et al. 1983a; Levin and Bessman 1983) and that these changes are associated with increased ploidy of the megakaryocytes (Odell et al. 1976; Paulus et al. 1979; Martin et al. 1983b). However, the majority of the evidence presented at this meeting in which the time relationships were studied indicates that the increase in ploidy occurs after the size change of the platelets has taken place (Corash et al. 1987; Warren 1988). Bessman (1984) has presented a strong argument for the concept that if megakaryocyte ploidy is increased, larger platelets are produced. This is an important point that requires further study.

In humans and animals with normal bone marrow, it appears that the circulating platelet mass regulates platelet production. A high platelet count with small platelets tends to equal the same platelet mass as a lower platelet count with large platelets. When the platelet count falls, the platelets that appear in the circulation are larger and thus restore the platelet mass even though the number of platelets is decreased. The mechanism that regulates platelet production and platelet size under these circumstances is unknown, and its significance in terms of platelet function is also not understood.

In studies with Wistar Furth rats, Jackson et al. (1988) have shown that there is a genetic control of platelet size because, in this type of rat, the platelets are twice as large as normal, but only one-third as numerous. In this condition, however, there is no significant difference in the average diameter or DNA content of the megakaryocytes, although their concentration in the bone marrow is only 30% of that of control rats (Jackson et al. 1988). Thus these rats provide at least one example of a control system that causes megakaryocytes to produce large platelets which is not associated with an increase in the size of the megakaryocytes or an increase in their ploidy. These rats would appear to provide an ideal situation for investigation of the question of whether large platelets are more functional than small platelets.

An unresolved question was whether the megakaryocytes form demarcation membranes and shed platelets in the bone marrow or whether platelets are formed in the blood by the process of binary division when the megakaryocytes hit bifurcations in the pulmonary circulation, as Trowbridge and colleagues have suggested (Trowbridge et al. 1982; Trowbridge 1988). Although theoretical calculations indicate that a fragmentation process in the pulmonary circulation could produce the distribution in platelet size that is seen with the circulating platelets, and megakaryocytes or megakaryocyte cytoplasm can be found in the pulmonary circulation, direct evidence that such a bifurcation process is a primary mechanism for platelet formation has not been obtained. In considering the question of platelet production, it must be remembered that circulating platelets are non-adhesive cells. Therefore when the demarcation membranes form in the megakaryocytes, the platelets must become non-adhesive and their separation must become relatively easy. Since a stationary thrombus, which is a form of platelet aggregate, can break up under the force of blood flow without having to hit a bifurcation, it is quite likely that the platelet mass formed in a megakaryocyte could break up under similar conditions. One of the interesting points, however, from the work of Trowbridge and colleagues is the possible consequence of a number of megakaryocytes entering the pulmonary circulation and not fragmenting readily. Are some diseases of the pulmonary circulation caused by megakaryocytes that do not fragment readily? The fragmentation of megakaryocytes into platelets is an interesting topic for further studies to answer some difficult questions, particularly the processes that result in the platelets becoming non-adhesive as they mature.

In general, studies of pathological processes in man show that there is a good correlation between platelet size and megakaryocyte size. Martin and Trowbridge have reviewed the evidence that subjects with clinical complications of coronary artery disease tend to have large platelets in the circulation and large megakaryocytes (Trowbridge et al. 1984; Trowbridge and Martin 1987). These size characteristics are probably related to the fairly well-established fact of shortened platelet survival and increased platelet turnover in these subjects (Kinlough-Rathbone et al. 1983). Early work in which we demonstrated shortened platelet survival in patients with clinical complications of atherosclerosis and showed that shortened platelet survival correlated with a family history of myocardial infarction (Murphy and Mustard 1962) was not well received when it was first presented to members of the American Society for the Study of Arteriosclerosis who, at that time, believed that cholesterol was the only cause of atherosclerosis. Subsequent observations by a number of investigators have now established the fact that platelets do contribute to the development of atherosclerosis and to its thromboembolic complications (Packham and Mustard 1986).

It is of interest that in the work of Martin and his colleagues with patients who had had a myocardial infarction, the bleeding time, which was shortened in acute myocardial infarction (Milner and Martin 1985), returned towards normal within two years of the initial studies. In interpreting this finding, it would be helpful to know whether these patients changed their habits in any way that would influence platelet survival. For example, did they stop smoking? Smoking shortens platelet survival and cessation of smoking restores platelet survival values towards normal (Mustard and Murphy 1963; Fuster et al. 1981).

The studies reported in this book by Martin and by Bessman about thrombocytopenia indicate that in circumstances in which the bone marrow is normal platelets show an increase in size when the platelet count is low. One of the key points that has to be taken into consideration, however, in studying platelet size during acute changes, is that in humans and other primates young platelets (which seem likely to be large platelets) tend to be sequestered in the spleen (Shulman et al. 1968) and under conditions of stress can be released and will therefore increase the proportion of large platelets in the circulation which have not been recently derived from the megakaryocytes. This problem, which can complicate some of the estimates of the survival of the larger platelets in man, is also a problem in considering size changes associated with changes in the platelet count in acute situations.

The studies that Martin and colleagues have described of an increase in the platelet count without an increase in platelet size when a cytotoxic agent such as vincristine was given in rats (Martin et al. 1981), although interesting, are difficult to interpret because of the possibility that these agents may have effects on other systems in addition to megakaryocytes and platelets.

Another example of a complicated problem is the effect of hypercholesterolaemia on platelets and megakaryocytes. Martin and colleagues found that in hypercholesterolaemic rabbits the megakaryocytes were larger after 12 weeks on the high-cholesterol diet, but the platelets were smaller (Martin et al. 1985). Winocour in my group has also demonstrated that platelets tend to be smaller in hypercholesterolaemia (Winocour et al. 1986); these smaller platelets are hypersensitive to thrombin, but not to ADP (Winocour et al. 1987). This hypersensitivity might be an effect of a change in the properties of platelet membranes caused by the incorporation of cholesterol, and although there may be increased platelet turnover in hypercholesterolaemia its effect on the megakaryocytes may lead to the production of smaller, hypersensitive platelets. Thus, a variety of conditions may modify platelet size and the platelets that appear in the circulation may differ in their characteristics from what one would expect under conditions of shifts in platelet counts in normal subjects.

An important question remains unresolved. Is platelet size unimportant or important for their function? At present we do not know whether the variation of platelet size is biologically important or is some chance circumstance of platelet production. It seems likely, however, that there is a physiological reason for the degree of heterogeneity that is unique to platelets. Perhaps this diversity has biological significance in maintaining the integrity of the vessel wall. Although there may be technical problems in bleeding time measurements there does appear to be a relationship between platelet mass and the bleeding time (Milner and Martin 1985). This relationship may involve the effect of platelet size on platelet function; this problem is certainly worthy of further study. Perhaps future experiments with the Wistar Furth rats described by Jackson and colleagues (1988) will help to answer the question of the importance of heterogeneity in platelet function.

The chapters in this book have shown conclusively that both the megakaryocytes and the agents to which platelets are exposed in the circulation contribute to platelet heterogeneity. It is also clear that when the platelet count falls the bone marrow tends to produce larger platelets. While we know that the properties of platelets can be changed as they circulate, we are uncertain about how platelet properties are changed as a result of their support of the integrity of the vessel wall. This question and the question of how the megakaryocytes function are probably the two most important unresolved problems in relation to this subject.

References

Aursnes I (1974) Blood platelet production and red cell leakage to lymph during thrombocytopenia. Scand J Haematol 13:184–195

Bessman JD (1984) The relation of megakaryocyte ploidy to platelet volume. Am J Hematol 16:161–170

Cairns JA, Gent M, Singer J et al. (1985) Aspirin, sulfinpyrazone, or both in unstable angina: results of a Canadian Multicenter trial. N Engl J Med 313:1369–1375

Cieslar P, Greenberg JP, Rand ML, Packham MA, Kinlough-Rathbone RL, Mustard JF (1979) Separation of thrombin-treated platelets from normal platelets by density-gradient centrifugation. Blood 53:867–874

Corash L, Tan H, Gralnick HR, Shafer B (1977) Heterogeneity of human whole blood platelet subpopulations. I. Relationship between buoyant density, cell volume, and ultrastructure. Blood 49:71–87

Corash L, Shafer B, Perlow M (1978) Heterogeneity of human whole blood platelet subpopulations. II. Use of a subhuman primate model to analyze the relationship between density and platelet age. Blood 52:726–734

Corash L, Chen HY, Levin J, Baker G, Lu H, Mok Y (1987) Regulation of thrombopoiesis: effects of the degree of thrombocytopenia on megakaryocyte ploidy and platelet volume. Blood 70:177–185

Dodds WJ, Raymond SL, Pert JH (1973) Isolated kidney perfusion: a model for testing platelet function. Proc Soc Exp Biol Med 144:189–194

Fuster V, Chesebro JH, Frye RL, Elveback LR (1981) Platelet survival and the development of coronary artery disease in the young adult: effects of cigarette smoking, strong family history and medical therapy. Circulation 63:546–551

Gimbrone MA, Aster RH, Cotran RS, Corkery J, Jandl JH, Folkman J (1969) Preservation of vascular integrity in organs perfused in vitro with platelet-rich medium. Nature 222:33–36

Guccione MA, Kinlough-Rathbone RL, Packham MA et al. (1985) Effects of plasmin on rabbit platelets. Thromb Haemost 53:8–14

Jackson CW, Hutson NK, Steward SA et al. (1988) The Wistar Furth rat: an animal model of hereditary macrothrombocytopenia. Blood 71:1676–1686

Jørgensen L, Packham MA, Rowsell HC, Mustard JF (1972) Deposition of formed elements of blood on the intima and signs of intimal injury in the aorta of rabbit, pig, and man. Lab Invest 27:341–350

Karpatkin S (1978) Heterogeneity of human platelets. VI. Correlation of platelet function with platelet volume. Blood 51:307–316

Karpatkin S, Charmatz A (1969) Heterogeneity of human platelets. I. Metabolic and kinetic evidence suggestive of young and old platelets. J Clin Invest 48:1073–1082

Kinlough-Rathbone RL, Packham MA, Mustard JF (1983) Vessel injury, platelet adherence, and platelet survival. Arteriosclerosis 3:529–546

Levin J, Bessman JD (1983) The inverse relation between platelet volume and platelet number: abnormalities in hematologic disease and evidence that platelet size does not correlate with platelet age. J Lab Clin Med 101:295–307

Lewis HD Jr, Davis JW, Archibald DG et al. (1983) Protective effects of aspirin against acute myocardial infarction and death in men with unstable angina: results of a Veteran's Administration Cooperative study. N Engl J Med 309:396–403

Martin JF, Francis P, Lee L, Shaw T, Macpherson J, Penington DG (1981) Differences in the volume of stress platelets and vincristine stimulated platelets. Thromb Haemost 46:410

Martin JF, Shaw T, Heggie J, Penington DG (1983a) Measurement of the density of human platelets and its relationship to volume. Br J Haematol 54:337–352

Martin JF, Trowbridge EA, Salmon G, Plumb J (1983b) The biological significance of platelet volume: its relationship to bleeding time, platelet thromboxane B_2 production and megakaryocyte nuclear DNA concentration. Thromb Res 32:443–460

Martin JF, Slater DN, Kishk YT, Trowbridge EA (1985) Platelet and megakaryocyte changes in cholesterol-induced experimental atherosclerosis. Arteriosclerosis 5:604–612

Mezzano D, Hwang K-L, Catalano P, Aster RH (1981) Evidence that platelet buoyant density, but not size, correlates with platelet age in man. Am J Hematol 11:61–76

Milner PC, Martin JF (1985) Shortened bleeding time in acute myocardial infarction and its relation to platelet mass. Br Med J 290:1767–1770

Murphy EA, Mustard JF (1962) Coagulation tests and platelet economy in atherosclerotic and control subjects. Circulation 25:114–125

Mustard JF, Murphy EA (1963) Effect of smoking on blood coagulation and platelet survival in man. Br Med J 1:846–849

O'Brien JR, Jamieson S (1974) A relationship between platelet volume and platelet number. Thromb Diath Haemorrh 31:363–365

Odell TT, Murphy JR, Jackson CW (1976) Stimulation of megakaryocytopoiesis by acute thrombocytopenia in rats. Blood 48:765–775

Packham MA, Mustard JF (1984) Normal and abnormal platelet activity. In: Lasslo A (ed) Blood platelet function and medicinal chemistry. Elsevier Biomedical, New York, pp 61–128

Packham MA, Mustard JF (1986) The role of platelets in the development and complications of atherosclerosis. Semin Hematol 23:8–26

Packham MA, Guccione MA, Kinlough-Rathbone RL, Mustard JF (1980) Platelet sialic acid and platelet survival after aggregation by ADP. Blood 56:876–880

Packham MA, Perry DW, Kinlough-Rathbone RL et al. (1985) Effects on the buoyant density of rabbit platelets of ADP and agents that increase the concentration of cyclic AMP. Blood 65:564–570

Packham MA, Kinlough-Rathbone RL, Mustard JF (1987) Thromboxane A_2 causes feedback amplification involving extensive thromboxane A_2 formation upon close contact of human platelets in media with a low concentration of ionized calcium. Blood 70:647–651

Paulus JM, Bury J, Grosdent JC (1979) Control of platelet territory development in megakaryocytes. Blood Cells 5:59–88

Rand ML (1983) Studies of changes in rabbit platelets as they age in vivo. PhD thesis, University of Toronto, Toronto, Canada

Rand ML, Greenberg JP, Packham MA, Mustard JF (1981) Density subpopulations of rabbit platelets: size, protein, and sialic acid content, and specific radioactivity changes following labeling with ^{35}S-sulfate in vivo. Blood 57:741–746

Reimers HJ, Kinlough-Rathbone RL, Cazenave JP et al. (1976) In vitro and in vivo functions of thrombin-treated platelets. Thromb Haemost 35:151–166

Shulman NR, Watkins SP Jr, Itscoitz SB, Students AB (1968) Evidence that the spleen retains the youngest and hemostatically most effective platelets. Trans Assoc Am Physicians 81:302–313

Somers DA (1984) The relationship among vessel injury, thrombus formation and platelet survival. PhD thesis, McMaster University, Hamilton, Ontario, Canada

Spurlock BO, Chandler AB (1987) Adherent platelets and surface microthrombi of the human aorta and left coronary artery: a scanning electron microscopy feasibility study. Scanning Microscopy 1:1359–1365

Thompson CB, Diaz DD, Quinn PG, Lapins M, Kurtz SR, Valeri CR (1983a) The role of anticoagulation in the measurement of platelet volumes. Am J Clin Pathol 80:327–332

Thompson CB, Love DG, Quinn PG, Valeri CR (1983b) Platelet size does not correlate with platelet age. Blood 62:487–494

Thompson CB, Jakubowski JA, Quinn PG, Deykin D, Valeri CR (1984) Platelet size and age determine platelet function independently. Blood 63:1372–1375

Trowbridge EA (1988) Pulmonary platelet production: A physical analogue of mitosis. Blood Cells 13:451–458

Trowbridge EA, Martin JF (1987) The platelet volume distribution: a signature of the prethrombotic state in coronary heart disease? Thromb Haemost 58:714–717

Trowbridge EA, Martin JF, Slater DN (1982) Evidence for a theory of physical fragmentation of megakaryocytes, implying that all platelets are produced in the pulmonary circulation. Thromb Res 28:461–475

Trowbridge EA, Slater DN, Kishk YT, Woodcock BW, Martin JF (1984) Platelet production in myocardial infarction and sudden cardiac death. Thromb Haemost 52:167–171

van Oost B, van Hien-Hagg IH, Timmermans APM, Sixma JJ (1983) The effect of thrombin on the density distribution of blood platelets: detection of activated platelets in the circulation. Blood 62:433–438

Warren CW (1988) Thrombopoiesis: the effects of platelet depletion. Eur J Clin Invest 18:A55

Winocour PD, Kinlough-Rathbone RL, Perry DW, Rand ML, Packham MA, Mustard JF (1983a) Changes in the properties of platelets from rats with experimentally induced shortened platelet survival. J Lab Clin Med 101:175–182

Winocour PD, Kinlough-Rathbone RL, Richardson M, Mustard JF (1983b) Reversal of shortened platelet survival in rats by the antifibrinolytic agent, epsilon aminocaproic acid. J Clin Invest 71:159–164

Winocour PD, Rand ML, Kinlough-Rathbone RL, Mustard JF (1986) Hypersensitivity to thrombin of platelets from hypercholesterolemic rats. Fed Proc 45:224

Winocour PD, Kinlough-Rathbone RL, Morazain R, Mustard JF (1987) The effect of dietary saturated fat and cholesterol in platelet function, platelet survival and response to continuous aortic injury in rats. Atherosclerosis 65:37–50

Discussion

Martin: I congratulate you. You were far more objective than I thought you would be. [laughter].

Mustard: It takes one to know one! [further laughter]

Martin: I would like to comment on two things. I think I would choose Dr Jackson's paper as the most elegant new science that we have seen. I was most impressed by it, but I do not want us to be misled by it. I think that there is an abnormality of cytoplasm in the megakaryocyte. I thought it looked like the May–Hegglin syndrome in the sense that some areas have large bunches of demarcation membrane system and other areas have none. This might mislead us if we adopted it as a model of true thrombopoiesis in man, giving the relationship between normal cytoplasm and normal platelets. For my second point, I have to disagree with you about the role of the spleen. You were implying that platelets might emerge from the spleen after thrombocytopenia and therefore give an artefactual result. That may be so, and I do take your point, but the evidence for large platelet sequestration in the spleen is sparse and I think the evidence against it is more than the evidence in favour of it. Simon Karpatkin investigated the effect of adrenaline in the rabbit. He suggested the spleen closes down with adrenaline to give larger platelets appearing in the population. I think that was in an era when Karpatkin was not distinguishing between density and volume. In addition, if you over-transfuse rats or rabbits with lots of platelets you get the converse result. Smaller platelets appear in the circulation. I do not think the spleen will be involved there. If one believes that there is a relationship between platelet size and count then one could say the opposite situation has occurred. Furthermore, I showed yesterday an instance of 36 days of change in hypoxia. I think that is fairly convincing. There is a slow change in ploidy and a slow change in platelet volume over that time. I do not think there is any evidence that the spleen was involved.

Mustard: Perhaps somebody else can comment on this. My perception is that sequestration in the spleen is relatively unimportant in rats and rabbits, but may be important in man. In the lectures yesterday, the comment was made several times that large platelets tend to go into the spleen and stay there for some time. When platelets are transfused into man one does have a sequestration process which is hard to control. This does not apply in the rabbit. As far as I know the sequestration is largely a spleen effect.

Corash: This is more of a question as well as a partial comment. I had a recent conversation with Leon Weiss, who is an expert in splenic anatomy, about this issue. In the mouse and rat the spleen is non-sinusoidal. I do not know if this applies to rabbit. In man and the sub-human primates it is sinusoidal, so the structure is different. Hence the pathophysiology of platelet circulation under those circumstances could be very different.

Mustard: If one considers the published literature about the pattern of radioactivity disappearance when one transfuses platelets of different densities into man, the most dense platelets show a rise and then a fall in time, which is compatible with large platelets entering the spleen and then leaving this organ. In contrast, the least dense platelets show a standard pattern of disappearance. In the one paper that I know that has been published, with cases of splenectomy, that rise associated with the most dense platelets did not occur. So I think you have to pay attention, Dr Martin, to the fact that primates may be a problem.

Thompson: In response to the problem associated with primates, I think that a large aspect of platelet heterogeneity and physiology in which we are interested is primarily applying platelet physiology to human pathology. So if we have a problem in studying primates in that endeavour then we shall have a problem in making any of our work applicable. On the other hand, there is the very real possibility that we need to use animal models to understand the realm or the range in which platelet physiology can vary. In that aspect, certainly, the rabbit model in which clearly you can demonstrate that density does decrease is important. However, I do not think that gives us the justification to say that primates might not be useful, particularly in this relatively applied field. I would like to make one comment on your summation, Dr Mustard, which I think was fair, based on the work that has been presented at this meeting. It is your bias that size may change with age. We certainly believe that function might deteriorate with age. Based on the data presented here at Graz, we cannot really resolve or conclude what the relationship of size to function is. I would agree that no one has really addressed adequately the role of platelet ageing and function in normal haemostasis, i.e. steady-state haematopoiesis. However, I would like to refresh everyone's memory about a paper that we published a couple of years ago. I think it is the only paper that addresses this issue. We wanted to be able to identify old and young platelets. This was done in baboons, a primate model therefore. I will accept the applied criticism that this model may have problems. We returned to the selenomethionine experiments (see Fig. 2.6). All problems that Dr Mustard identified with the peak yesterday (see Discussion after chapter 3) are valid, but one assumption can be made. I think you can say the radioactivity which is present in platelets on the second day is all in the young population of cells. Platelets do not make proteins at any meaningful rate, so therefore if we believe the survival is at least 7–10 days, on average, in the baboon, then on the second day after a selenomethionine impulse all of this radioactivity is in young platelets. In contrast, using the best analysis we have available, particularly if you consider the slopes of these declines which look like survival curves, compared to our other labellings the 50% downpoint on the decay curve, which roughly corresponds to day 9, represents a relatively older population of cells. Now one can investigate the functional characteristic of young and old platelets by studying what happens to the radioactivity in a functional assay relative to the total population in steady-state haematopoiesis. One can do aggregation experiments. We initiated the aggregation response with a set dose of agonist and then arrested it at some fixed change in the total scale of absorption. We stole this idea from Haver and Gear.

In Fig. D2.1 you can see we allowed for a 20% change in the aggregometer tracing; we then arrested the platelets by fixation at that point, in single cells or as aggregates. We then spun out the aggregates, by a fixed time and a set centrifuge, and assayed the amount of radioactivity which was present in those aggregates. The number of platelets in the aggregates in an unseparated population was identical, both at day 2 and day 9, but the amount of radioactivity was not identical: there was almost a 50% decrease in the radioactivity at day 9. This suggests that in normal steady-state haematopoiesis there is clearly a decline in platelet function as platelets get older. I think we are all biased in that direction. It would certainly fit the idea that glycoproteins are processed on the surface, and those are important for interactions. How is this related to size? We also did the same experiment with our size-separated populations. Table D2.1 shows the summary of the baseline data that we accrued to make this point. They are the same volume fractions I showed in my lecture, the same mean platelet volumes. There are no differences in our separation abilities between day 2 and day 9. The radioactivity roughly mimics the activity curves I showed in my lecture. One has about the same amounts of radioactivity on both the upslope and downslope of the same distribution. One allows for a 20% change in the aggregometer tracing after stimulation. Then the aggregates are removed. The same percentage of platelets is left unsuspended but about 40% are removed with the aggregates. We then investigated whether there was a difference in the percentage in each population at day 2 compared to day 9. The amount of radioactivity of the

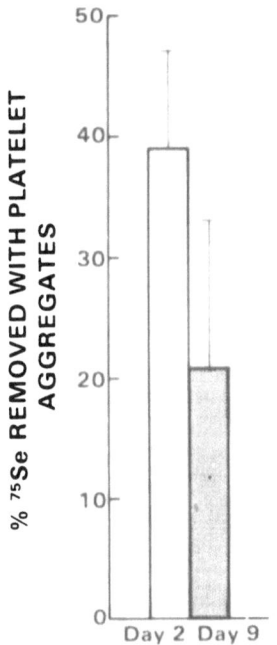

UNFRACTIONATED
PLATELETS

Fig. D2.1. Percentage ^{75}Se removed with aggregates (Day 2 versus Day 9) during thrombin (2 U/ml)-induced aggregation.

Table D2.1. The mean platelet volume, ^{75}Se content, and response to thrombin (2 U/ml) of size dependent baboon platelet subpopulations

Day 2 Fraction no.	MPV (μm^3)	^{75}SE/10^9PLT (cpm/10^9PLT)	Particles remaining after aggregation (%)	Time to 20% agg. (min)
1 2	4.23±0.62	50.6±15.0	68.3± 6.6	1.97±0.22
3	5.30±0.70	61.4±13.7	63.6± 5.9	1.20±0.19
4	6.09±0.83	70.4±16.8	60.4± 3.1	0.98±0.16
5	6.60±0.62	85.5±18.2	59.7± 5.5	0.89±0.12
6 7	7.03±0.51	100.0±14.2	63.7±13.2	0.73±0.18
Original	6.35±0.63	80.8±15.7	47.7± 7.1	1.12±0.24

Day 9 Fraction no.	MPV (μm^3)	^{75}SE/10^9PLT (cpm/10^9PLT)	Particles remaining after aggregation (%)	Time to 20% agg. (min)
1 2	4.24±0.44	68.9± 5.5	60.1±10.8	2.04±0.72
3	5.04±0.75	97.4±12.5	67.3± 7.6	1.31±0.51
4	5.89±0.74	113.3±30.9	67.0± 8.2	0.97±0.18
5	6.65±0.60	125.6±14.7	62.6±12.7	0.84±0.20
6 7	7.08±0.67	148.8±13.6	56.5± 8.7	0.85±0.15
Original	6.32±0.61	109.7±10.6	50.4±11.5	1.06±0.34

selenomethionine that was present in the aggregates had been spun out before we did those counts. In addition, what we have said before about aggregation holds true. The amount of time that it took to get to a 20% change in the aggregation tracing was over twice as long in the small platelet population compared to the large platelet population. So at least the rate at which the smaller platelets aggregate is much slower than the larger platelets. The ratio in radioactivity in each of the populations is shown in Fig. D2.2. In every population there has been a decline in the amount of radioactivity that is present in the aggregates. There is no real statistical difference in these ratios, based on standard statistical arguments for our value of n, which was only 3. Nevertheless, when they are combined the results are highly significant statistically and suggest that platelet function is declining in each of the populations but does not correlate with the relationship of size. So I think size and age both determine function, but determine it independently.

Born: I think they are a very interesting experiments. They cannot be criticized on technical grounds. Do you know whether any known biochemical component on the platelet surface involved in aggregation declines with platelet age? For example, do they have a reduced GPIIb/IIIa complex with age?

Mustard: I am not aware of anybody having really systematically studied that. Does anybody else know?

Corash: There is a paper by Blajchman [Blajchman MA, Senyi AF, Hirsh J, Genton E, George JN (1981) Hemostatic function, survival, and membrane glycoprotein changes in young versus old rabbit platelets. J Clin Invest 68:1289–1294] from McMaster University in which he looked at the glycoprotein composition of platelets from rabbits that had been irradiated to shut off platelet production. I believe that he found minor glycoprotein changes. Was that a study involving Jim George?

Thompson: Jim George was an author. Yes, they found changes in spots on

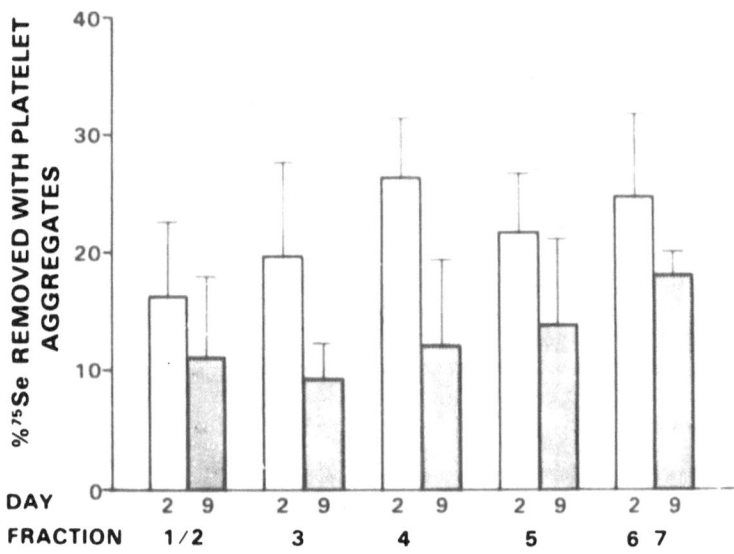

Fig. D2.2. Percentage ^{75}Se removed with aggregates (Day 2 versus Day 9) during thrombin (2 U/ml)-induced aggregation.

gels, but that was prior to the time when we could adequately identify the differences in the protein composition.

Corash: So I do not think that we have seen convincing changes in this area.

Packham: You might not see a change in the absolute number of GPIIb/IIIa receptors but the platelets may have changed in their ability to mobilize those receptors, because they are not normally available and the platelets have to be stimulated to make them available.

Born: Yes, that's right.

Mustard: Another problem is that the survival of platelets can be shortened by slightly modifying the glycoproteins, they do not have to be lost. Hence, we may be dealing with very subtle modifications of membrane glycoproteins in terms of the problems that we are discussing.

Trowbridge: Can I take us back to the spleen and platelet size and count and get away from the receptor sites and biochemistry. I do not feel completely happy with that. The evidence associated with humans suggests that they behave in the same way as the animals, irrespective of whether or not you have sinuses in the spleen. The cardiopulmonary bypass experiment indicates that you get an increase in mean platelet volume. It is only small, but it must be remembered that the drop in platelet count was only 30%. There is a mixing with 70% of the platelets that were there previously. Therefore, the actual increase in size in that system is higher than the measured 6%. So the human platelets are behaving the same as the rat platelets after a single injection of anti-platelet serum (APS). Secondly, according to our experiments there is an increase of about 65% in platelet volume for rats after a single injection of APS. That would be difficult to explain totally in terms of splenic involvement. Let us consider the relationship between platelet count and volume in normal humans and the fact that when the count goes up the volume goes down and vice versa. Thinking in a very simple-minded way, if one has a total mass of megakaryocyte cytoplasm, and there is not too much change in that variable in normal people, then in a production process in which the megakaryocyte is fragmenting, irrespective of how it happens, and the number of fragmentation steps is decreased slightly then the volume of platelets goes up and the count goes down. It has to happen like that. That is a very simple explanation for the differences in counts and volumes and why they fit together. Thirdly, I think we have to be very careful about distinguishing between the larger platelet volumes within the distribution, i.e. in the tail of the volume distribution, and the changes that are seen in mean platelet volume. Those two things are totally different for a perturbation or experimental manipulation. So when Dr Thompson is considering large platelets as sub-populations of a volume distribution, that is totally different from investigating changes which are reflected in increases or decreases of mean platelet volume.

Mustard: I think I should make one comment. My reference to the spleen was not in relation to your longer-term studies, Dr Martin. It was related to two specific points. In sudden acute stress giving an increase in platelets, as I recall the old data with which I am familiar in primates, there is a significant spleen contribution. The second issue is that when you re-infuse platelets into humans you can get a sequestration process in which platelets gradually come back into the circulation. This does not occur in splenectomized people. Therefore, when you are trying to study the survival patterns of cohorts of so-called older and younger platelets, if indeed the spleen tends to sequester larger platelets, as was mentioned in the earlier lectures several times, then that is a contaminating factor in those acute experiments. I do not think it is relevant to longer-term experiments. I think your arguments are quite sound in an equilibrium situation.

Bessman: Fortunately Dr Mustard answered the first comment. I agree completely with Dr Trowbridge on his third point. That is, the bigger platelets in a given population are entirely different from a person having bigger platelets, and likewise for smaller platelets. However, on his second point about a given megakaryocyte cytoplasmic mass fragmenting a bit more or a bit less, and thus making bigger or smaller platelets, I think that the product of platelet size and count, even within just the normal range, is not at all constant. That is, using EDTA anticoagulation the average mean platelet volume at a platelet count of 400×10^9 platelets/l of blood will be about 8.0 fl. At 200×10^9 platelets/l of blood it will be about 10.0 fl. That is not a constant product. That is a gross nominal impedance volume. Actual volume minus the canalicular contents and so forth may be very different. It could conceivably, although I doubt it, be constant. If that is not constant, presumably, something else is, although I cannot say what it is – perhaps some particular glycoprotein or some particular cytoplasmic content. The same distinction would be true using acid–citrate–dextrose (ACD) anticoagulation, just with a slightly different number scale. The nominal mass would not be the same at 200×10^9 and 400×10^9 platelets/l of blood.

Trowbridge: I do not think one should expect to get exactly the same number associated with the mass. One might expect there is some randomness associated with it. The major determinant of biomass is always going to be platelet count. The platelet volume does not change sufficiently to account for the changes you see in biomass. There will be a variation in megakaryocyte cytoplasmic volume throughout the normal population and the differences seen in platelet volume and count are just a perturbation on that particular feature. I do not think it is that desperately important. It is just the normal spread associated with people in the same way there is a variation in height and weight in normal circumstances.

Paulus: I would like to refer to Chapter 6 by Dr Jackson, who studied the rats with macrothrombocytosis. The same kind of anomaly has been found in humans around 1975. This was called, because no other words were available, Mediterranean macrothrombocytopenia or macrothrombocytosis [von Behrens WE (1975) Blood 46:199]. It is very similar to what Dr Jackson described. We studied ten people with moderate thrombocytopenia (see Table D2.2). The average platelet count was 117×10^9 platelets/l of blood, ranging from 80 to 150×10^9 platelets/l of blood. The mean platelet volume was about double the normal value. The thrombocytocrit was virtually the same as in normals: 0.19 or 0.88/100 ml of blood. In that group of ten subjects platelet mass was maintained at the same level as non-Mediterranean subjects (ignoring the splenic pool). There was another difference in these people. When you measured the platelet survival it was normal, but the recovery was decreased. In other words, in normals there are about 60% of the platelets circulating after infusion of chromium-labelled platelets. In these people one finds only about 40%. The spleen has been measured by von Behrens using radiographic techniques, and a moderate increase in spleen size was found, but apparently not enough to explain that increased pooling of platelets [von Behrens WE (1975) Scand J Haematol 14:258]. Finally, in the humans evidence of heredity could not be found; however, if the anomaly was hereditary then it was not dominant.

Table D2.2.   Kinetic and size parameters in normals and in Mediterranean macrothrombocytosis

	Mediterranean group	Control group	p
Platelet count (/μl)	117 700±25 700 (10)	274 800±65 200 (50)	<0.01
Platelet volume (fl)	16.4 ±4.3 (10)	6.6 ±0.9 (50)	<0.01
Thrombocytocrit (ml/100 ml)	0.19±0.06 (10)	0.18±0.05 (50)	NS
Mean platelet life-span (days)	6.6 ±1.6 (10)	6.6 ±1.6 (10)	NS
Mean platelet age (days)	4.3±0.6 (10)	4.3 ±0.3 (10)	NS
Platelet recovery (%)	40.9 ±6.2 (10)	61.6 ±6.0 (10)	<0.01
Spleen/liver ratio	4.3 ±2.9 (9)	1.8 ±0.7 (10)	<0.05
Platelet production (cells/μl/day)	43 600± 8600 (10)	60 300±14 600 (10)	<0.01
Platelet mass produced (ml/100 ml/day)	0.072±0.018 (10)	0.039±0.012 (10)	<0.01

All results are expressed as mean ± 1 standard deviation. Numbers in parentheses refer to the number of subjects studied.
NS indicates non-significant *t* test at the 5% level.

Martin: I disagree with Dr Paulus on two counts. Firstly von Behrens did not look at the megakaryocytes of his patients. We assume that they were normal. In contrast the megakaryocytes in the rats studied by Dr Jackson were abnormal. Secondly, von Behrens showed that there was no change in platelet volume with subject age. So I think Dr Jackson's model is a model of abnormal fragmentation of megakaryocyte cytoplasm whereas Mediterranean macrothrombocytopenia is a different setting of the control mechanism in some way within that population.

Jackson: I guess I would disagree with Dr Martin on that last part because I think they are both models of some abnormality in subdivision of cytoplasm. I think Dr Paulus and also von Behrens looked at the megakaryocytes from

Mediterranean macrothrombocytopenia patients and found the same abnormalities – the same type of membrane complex. Is that correct?

Paulus: We measured ploidy but did not find any differences, and looked at electron micrographs on only three patients, so we cannot really draw any conclusions. However, we did not see these big interesting membrane complexes, which are an association of demarcation membrane and endoplasmic reticulum. They apparently appear normally in megakaryocyte maturation, but usually disaggregate rather rapidly. However, they persist in these subjects in thrombocytopoiesis. Such persistence may be a sign that demarcation proceeds properly.

Jackson: I would like to touch on one or two points and then return to the Wistar Furth rat. The first relates to the spleen question in humans introduced by Dr Mustard. I think one of the nicest studies that was done along that line does not address the platelet size problem, but it does indicate that the spleen is removing probably young platelets that are just released. This study was carried out [Shulman NR (1968) Trans Assoc Am Physicians 8:302] several years ago. He performed reciprocal platelet transfusion studies between asplenic and eusplenic patients. When he transfused platelets from a patient with an intact spleen into an asplenic patient there was no platelet sequestration. When he transfused platelets from eusplenic patients into eusplenic patients there was very little sequestration. However, when he transfused platelets from asplenic patients into patients with intact spleens then there was significant sequestration, or a longer sequestration is what I should say, of a higher proportion of the populations. This suggests that normally in humans the spleen does remove a sizeable proportion of young platelets for some time. I think it could be done more elegantly today, but it is a classical study that should be remembered. On the question of what is being regulated, platelet mass or whatever, you probably recall that in 1977 [Jackson CW, Edmunds CC, Br J Haematol 36:97] we did an experiment with vincristine similar to the one Dr Martin reported in his lecture. Up to that time, it was thought that low doses of vincristine induced a thrombocytosis by causing some damage to the marrow and this was then followed by a rebound. Because Choi [(1974) In: Baldini MG, Ebbe S (eds) Platelets: Production function, transfusion and storage. Grune & Stratton, New York, p. 51], who was working with me at that time, could not demonstrate a significant decrease in megakaryocytes or in megakaryocyte parameters within the first 24 hours after vincristine administration, we tested an alternative hypothesis. That was vincristine might be altering some platelet function that is really the function that is monitored for platelet regulation. Nobody knows, of course, what that is. The experiment was a simple one. We gave rats 1–10 mg/kg of vincristine, then 2 hours later we either transfused them with normal platelets, one body-equivalent of normal platelets, or one body-equivalent of platelets from vincristine-treated rats. Then we studied the megakaryocytes 2 days later when the greatest change in megakaryocyte volume, and so on, occurs, after vincristine administration. The rats transfused with the normal platelets did not show an increase in megakaryocyte size and increase in tritiated thymidine labelling index that one normally sees associated with vincristine administration. The rats given platelets from vincristine-treated animals did show the increase, as though we had not transfused those vincristine-treated platelets. This suggests that vincristine was affecting some platelet function, the real platelet function that is monitored in daily regulation. It is probably related to platelet mass in some way, but is not platelet mass itself.

Martin: Just one point about vincristine, Dr Jackson: I remember your very elegant paper in the *British Journal of Haematology* that you have just described. However, can I suggest there may be two effects of vincristine on thrombopoiesis. I did not show the diagram of platelet count after intravenous vincristine administration, but it occurred slightly after the change in ploidy. What I want to say concerns the nature of ploidy. These are my ideas, but I quote from the elegant monograph of Nagl, which you might know. He states that ploidy in insects and plants is an increase in DNA within a round nucleus. It is a very primitive mechanism, wherein one puts gene by gene, or chromosome by chromosome. Mammalian polyploidy is essentially megakaryocytic. I think the megakaryocyte is different from all other cells, because it is the nature of the mature cell to be polyploid. One finds that nowhere else in the mammal and there is a large lobulated nucleus. If one takes the root of the onion and treats it with colchicine you can produce an increase in DNA with a large lobulated nucleus. Nagl proposes that in this case a problem arises in telophase caused by the colchicine binding to the unpolymerized α- and β-tubulin, so that the chromosomes cannot pull apart. Therefore one gets an increase in chromosomes hanging apart in the same nucleus and the DNA is increased. He calls this the restitution cycle and proposes mammalian megakaryocyte ploidy may be a restitution cycle. So there is a genetic defect in telophase that is keeping the chromosomes within the same nucleus. If that is so and if the colchicine onion root experiment is correct, then could not giving vincristine at a certain concentration (I think we both found that there was only a very small window that could be used) produce two effects? One, as you suggested, Dr Jackson, on the recognition of circulating platelets, but a possible additional one of binding to tubulin and causing a restitution cycle problem, so mimicking normal ploidy. My final point: if that is so, then could it be that the control of ploidy, about which I know nothing, is in some way related to tubulin polymerization? If we are seeking hormones, it might be interesting to look for one that might influence that characteristic.

Jackson: I feel that the experiment involving the transfusion of the normal platelets into the vincristine-treated animal where we prevent the increase in megakaryocyte size, and tritiated thymidine labelling index, suggests that we were not having this restitution cycle. We did not see the increase in megakaryocyte size after vincristine, if we gave one body-equivalent of normal platelets. In contrast we did see it if we gave back one body-equivalent of vincristine-treated patients. We did not study megakaryocyte nuclear DNA content in these experiments.

Martin: Do you recall what your concentration of vincristine was?

Jackson: The concentration was 0.1 mg/kg of body weight. Going back to the Wistar Furth rat, and particularly the membrane mazes, you may recall the study [Bentfeld-Barker ME and Bainton DF (1977) J Ultrastruct Res 61:201] of the effects of anti-serum-induced thrombocytopenia on rat megakaryocytes, in which these types of membrane complexes were found, also with prolonged thrombocytopenia. I do not remember what "prolonged" was in detail, but 3 or 4 days in their case, I think. So, I agree with Dr Paulus' comments that these membrane complexes may be a normal part of megakaryocyte maturation. I think we would all agree that there is some defect in the Wistar Furth rat, in the membrane formation perhaps, but this type of membrane complex does form in the normal animal, at least in prolonged thrombocytopenia and to a lesser extent as part of normal megakaryocyte maturation, as Dr Paulus said.

As Dr Martin pointed out, there is a difference in platelet size with age in the

Wistar Furth rat compared with that seen in Mediterranean macrothrombocytopenia. There is an increase in mean platelet volume and a decrease in platelet count with the age of the rat. I do not have any ideas, which explain this observation and would welcome any proposals.

Trowbridge: Dr Martin and I performed a study with neonates and the platelet volume of the children tends to be much smaller – less than 6 fl – than that associated with adult normals and the platelet count is increased to about 350 × 10^9 platelets/l of blood. That might be the same feature that is seen in the rats.

Jackson: But in the Long–Evans rat we did not see any increase in platelet mean volume with age.

Thompson: I wish to comment on Dr Jackson's very nice vincristine study and relate that to our definition of platelet mass. We think it is a functional component linked to the platelet mass, rather than the platelet mass itself, which is regulated. It is important to draw an analogy with red cell mass. It is not the mass of red cells which is regulated but the oxygen-carrying capacity. I think Dr Jackson's study identifies the fact that it is probably some function associated with the platelets that is regulated and maintains a normal steady-state platelet mass under normal physiological conditions. When one alters that physiological ability, in the way you can with carboxyhaemoglobin in the red cell mass, one can then force a physiological alteration in the total platelet mass produced. Your study is an important confirmation that there is something such as the functional platelet mass. We need to be searching for that regulation. We have thought long and hard about what that might be, and have toyed with the idea of performing some studies, but as yet have nothing.

Paulus: On the same subject, one candidate that might regulate platelet concentration could be β transforming growth factor (TGFβ). In culture it has been observed that serum was much less efficient in promoting megakaryocyte colonies than plasma. On seeking the substances which inhibit megakaryocyte colony formation it was found that TGFβ, which is extremely abundant in platelets, was one of them [Ishibashi T, Miller SL, Burstein SA (1987) Blood 69:1737–1741]. I believe vincristine inhibits cellular secretions. Suppose vincristine, in the way you administered it, inhibited secretion of a substance, such as transforming growth factor. Obviously that needs to be verified.

Jackson: I share a lot of these ideas. My feeling is that the platelet function which is monitored must be something which is analagous to the red cell function. I think it must be some small molecule which is involved, but we have no good idea what that is. I would agree with one point that Dr Paulus made. I think there are many things secreted by platelets into serum that will inhibit megakaryocyte colony formation: TGFβ is one [Mitjavila MT, Vinci G, Villeval JL et al. (1988) J Cell Physiol 134:93–100]. One or two more have been described as well [Dessypris EN, Gleaton JH, Sawyer ST, Armstrong OL (1987) J Cell Physiol 130:361–368]. Some people say platelet-derived growth factor also inhibits megakaryocyte colony formation in vitro. I think we are talking about α-granule constituents here, for example TGFβ. I have trouble in understanding the physiological significance of those in vitro cultures because to quote an elegant statement by some pathologist, "We do not really have serum circulating in vivo!"

Martin: I think it is dangerous to use the analogy of the red cell. It led us astray in platelet kinetics in the mid-1970s. We must remember that red cells, although they are anucleate in the circulation, do have a nucleus that they lose. In contrast the platelet has two unique properties. Firstly, it is not produced by mitosis, it is produced from a polyploid cell. Secondly, it is produced by a process where one cell gives rise to a thousand new cells. Red cells occur in lower orders of animals, in birds and reptiles, but platelets do not. Therefore, there is probably going to be a unique control mechanism and possibly a unique sensing mechanism. It may be related, as Dr Thompson said, to platelet mass and perhaps some functional aspect. I think we all believe that, but it is dangerous to use the analogy of the red cell.

Mustard: In thinking about control mechanisms, it is also important to consider the primary role of the platelet. If you ask yourself what are the functions of the platelet and consider what its primary function surely must be, it is maintaining the integrity of the lining of the blood vessels, which is a huge surface area. The size of the platelet is such that in flowing blood it is distributed close to the surface of the blood vessel, so it is positioned uniquely. If you make an animal absolutely thrombocytopenic, which is possible, then within 24 hours there is massive evidence of breakdown of the microvascular circulation in terms of extrusion of red cells, which can be detected in the tissues and the lymph. Secondly, 60% of the animals will die within 48 hours. There is massive bleeding into the gastrointestinal tract or into the brain. So the platelets are fairly crucial for maintaining the integrity of the vascular system. How they do this is the question that I think has to be asked. Perhaps somebody has the answer to it. However, I am going to tell you what I think takes place. When you put platelets back into a thrombocytopenic animal, the platelets must contribute something to the vessel wall. I doubt very much that the platelets are releasing anything, because I do not know of any biological evidence that the junction sites between endothelial cells induce the platelet release reaction. If you are going to look for something, it has to be something that is on the surface of the platelets. If you think about the surface properties of platelets, you have the glycoproteins, but you also have glycosaminoglycans associated with the surface. They may be internal, but they may be with the surface. Dr Packham published one paper in which she showed ^{35}S was lost from rabbit platelets that had been prelabelled with ^{35}S and aggregated by ADP, which I thought was a surface phenomenon, but she suggests it may be coming from the α-granules. Be that as it may, glycosaminoglycans play a very critical role in vessel wall function. How that works we do not know, but it may just be possible that the platelets' function in maintaining the integrity of the endothelium is totally different from that which we ordinarily accept. It may be almost a "kissing" function, if I can describe it that way, with the surface, which contributes something to the endothelial surface. I wonder if anybody has any better evidence than the speculation I am giving you, because it seems to me this is the crucial question when we are trying to consider the platelets and their function. The role of platelets in haemostasis is important if a large vessel is cut, but that does not occur very often. Arterial thrombosis is an episodic process in atherosclerotic vessels, but the chief function of platelets in normal biology is maintaining the integrity of that wall. What kind of process is taking place?

Born: That experiment by Dr Packham was very nice and if you remember there was a similar experiment undertaken by Wilbrandt in Berne and she obtained the same result as Dr Packham. Something remains to be explained: there is some kind of transfer of some substance which labels with ^{35}S.

Thompson: I would like to play the devil's advocate even further. If one considers the problem rigorously and scientifically I do not think there is any adequate demonstration that platelet interaction with endothelium is the function that allows you to survive the kind of vascular injuries that Dr Mustard has been talking about. One could make an equally good hypothesis, based on all the known functions of the platelet, that it may be something that the platelet releases systematically. This substance then interacts with the endothelium. One could make an alternatively good hypothesis that, in fact, it may be something that the platelet selectively takes up and removes from the circulation. This substance would then be prevented from interacting with the endothelial cells. Certainly an example of that would be serotonin (5-hydroxytryptamine, 5-HT). Platelets are probably the major physiological regulator of the free 5-HT levels that are circulating.

Born: May I just make a comment on that point. This is a very interesting statement that is often made. In fact, by far the greatest quantitative sink for 5-HT in the circulation is not the platelet, but the red cell. We produced a paper in 1967 where this was evaluated. The red cell does not have an uptake system, but the 5-HT just diffuses in according to the Donnan equilibrium. The actual sink in the red cell, quite apart from what actually leaves the circulation elsewhere, is far, far larger than quantities found in the platelet. I just wanted to get that point straight.

Thompson: I agree with you entirely, Professor Born. We also have looked at prostaglandin metabolism, as you remember. We reported in the *British Journal of Haematology* a similar function for red cells, in that they are providing a sink, not because of a specific uptake, but because simply they have so much lipid there. I think it is true for acute physiological changes, where you are probably correct, but at constant steady-state levels there may be a different phenomenon. All that I am suggesting is we may need to look broader and wider for what the physiological functions of platelets are; I am not saying it is any one thing. As Dr Mustard suggested, it may not be simply the haemostatic function of making a platelet plug in a large rent that is going to be important in the normal physiological control of platelets.

Jackson: To follow up Dr Thompson's comments. I would ask you to remember that patients with Glanzmann's thrombocythaemia, who have not had multiple transfusions, seem to have normal platelet production, but they are lacking GPIIb/IIIa receptor sites in the classical case. Hence, it does not seem to be the IIb/IIIa receptor that is interacting with something. On Dr Mustard's question relating to more direct evidence for platelet support of endothelium, I cannot quote the paper well, but the observation [Kitchens CS (1975) Blood 46:567] from both animal studies and in thrombocytopenic humans [Kitchens CS (1986) Blood 67:203] is that there is dilation of capillaries I believe, or maybe the junctions, I cannot really remember now.

Unidentified voice from audience: Junctions.

Jackson: Junctions, is that right? Yes. So in thrombocytopenic individuals one does see a difference in the vasculature.

Dickinson*: I have found this all very interesting. The reason I have come to this meeting was because Dr Martin and I wondered whether, in fact, the impaction of large platelet clumps in axial streams in the digits might be the cause of clubbing through the release of platelet-derived growth factor [Dickinson CJ, Martin JF (1987) Lancet *ii* 1434–1435]. If the process of fragmentation in the

---

*Professor John Dickinson, St. Bartholomew's Hospital Medical College, London, UK.

lungs is actually correct, then one could also hypothesize that a large right-to-left shunt would let through large particles. These would also pass in an axial stream and impact in the finger tips and produce clubbing by the same mechanism, thus unifying possible causes of clubbing. I have been very interested in the revelations of platelet physiology. I agree with Dr Mustard, it does seem as though the platelet is contributing some measurable stuff which is lost when it contacts the vessel wall. I have no idea whether this is part of the platelet membrane so that it loses density with time, which it appears to do, or whether it is perhaps some internal procedure. The regulation goes wrong clinically, does it not, in splenectomized patients. They have platelet counts twice those of normal subjects. So one wonders whether the spleen has some part in the regulation process, and whether the spleen measures whatever this platelet function is which is necessary to restore the vascular endothelium. I find it difficult to believe that the spleen is just a reservoir for platelets and only destroys them. One would think it is probably contributing some other function.

12　Chairman's Commentary

G. V. R. Born

Thank you for inviting me to provide a short commentary to the proceedings. As one who has had little experience in the field of platelet heterogeneity I am sure that I have learnt much more than anybody else at this meeting. I believe that it is the first of its kind. It raises fascinating questions all the way from molecular biology and the uniqueness of mammalian platelets to the possible role of platelet heterogeneity in disease. I would like to divide my commentary into technical and basic questions.

Technical Questions

The technical questions may all have answers and may indeed have been answered already. However, they highlight some problems which appear to me to matter.

The first question concerns the general reliability of the measurement of platelet volume. As I understand it almost everybody here uses the impedance principle or some variant of it. It is likely that the platelet volume distributions obtained by this method are mostly correct, but I still remain sceptical. Some time ago I showed that apparent increases in platelet volume as measured by the Coulter system could be attributed to the extrusion of processes associated with activation. Activated platelets are not able to pack so tightly when spun at high centrifuge forces. I would suggest that people check the volume distributions obtained with aperture impedance systems against other types of quantification such as morphometric measurements on electron microscope pictures.

The tail on the platelet volume distribution curve can be explained in principle by some log-normal law, possibly through the mechanism proposed by Dr Trowbridge or by some other process. A biological system which does not produce a Gaussian distribution is a serious intellectual puzzle.

The second technical point concerns platelet aggregation. This should always be quantified by dose–response curves, never by single-dose effects. The best measurement is the velocity of aggregation. This can be interpreted because we have related aggregate size distribution to the optical changes.

A third technical point concerns the hypothesis proposed by Dr Trowbridge. It is certainly a stimulating proposal. Pulmonary platelet production presumably depends on the break-up of megakaryocytes. This suggests some experiments that appear feasible. If megakaryocytes of various ploidies can be harvested, perhaps by differential centrifugation, then their fragilities could be measured. So it is necessary to understand and quantify fragility. This may not be easy. Fragility may be related to size and other parameters, but the physics of cell fragility is not properly understood. In addition, the methods for collecting and counting megakaryocytes in central venous and arterial blood should be refined.

The fourth and last technical point concerns the slicing of suspension gradients in centrifuge tubes discussed by Dr Corash. While listening to this discussion I wrote down "The best thing since sliced bread is a sliced centrifuge tube". I think there must be methods for getting materials from the slices which are known in California that we are not aware of in London. Slicing is probably the best way if one can minimize artefacts. We should be aware how much of our art depends on tiny ponts of technique.

Basic Questions

The main basic question on the heterogeneity of platelets is surely whether it is a first- or second-order phenomenon in medicine. In other words, is heterogeneity reflected in differences in actual disease processes or incidences? This was the background to the entire discussion. Normally one would expect to find in the blood a distribution of platelets of all ages. These platelets will have certain mean properties with appropriate dispersions measurable by standard deviations.

So, what are the major diseases in which platelets matter? Dr Mustard has referred to bleeding disorders associated with thrombocytopenia. This is comparatively uncommon but extremely important in radiation injury. There is also the form still known as idiopathic, with no established mechanism.

The disease in which I am now mainly interested is atherosclerosis as the predisposing cause of heart attacks and strokes. Dr Martin has demonstrated differences in platelet heterogeneity and behaviour after myocardial infarction. In this area I can be rather more certain. When Vane and Moncada discovered prostacyclin they formulated the hypothesis of a balance between thromboxane and prostacyclin. They suggested that whether you or I had a thrombosis depended on this balance. I said from the beginning that I did not believe this hypothesis and I think in the event I have been proved correct. The amount of prostacyclin that coronary arteries produce is irrelevant in relation to the actual mechanism of coronary thrombosis. What really matters is the disaster of an acute pathological event which, in over 90% of cases, has proven to be fissures of an atheromatous plaque. This unpredictable change is the initiating event and the consequent thrombosis depends on many factors. The classical risk factors including cholesterol and, more recently, fibrinogen and factor VII in the blood evidently come into one or other or both of the two pathological processes. In view of the results on heterogeneity it may be that platelets are also a risk factor. Thus, large epidemiological studies may reveal that certain types of platelets are associated with high incidence of coronary thrombosis in the same way that fibrinogen, factor VII and blood cholesterol are. Smoking is another undoubted risk factor which may affect not only fibrinogen but also platelets. This may be worth investigating.

Finally I come to the bleeding time. Platelets are certainly a primary determinant of bleeding time, but there are, of course, other factors too. I wonder whether there are any local hormones that influence platelets and vascular contractility. Bleeding time results are difficult to interpret, so I was interested when Dr Martin suggested that perhaps we could forget bleeding time and concentrate on platelet mass. Then bleeding time could just be considered as a clinical corollary to platelet mass.

In conclusion I have to say that I have found the meeting enormously stimulating, so that I hope that it can be repeated in the future.

Subject Index